Immunobiology of the Tumor–Host Relationship

Perspectives in Immunology

A Series of Publications Based on Symposia

Maurice Landy and Werner Braun (Eds.)
IMMUNOLOGICAL TOLERANCE
A Reassessment of Mechanisms of the Immune Response
1969

H. Sherwood Lawrence and Maurice Landy (Eds.)
MEDIATORS OF CELLULAR IMMUNITY
1969

Richard T. Smith and Maurice Landy (Eds.)
IMMUNE SURVEILLANCE
1970

Jonathan W. Uhr and Maurice Landy (Eds.)
IMMUNOLOGIC INTERVENTION
1971

Hugh O. McDevitt and Maurice Landy (Eds.)
GENETIC CONTROL OF IMMUNE RESPONSIVENESS
Relationship to Disease Susceptibility
1972

Richard T. Smith and Maurice Landy (Eds.)
IMMUNOBIOLOGY OF THE TUMOR—HOST
   RELATIONSHIP
1974

Immunobiology
of the
Tumor–Host
Relationship

Edited by
Richard T. Smith

University of Florida
College of Medicine

and

Maurice Landy

Schweizerisches
Forschungsinstitut

Proceedings of an International Conference
Held at the Sormani Palace
Milan, Italy
January 14–18, 1974

Academic Press
New York   San Francisco   London   1975
A Subsidiary of Harcourt Brace Jovanovich, Publishers

ACADEMIC PRESS, INC.
111 Fifth Avenue, New York, New York 10003

United Kingdom Edition published by
ACADEMIC PRESS, INC. (LONDON) LTD.
24/28 Oval Road, London NW1

Library of Congress Cataloging in Publication Data
Main entry under title:

Immunobiology of the tumor-host relationship.

    (Perspectives in immunology)
    Bibliography: p.
    Includes indexes.
    1.   Tumors–Immunological aspects–Congresses.
2.   Immunochemistry–Congresses.   I.   Smith, Richard
Thomas, (date)   ed.   II.   Landy, Maurice, ed.
[DNLM: 1.   Neoplasms–Immunology–Congresses.   QZ200
I335 1974]
RC254.I43   616.9'92'079   74-28342
ISBN 0–12–652260–X

CONTENTS

CONFEREES

Peter Alexander, Chester Beatty Research Institute, Belmont, Sutton, Surrey, England

Fritz H. Bach, University of Wisconsin, Madison, Wisconsin

Robert W. Baldwin, University of Nottingham, Nottingham, England

Arturo O. Carbonara, Universita di Torino, Torino, Italy

Ruggero Ceppellini, Basel Institute for Immunology, Basel, Switzerland

Jean-Charles Cerottini, Swiss Institute for Experimental Cancer Research, Lausanne, Switzerland

Luigi Chieco-Bianchi, Universita di Padova, Padova, Italy

Melvin Cohn, Salk Institute for Biological Studies, San Diego, California

Robert E. Cone, Basel Institute for Immunology, Basel, Switzerland

Giuseppe Della Porta, Istituto Nazionale per lo Studio e la Cura dei Tumori, Milano, Italy

Robert A. Good, Sloan-Kettering Cancer Center, New York, New York

Joseph G. Hall, Chester Beatty Research Institute, Belmont, Sutton, Surrey, England

Jonathan C. Howard, A.R.C. Institute of Animal Physiology, Babraham, Cambridge, England

Robert Keller, University of Zurich, Zurich, Switzerland

Eva Klein, Karolinska Institutet, Stockholm, Sweden

George Klein, Karolinska Institutet, Stockholm, Sweden

Francois M. Kourilsky, Hôpital Saint-Louis, Paris, France

Maurice Landy, Schweizerisches Forschungsinstitut, Davos, Switzerland

George B. Mackaness, Trudeau Institute, Saranac Lake, New York

Ralph Mannino, Biozentrum, University of Basel, Basel, Switzerland

W. John Martin, National Cancer Institute, Bethesda, Maryland

Abner L. Notkins, National Institute of Dental Research, Bethesda, Maryland

Peter Perlmann, Wenner-Gren Institute, Stockholm, Sweden

Benvenuto Pernis, Basel Institute for Immunology, Basel, Switzerland

Carl M. Pinsky, Sloan-Kettering Cancer Center, New York, New York

Richmond T. Prehn, Institute for Cancer Research, Philadelphia, Pennsylvania

Geoffrey R. Shellam, University College London, London, England

Hans O. Sjögren, University of Lund, Lund, Sweden

Richard T. Smith, University of Florida, Gainesville, Florida

Jan Stjernswärd, Swiss Institute for Experimental Cancer Research, Lausanne, Switzerland

Osias Stutman, Sloan-Kettering Cancer Center, New York, New York

William D. Terry, National Cancer Institute, Bethesda, Maryland

Jonathan W. Uhr, Southwestern Medical School, Dallas, Texas

Jan Vaage, Pondville Hospital, Walpole, Massachusetts

David W. Weiss, The Hebrew University, Jerusalem, Israel

Hans Wigzell, University of Uppsala, Uppsala, Sweden

PREFACE

Just 15 years have elapsed since the work of Richmond Prehn, George Klein, and Lloyd Old, among others, undermined the long-standing concept of the tumor–host relationship as autonomous tumor growth in a supplicative and supportive host. This old concept still provides the rationale for most therapeutic approaches to cancer today. Gradually, it has been replaced by a much more dynamic and biologically sound set of ideas involving active and specific resistance on the part of the host, tightly interlocked with other functions of the lymphoreticular system.

The supporting data-base is still distressingly small and restricted in content directly relevant to tumor biology. However, it has generated a conviction on the part of many investigators that full understanding of the immunobiology of the tumor–host relationship provides the most logical and sanguine of all current approaches to many unsolved problems of cancer. This conviction was shared by most, but not all of our colleagues who gathered in Milan to cope with the implications of the rapidly growing mass of new and pertinent data. The goal was to assess, to integrate, and to synthesize these data as testable hypotheses, and to evaluate them as potentially applicable to clinical problems in man.

The central paradox of the tumor–host relationship from the point of view of the tumor biologist is still embodied in the unrelenting, lethal growth of primary malignant neoplasms, despite amply documented evidence of a specific, strong, and multicomponent immunologic response to the tumor. The conferees in Milan can be said to have failed in their mission, since this paradox certainly has not been resolved, at least not in any terms which prescribe novel immunotherapeutic approaches in man. On the other hand, they did succeed in bringing to light for the first time several important and relevant lines of evidence which further define the dynamics of the tumor–host relationship. They also fabricated, in discussion of these data and by agreement on interpretations, some new and likely useful conceptual lattices on which to build future efforts.

Among such developments, several warrant emphasis here. Evidence came from many sources indicating that the uncomplicated idea of a single tumor-specific antigen is no longer viable. Immunogenic tumor-borne structures are probably large in number, and can include components usually defined as "self," including at the least enzymes, alloantigens, differentiation, and embryonic structures. The suggestion was that the immune response to such tumor antigens is not irrelevant to the relationship, even though such structures alone do not seem to provide targets in transplantation tests. Tumor antigens were in fact shown to be a controlling element in the relationship, either acting alone or complexed with antibody. As targets for immunologic attack on tumor cells, these structures appear much more capricious than previously thought. These structures may respond to antibody-mediated attack, for example, by aggregating on the cell surface (''capping''), or by exocytosis (''shedding'') into their environment as antigen–antibody complexes having potent biologic effects on attacking lymphoid cells. In either case this can leave the tumor cell functionally naked (''modulated'') in terms of providing a proper attack point for potentially cytotoxic cells or antibody. Moreover, the first evidence was presented that this process can actually occur *in vivo*, both in terms of capping and shedding.

Much attention was given to the effector systems potentially capable of specific tumor cell destruction. Here it became quite clear that T lymphocytes are not the only ''killer'' cells, but that both B cells and other antibody-armed lymphoid cells share this property. Macrophages were shown to have even more power and significance in this role both *in vitro* and *in vivo* than previously envisioned. But macrophage involvement in tumor destruction has a paradoxical quality. Tumors were described that grow and kill the host, despite containing in their intracellular matrices up to 50% of macrophages. Moreover, evidence was considered that restricts the mechanisms involved in the general depression of delayed-type hypersensitivity observed in the tumor-bearing host to effector system malfunction, probably involving macrophages, rather than the T-lymphocyte deficit previously postulated.

The concept of immune surveillance emerged battered from the siege, but usefully transformed after a thoroughgoing reexamination. Crucial here was evidence for specific immunological effects involving cells or antibody, which stimulate or support tumor growth. Also germane were data demonstrating that the putatively T-deficient nude mouse is not without immune defenses to tumor growth. This provided but one element suggesting that a significant and important change in emphasis may be occurring in the direction of work of those involved in immunobiology. A gradual shift is perceived, from a preoccupation with experiments that employ tumor systems to explore basic immunobiologic problems, to studies which are primarily relevant to tumor biology. This conference, and the volume to which it has given birth, hopefully will give further impetus to this new direction.

RICHARD T. SMITH

MAURICE LANDY

ACKNOWLEDGMENTS

The Conference Organizing Committee, consisting of Ruggero Ceppellini, Maurice Landy, and Richard T. Smith, gratefully acknowledges the invaluable assistance of the many individuals and the generous financial support of the four organizations which made this Conference possible. Thanks go to: Consiglio Nazionale Delle Ricerche (Italian Research Council), Fondazione Giovanni Lorenzini, Gruppo Italiano Ricerche Farmaceutiche (GIRF), and the World Health Organization (Immunology Unit).

Special acknowledgment is made to Dr. Luigi Gorini, Director, to Angelina Perroni, his efficient secretary, and to the staff of the Lorenzini Foundation, for the key role they played as Conference Secretariat, and for making all local arrangements, including a unique and enjoyable cultural and social program.

Thanks, also, for the expert services of Eugene Wallach and his assistants, who so effectively retrieved, by stenotypy, an entire week of animated discussions, and to Mrs. Ruth Ceppellini and Mrs. Reba A. Landy, for volunteering their services in separating each day's mass of conference transcript into individual segments for prompt editing by the conferees.

And to Ms. Linda Mannooch, Dept. of Pathology, University of Florida, the editors and the conferees express their gratitude for the help she extended in the preconference planning phase and in the preparation of the manuscript for publication.

Immunobiology of the Tumor–Host Relationship

SESSION I

TUMOR ANTIGEN AS THE CONTROLLING ELEMENT IN THE TUMOR–HOST RELATIONSHIP

Multiplicity of tumor antigens and their relationship to self-components—F_1 Parental interaction in the MLC—Cross reacting versus specific tumor neoantigens—Alloantigens and embryonic structures as tumor antigens—Production and shedding of tumor antigens—Evidence for capping *in vivo*—Relationship between shedding, capping, and modulation—Occurrence of non-immunogenic tumors.

1

CHAIRMAN SMITH: The tumor-bearing host is perfused continuously with tumor membrane proteins, fragments, and even whole cells (reviewed in Smith, *New Eng. J. Med.*, **287**, 439, 1972). This antigenic barrage initially engages specific recognition receptors, leading to proliferation of lymphoid cell subsets, secretion of antibodies, and generation of cytotoxic cells. The intensity of the immune responses generated is such as to be indicative of hyperimmunity directed toward the various tumor membrane structures. This hyperimmune state is unique in that it is usually concurrent with the continuous circulation of the tumor membrane antigens which generates it. Paradoxically it is usually impotent in destruction of the established primary autochthonous tumor which gave it birth.

In beginning this session, I shall focus upon the nature of the tumor membrane structures, their possible sources, production, and distribution. Most of these structures are not of viral origin; thus, most are properly categorized as expressions of ''self,'' and the responses they elicit arise from ''self-recognition.''

Table 1 concerns the heterogeneity of membrane structures presented by tumors. Solid evidence supports the concept that single tumor cells may also express, in their membrane, structures of direct or indirect viral origin. Any of the so-called ''self-components''—those associated with embryonic development, organ or tissue specific differentiation structures, structures present at specified phases of the cell cycle, or structures novel because they represent degraded membrane products—may be immunogenic to the lymphoreticular system. Boyse (in *Immune Surveillance,* Smith and Landy, eds., p. 5, Academic Press, N.Y., 1970) has postulated that another rich source of unique structures may result from alloantigen matrix concatenations in the cell membrane, although no direct experimental evidence for this is known.

It should be obvious that most of the membrane structures comprising this are those usually defined as ''self.'' Some other rather precise gene-locus products—structures determining histoincompatibility with respect to allogeneic hosts—are another possibility of polymorphic structures on tumors potentially

TABLE 1

Some Sources of Individual Membrane Structures
Potentially Stimulating to Cell Recognition Systems

Virion – tumor-associated or passenger virus
Virus directed or indirect structures
Differentiation directing or fetal structures
Cell cycle specialization structures
Cell membrane degradation products
Matrix or grid concatenations (Boyse)
Allotypic structures – universal or organ representation

TABLE 2
Specificity of F_1 Hybrid Subsets
Stimulated by Parental Cells in One-Way MLC

Source of reacting cells	Source of 1° mitomycin-blocked target cells	Source of 2° mitomycin-blocked target cells	³H-thymidine incorporation (mean CPM ± SE)
(C57BL/6 × CBA)F₁	–	–	376 ± 42
(C57BL/6 × CBA)F₁	(C57BL/6 × CBA)F₁	(C57BL/6 × CBA)F₁	210 ± 18
(C57BL/6 × CBA)F₁	CBA	CBA	408 ± 74
(C57BL/6 × CBA)F₁	CBA	C57BL/6	3025 ± 218
(C57BL/6 × CBA)F₁	C57BL/6	C57BL/6	645 ± 87
(C57BL/6 × CBA)F₁	C57BL/6	CBA	2097 ± 109

affecting the tumor-host interaction. Three lines of investigation in our laboratory have led us to focus upon such antigens as a source of tumor-associated antigens, giving rise to (1) self-reacting clones, (2) antibodies, and (3) competing, perhaps suppressive, elements in tumor-host relationships.

Classical approaches to tumor immunobiology have centered on the elimination of residual heterozygosity in order to define TSTA through use of highly inbred animals. I should first like to show how heterozygosity may conceivably be a self-generated source of immunologically significant membrane structures in the tumor-bearing host. The critical element would be to demonstrate self-recognition clones for H-2–linked membrane structures in the mouse. In observations made over the past five years in our laboratory, and confirmed in several others, F_1 hybrid mouse lymphocytes, whether from thymus, spleen, or lymph node, were shown to proliferate significantly in one-way MLC with parental peripheral lymphocytes (Table 2). Recognition, signified by such proliferation, has all the characteristics we have defined for allogeneic cell combinations: alloantigen specificity, probable T dependency, augmentation by tumor-bearing, and B-cell triggering. Through "suicide"-type experiments, Gebhardt *et al. (J. Exp. Med.,* in press) have shown that different subsets or clones of cells in the F_1 hybrid spleen or lymph nodes proliferate in response to each parental target cell. Work in congenic lines further defines the stimulating structures on parental cells as being products of, or determined by, the MHC locus or by genes closely linked to it. The data do not disclose whether the stimulatory structure is LD-like, SD-like, the product of a latent virus-activating gene, an Ir gene product (Ia-1 locus?) or some unknown product of the H-2 locus. The data imply also that the recognition receptors on responding cells are not expressed codominantly as are SD locus products. Interpreted literally, the data signify that F, recognition of parent is clonal. Further, they infer that lymphocyte recognition subsets or clones, detectable only in the unique circumstances of *in vitro* culture of a coherent heterozygote, an F_1 hybrid between congenic

4

strains, may possibly also exist for similar "self"-membrane structures in outbred or noncoherent heterozygotes. Such self-recognition subsets must obviously be under effective steady-state control *in vivo*—"blocked," defused, or tolerant—thus prevented in some way from proliferating or expressing cytotoxicity. They are detectable only *in vitro* and in those circumstances in which the alloantigen recognition subset augmenting effect of tumor-bearing stimulates their proliferation, as we shall discuss later (Session V, pp. 309–310). Caution is urged in accepting without reservation this conceptual fallout of the data described because the phenomenon is limited to mouse cells at present; Wilson could find no evidence for the effect in PBL of rats. (Darcy Wilson, personal communication.)

A second line of evidence for elements of the histocompatibility complex having significant contributions to the tumor-host relationship is derived from experiments in which novel antigens are detected on tumor cells by anti-SD sera raised against normal cells. Lymphoblastoid cell lines derived from healthy human donors (HuLCL) and from infectious mononucleosis (IM) patients have been tested for cytotoxicity with a variety of supposedly monospecific anti-HL-A sera (Tables 3 and 4). Multiple positive reactions are found in the lines for determinants not represented in the donor's phenotype. Some, but not all, of these reactions are absorbed by donor cells. Moreover, in a series of over 50 congenic MCA tumors developed in our laboratory, Klein has found that multiple H-2 specificities, both "public" and "private," are detected by oligospecific anti-H-2 determinant antisera but are not represented in the phenotype detected in normal cells of the donor strain (Table 5). Absorption studies suggest that these, too, are not absorbed by normal cells. Other explanations of the phenomena are conceivable, we readily concede. These findings are, however, consistent with the hypothesis that some of the multiple membrane structures on the tumor cell are immunogenic components of normal cells but only readily detectable when expressed in tumor cells.

The third element in evidence for an immunologic activity toward histo-

TABLE 3
Comparison of Cytotoxicity Patterns of Anti-HL-A
Typing Sera on Three LCL from a Single Donor

| | Putative specificity of sera | | | | | | | | | | | | | |
	1	2	3	9	10	11	4C	5	7	8	W10	12	13	4A/12
Donor				+		+	⊞					+		+
Line − 7A	⊞		⊞	+	+	+	⊞		⊞	+		+	⊞	+
− 7B				+	+		⊞		⊞	+		+	⊞	+
− 7C		⊞		+	+	+	⊞			+		+	⊞	+

5

TABLE 4

Cytotoxicity Comparison of Anti-HL-A
Typing Sera on LCL and Respective LCL Donors

Donor	Line	Concurrent cytotoxicity	Disparate positives	
			Donor	Cell line
1.	B-6	19	0	9
2.	B-7	20	0 (1±)	7
3.	B-8	21	0	7
4.	B-9	13	0 (1±)	15
5.	B-10	24	0 (1±)	3
6.	B-11	10	0 (2±)	9

TABLE 5

Comparison of Cytotoxicity Patterns of
Anti-H-2 Sera on Congenic MCA Tumors

Cells tested	Putative H-2 specificity of sera								
	15	52,53	23	31,34	33,53,54	8	11,25,54	16,34,35,41	4
C57BL/10·spleen		+			+		+	+	
C57BL/10·M2 tumor	+	+		+	+	+		+	+
C57BL/10·A·spleen		+	+			+	+	+	+
C57BL/10·A·M1 tumor	⊞			+	+	⊞		+	⊞

compatibility structures involved in tumor-bearing is the confirmation, in our laboratory, of Haywood and McKhann's *(J. Exp. Med.,* **133,** 1171, 1971) experiments showing inverse correlation between the detectability of H-2 specificities on tumor cell membranes and tumor immunogenicity. We found that the stimulating capacity of soluble tumor antigens has roughly an inverse relationship to the immunogenicity of the tumor from which it was obtained.

If membrane structures we have come to know as "histocompatible" antigens contribute in a major way to the tumor-host immunologic interaction, an obvious corollary is that "self" and "non-self" no longer carry the significance enshrined by our immunologic gurus. Self-tolerance would be a necessary, normal characteristic of a fragile, balanced system, a balance disturbed by the exceptional demands for disposal of membrane components, presented to the host by injury or by tumor bearing.

Next, I want to turn to a consideration of our concept of cross-reacting TSTA as being wholly different from TSTA or tumor-unique antigens. The original experiments establishing TSTA demonstrated that chemically induced tumors have a unique transplantation antigen, whereas virus-induced tumors cross react regardless of the organ system. Studies of the MTV system by our colleague Vaage indicated that some tumors have both types of antigenicity.

TABLE 6

Apparent *in Vitro* Cross Reactions
among MCA Mouse Tumors[a]

LNC source by immunizing tumor	Colony inhibition of target tumor (%)	
	49	81
32	26.1	0
33	26.1	45.3
35	19.4	
44	11.6	
47		5.5
49	18.4-89.5 (4)	
51	19.4	0
53	33.0	
61	25.5	16.8
67		18.8
74	45.8	
81		26.5-91.8 (6)

[a]Calculated from data of Hellström, I, *et al.*, 1968.

TABLE 7

In Vitro Cytotoxicity of Congenic
Anti-MCA Tumor Sera

Serum (1-5)	Target cell (C.I.)	
	B10·M2	B10·A·M1
B10 anti-B10·M1	0.75	0.66
B10 anti-B10·M2	0.51	0.35
B10·A anti-B10·A·M2	0.60	0.27
B10·BR anti-B10·BR·M1	0.57	0.47
B10·BR anti-B10·BR·M2	0.58	0.41

As *in vitro* assays are used extensively in studying chemically induced tumors, it becomes clear that whether tested by colony inhibition (Table 6), cell, antibody-mediated cytotoxicity (Table 7) or, as I shall describe, by stimulation assays for solubilized membrane structures, cross reactions are nearly universally encountered between chemically induced tumors.

These cross reactions are usually interpreted to signify that common or *shared* antigens exist in addition to the unique TSTA disclosed by transplantation tests. Hellström's data, shown in Table 6, are exemplary in this context.

In order to analyze so-called cross reactions in greater depth, Forbes, Nakao, Blackstock, and I have tested responses of various lymphoid cell subpopulations to soluble antigens from about 50 tumors, grown in 10 strains of mice (*Fed. Proc.*, **32**, 1020, 1973; manuscripts in preparation). We compared proliferative responses of spleen, PBL, and/or lymph node cells to a wide dosage

7

range of KCl-solubilized tumor and normal cell membranes, at varying intervals after tumor inoculation. Evidence which I will summarize, is interpreted to mean that different subsets of lymphoid cells are responding to *multiple* stimulatory components of the tumor membrane rather than a single large homogeneous subset responding to a single or a few shared antigens. Moreover, recognition subsets responsive to membrane structures present on normal muscle cells are stimulated and proliferate in the later period of tumor bearing in most animals.

When a typical stimulation pattern for peripheral blood cells (Fig. 1) or lymph-node cells (Fig. 2) is expressed as incorporation per 10^6 cells, an interesting effect is observed. Proliferating nodes or spleen show high unstimulated incorporation and this high level is inhibited—reduced toward control background levels, with *very* low amounts of the antigen—on the order of 0.1–0.5 μl/culture. Stimulation supervenes as more antigen is added, and peak stimulatory values are usually in the 10-50 μl/culture range. While the mechanism of inhibition is not understood as yet, it is tumor specific and appears to be mediated by a relatively low molecular weight component of the antigenic mixture. Based upon considerations detailed elsewhere (Smith and Konda, *Int. J. Cancer,* **12**, 577, 1973; Konda, Nakao and Smith, *Cancer Res.,* **33**, 2247, 1973; Konda and Smith, *Cell. Immunol.,* in press) expression of data per 10^6 cells fails to account for the occurrence of major changes in cell mass. Expression for cell mass *per se,* provides a more meaningful basis for comparisons (Fig. 3) between normal or nonregional node masses which have variable total cell numbers.

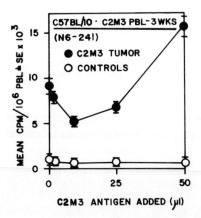

Fig. 1. Stimulation of ^{3}H-TdR incorporation of PBL, taken from C57BL/10·A mice, bearing C57BL/10·A C2M1 tumors of two weeks duration, by varying amounts of a KCl-solubilized C57BL/10 C2M1 tumor membrane preparation. Data are expressed as cmp/10^6 PBL ± SE. These and data in Figs. 2, 3, 4, 5, and 6 are taken from Forbes, Nakao, and Smith (manuscript in preparation).

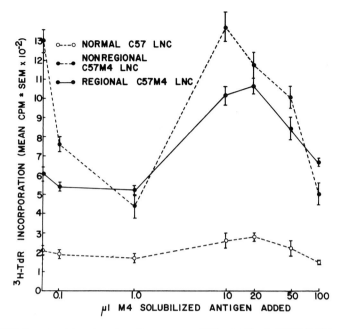

Fig. 2. C57BL/6 regional lymph node cell response to KCl solubilized C57BL/6-M4 antigens, 22 days after inoculation of 1×10^5 C57BL/6 M4 tumor cells.

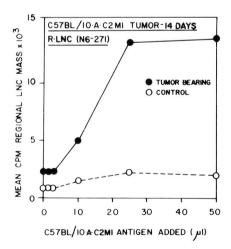

Fig. 3. Dose-response relationship between amount of C57BL/10 · A   tumor antigen and [3]HTdR incorporation by regional LNC taken from mice bearing that tumor for 14 days. Data are expressed as cpm/R-LNC mass, as compared to effect of antigen on normal LNC.

9

Peak stimulated incorporation per spleen elicited by the KCl-solubilized-tumor-membrane preparation is shown on the horizontal axis in spleen cells taken from mice which have borne the tumor indicated on the vertical axis at 14 or 28 days after inoculation of 1×10^5 tumor cells s.c. The antigens indicated as C and S are KCl-solubilized cardiac or skeletal muscle membrane, respectively. The filled-in boxes represent stimulation two times or more than that in the normal controls and above background in the tumor bearer. Those tests indicated by the asterisk were not done (from unpublished data of Forbes, Nakao, and Smith).

The membrane preparations we have used are heterogeneous in net charge and molecular size. The greatest stimulatory activity is contained in a fraction of 30–40,000 MW.

The question of cross reactions has been examined in two ways: (1) by using multiple membrane preparations as stimulants of cells from a single tumor-bearing animal (Figs. 4a, b) or (2) using a single antigen on cells taken from different animals which have borne syngeneic tumors. Figure 5 shows that cells from two of the tumor-bearing animals were stimulated by the tumor membrane used—those from the homologous tumor bearer and those from one other. This differential effect is a temporal variable, however, since responses shown in cell subpopulations taken earlier in the course of tumor bearing are often specific exclusively for the homologous tumor. The so-called cross-reactive reactions may greatly exceed the specific one in subpopulations taken later. Moreover, later in the course of tumor bearing, reactions to normal muscles were frequently observed.

In similar studies, we compared sequential responses to homologous and other syngeneic preparations in spleen and regional and nonregional lymph nodes. The results are illustrated in Fig. 4. In this experiment, stimulation elicited by antigen prepared from the homologous tumor was strongest in the spleen cell subpopulation, while at the same time a syngeneic antigen preparation stimulated the lymph node cells. Figure 6 illustrates an experiment in which extensive "checkerboard" titrations were made at two intervals, again suggesting an extensive overlapping of antigenic specificities.

To generalize from many experiments of this type, both time and subpopulation variables are observed. Homologous tumor preparations are uniquely stimulatory in regional lymph nodes, starting 5–10 days after tumor inoculation. As the tumor grows, what appears to be a broadcasting of responsiveness to the specific tumor occurs, with responses being elicited in the spleen, then in nonregional nodes. Very soon (10–20 days) preparations from syngeneic nonhomologous tumors are detected, first in the regional lymph nodes, then the spleen, then the nonregional lymph nodes. Frequently responsiveness to the homologous tumor disappears in the regional node after 15–20 days. Thus conclusions regarding specificity or nonspecificity of the tumor system depend upon: (1) time of assay, (2) cell mass assayed, and (3) antigen dose used.

10

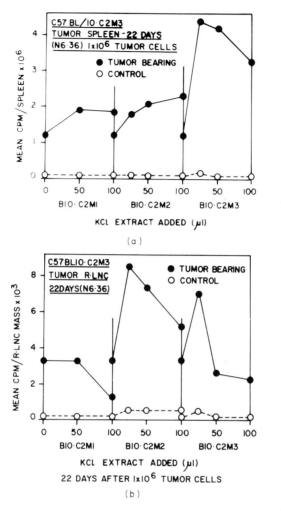

Figs. 4a, b. ^{3}H-TdR incorporated by spleen (a) or LNC (b), taken from the same C57BL/10 mice bearing C57BL/10 C2M3 tumor for 22 days, upon addition of the indicated C57BL/10 KCl-solubilized tumor membrane preparation indicated on the abscissa. Note the differences in peak stimulated incorporation elicited by the 3 preparations in the spleen and LNC.

A reasonable interpretation of these data is that the lymphoreticular system is responding to multiple membrane antigens on tumor cells which vary in size of responding clone and in susceptibility to detectable stimulation, and which differ by interval and setting. The checkerboard experiment shown in Fig. 6 involved ten tumors and ten sets of tumor-bearing animals. At two or four weeks, the pattern of peak stimulated incorporation in the spleen appears to support the generalization that differing subsets are involved.

11

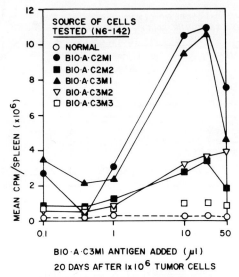

Fig. 5. ³H-TdR incorporation stimulated by addition of varying amounts of a C57BL/10·A C3M1 tumor KCl-solubilized preparation in spleen cells, taken after 20 days of bearing one of the indicated C57BL/10·A tumors of normal C57BL/10·mice. Data are expressed in terms of cpm/spleen × 10⁶.

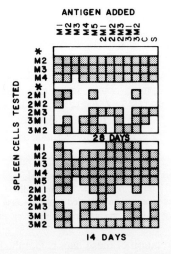

Fig. 6. Peak stimulated incorporation per spleen elicited by the KCl-solubilized tumor membrane preparation, shown on the horizontal axis, in spleen cells taken from mice which have born the tumor, indicated on the vertical axis, at 14 or 28 days after inoculation of 1 × 10⁵ tumor cells s.c. The antigens indicated as C and S are KCl solubilized cardiac or skeletal muscle membrane, respectively. The filled-in boxes represent stimulation 2 times greater than that in the normal controls and aforementioned background in the tumor bearer. Those tests indicated by the asterisk were not done.

12

Our interpretation is that multiple membrane structures represented on the tumor cell induce unique subsets of responding cells rather than a single large subset responding to a single broadly represented or so-called cross-reacting antigen. If this is correct, a hypothesis can be developed to relate the cross reactions we detect in *in vitro* tests and the unique immunogenicity observed in transplantation tests.

The hypothetical tumors shown in Table 8 have in their membrane structures A,B,1,2, etc., representing common antigens detected by *in vitro* tests such as colony inhibition. The numbers represent other similar structures, but not those shared by syngeneic tumors of this line. Any of the indicated structures may stimulate a subset of responding cells at one time or in one setting, as we have suggested. The summation of effects of all of these subsets would be required to prevent growth of the test inoculum of tumor cells used in the usual *in vivo* assay.

The nonhomologous tumor would elicit its own large number of specific subsets, but too few of these would be directed toward antigens shared by the specific tumor to give detectable *in vivo* tumor inhibition. Yet *in vitro* tests of sufficient sensitivity are positive whenever any antigenic structures are shared. This hypothesis predicts that an occasional MCA tumor will show cross immunogenicity in transplantation tests, and such exceptions observed by ourselves and others can be considered as favoring this construct. In the case of virus-associated tumors, such as the MTV tumor example also illustrated, the hypothesis could account for both the unique and cross-reacting immunity observed in this system.

The role of self-responding subsets directed toward histocompatibility structures in the response to tumors is essentially unknown. The most probable effect on the tumor-host relationship would be by preemption of rejection through a dominant, active tolerance state to self-antigens. Haywood and McKhann's data might be taken as favoring this idea.

TABLE 8
Hypothetical Explanation for TSTA Specificity

Tumor	Tumor-specific membrane structure complex	Transplantation test results	*In vitro* test results
MCA 1	ABCD-1,2,3,4,5,6,7...	"Specific"	"Cross react"
MCA 2	ABCD-11,12,13,14,15 ...	"Specific"	"Cross react"
MCA 3	AB-1,2,3,19,20,21. . .	"Specific"	"Cross react"
MTV 1	ABC EFG 1,2,3,4,5,6,7,8,9,10. . .	"Cross react"	"Cross react"
MTV 2	ABC EFG 11,12,13,14,15,16,17. . .	"Specific"	"Cross react"
MTV 3	ABC EFG 1,2,3,4,5,6,18,19,20,21. . .	"Cross react"	"Cross react"

ABCD: antigen mosaic detected by *in vitro* tests.
EFG: "strong" virus-directed antigen system.
1,2,3 ... : Other antigenic membrane structures expressed on tumor surface.

These ideas are offered to provoke a deeper probe into the biologic nature of membrane structures found on tumors and their relationships to what we now consider ''normal'' or ''self'' membrane structures. We should especially bring into consideration those components we have learned to consider ''self'' in terms of the consequences of self-recognition. We should evaluate the possibility that tumor bearing, in part at least, represents a problem in controlled self-destruction. There is, within this area alone, sufficient fuel for our intellectual fires and grist for our analytic and speculative mills.

PREHN: All of the *in vitro* tests of whatever type, even those based on cytotoxicity, seem to give greater cross reactivity than the *in vivo* test. *In vitro* tests based upon killing cells should have the same quantitative receptor requirements as the *in vivo* tests. I fail to see then, why a cytotoxicity test *in vitro* is necessarily more sensitive and thus more able to pick up cross reactivity than are the *in vivo* tests.

CHAIRMAN SMITH: Prehn's point is well taken. *In vivo* discrimination is the difference between a positive and negative test, and it depends on the number of tumor cells which do or do not seed a growing tumor in the host which has previously experienced the homologous or nonhomologous syngeneic tumor. In weakly immunogenic tumors the spread between these numbers may be 10- to 50-fold—two test increments. I can speak only of stimulation tests which are positive or negative at 2- to 3-fold increments over background. They also have the capacity to measure degrees of positivity, which makes such tests more discriminatory of quantitative differences in response.

MARTIN: Prehn's point is important: Do cytotoxic assay data *in vitro* have any correlation with the *in vivo* behavior of cross reactions and the non-cross-reacting tumors?

CHAIRMAN SMITH: If cross reactivity could never be demonstrated in MCA systems *in vivo*, I would agree completely. But actually, Prehn's own data show a degree of cross reactivity in *in vivo* tests, and others have reported, as well, the occurrence of some cross immunogenicity when large groups of tumors are tested.

BACH: How is cross reactivity tested *in vivo*?

CHAIRMAN SMITH: Evidence of cross reactivity in the *in vivo* systems is derived by showing that growth of one MCA tumor, followed by removal, will cause a rejection or less rapid growth of a second syngeneic tumor.

BACH: Has that been tested with very low numbers of tumor cells in the secondary challenge?

CHAIRMAN SMITH: Usually that challenge is made with large numbers of tumor cells, but broad $\log_{10}$ titrations are usually performed.

BACH: Use of high numbers of tumor cells would explain the findings.

CHAIRMAN SMITH: The way these tests are usually performed, an interval is observed after tumor removal, prior to challenge, so that any residual blocking tumor antigen is probably gone. The only immediate source of tumor antigen is the challenge tumor—usually in the order of 10^5–10^7 cells.

DELLA PORTA: I agree with Prehn that perhaps in the *in vitro* tests we are seeing something that we cannot yet correlate with *in vivo* data or even explain. Even in *in vivo* experiments with chemically induced tumors involving the usual growth-excision type of immunization and an *in vivo* challenge, we identified cross-reacting antigens. Actually such antigens were more frequent in tumors which had been transplanted for several generations. We found a cross reaction among them with cell-mediated cytotoxicity *in vitro*, but cross reactions were also seen as detected by enhancement *in vivo*.

STUTMAN: We did some work with 3M KCl-soluble antigens from MCA tumors; one of the major problems we experienced was endotoxin contamination of the antigens. Such contamination gave us false cross reactivities, and we had to add normal cells as controls for the *in vitro* stimulation experiments.

CHAIRMAN SMITH: How did you assay for endotoxin?

STUTMAN: We measured pyrogenic response in rabbits.

CHAIRMAN SMITH: This is a problem that worried us at one time, and we still cannot say with finality that one never gets endotoxin contamination. On the other hand, with the solubilization method we use, this is highly unlikely. Moreover, the solubilized antigens do not stimulate normal cells in *in vitro* systems designed to maximize the mitogenic effects of endotoxin. The *in vitro* test you describe—using normal lymph node cells—does not detect LPS stimulation optimally.

CEPPELLINI: Smith gave evidence that antigens which are not present in normal peripheral lymphocytes of man are present in lymphoblast cell lines derived from that donor. Only a minority of these antigenic determinants may be new antigens. For one thing, it very often occurs in 3,9,13, and W-5 that cross-reacting specificities are frequent. These reactions do not detect new antigens but just a higher sensitivity of the lymphoblast line. The same thing is true for PHA blasts. One should, therefore, be cautious that one is not detecting false new antigens.

CHAIRMAN SMITH: Some of these aberrant HL-A or H-2 specificities can be absorbed out with normal autochthonous lymphoid cells but *not* all of them. We agree that caution is warranted in interpreting such data, for we simply do not know the significance of the extra specificities detected. The fact that they are raised in response to normal cells and are expressed either *de novo* or in a form more susceptible to histotoxicity on tumors probably is indicative of an antigen significant to the tumor–host relationship. It was in the context of such self-resembling components of the tumor antigen complex that these data were described.

ALEXANDER: In trying to analyze the different antigens on tumor cells, why do it with cell-mediated tests when serological techniques are available? For example, Thomson has characterized two tumor antigens from a rat sarcoma by affinity chromatography. One of these is TSTA, unique to the individual sarcoma, and the other a cross-reacting fetal antigen. There is no need to talk about these substances in ill-defined terms.

CHAIRMAN SMITH: Other than doing things the hard way, which is what Alexander means, there is a good reason for examining cell response to these antigens. It represents a view of reality which is different from that obtained by the serologic test he describes. These studies are all done in the context not only of what is happening with respect to the tumor-specific response in each lymphoid mass, but in respect to the numbers of cells carrying various immunoglobulin markers, theta and other T cell markers, and the susceptibility of such cells to various mitogens and alloantigens. The tumor specificity studies are a fallout of the total cellular ecologic approach we have taken.

BACH: I believe cellular models are of greater value than using only serology. If we relate to the normal histocompatibility situation, we now have to face the possibility that there are "alloantigenic" differences which are not easily defined serologically. These differences can lead not only to *in vitro* reactions such as the MLC, but also to *in vivo* reactions including GVH, runt disease, and skin graft rejection. Thus despite my hesitation in accepting some of the preliminary data Smith has shown us, I do not concur with Alexander, that serology is a much easier and more direct way of looking at things. We may be looking at different things, both of which are probably important.

ALEXANDER: I just thought that, as in work on transplantation antigens, one got the serological data first and then the cell-mediated data. That being the case, this would seem to be the way to proceed in the tumor field, because I doubt whether we have the degree of understanding of the different antigens and their responsiveness, even now, in the transplantation situation. Had it not been worked out serologically first, had we gone first into mixed reactions, I think life would have been a great deal more difficult.

MARTIN: I would like to comment on the apparently anomalous cytotoxic activity of congenic antisera against tumors but not splenic target cells shown by Smith. These antisera may contain other antibodies, in addition to those directed against the serologically defined H-2 antigens. If we are to conclude that these anomalous antigens are not present on normal tissues, it may be worthwhile to test by absorption rather than by direct cytotoxicity and include normal fibroblasts and other normal tissues in such absorption studies.

CHAIRMAN SMITH: Martin is right. These data need to be expanded. As I indicated, they are quite preliminary. The absorption studies are being done.

VAAGE: With reference to the discrepancies between *in vivo* and *in vitro* studies of tumor antigenicity, discrepancies also exist *within in vivo* systems testing for tumor-specific antigenicity. If, for example, one compares the resistance of immunized mice to subcutaneous versus intravascular challenge, immune resistance is more strongly expressed against tumor cells injected intravascularly than against tumor cells injected subcutaneously. This probably has several explanations. Within the circulation, immune resistance elements are probably more available to destroy tumor cells than in subcutaneous implantation sites. Structural or physiological differences may also exist between visceral organs and subcutaneous implantation sites. For example, unsensitized mice are protected against a syngeneic fibrosarcoma with transferred antiserum if the challenge is intravascular, but not if it is subcutaneous. A second example is that established tumor immunity in mice can be abrogated by injecting tumor antigen preparations and challenging subcutaneously, but so far this has not been observed when challenged by the intravascular route.

TERRY: Intepretation of the experiment Smith showed, where MCA-induced tumors demonstrate unexpected H-2 specificities, depends upon the specificity of the typing sera used. Recent information concerning anti-H-2 typing sera makes it necessary to carefully question previous assumptions of monospecificity. Antigens may be detected by anti-H-2 typing sera, but do not represent conventional H-2 antigens in that they map in the Ir region and appear to be expressed preferentially on B cells. One specificity of this class was reported by

17

Sachs and Cone and referred to as β-antigen (*J. Exp. Med.*, **138**, 1289, 1973). Agreement has been reached to refer to these antigens as Ia antigens. It is clear that many antisera, previously considered monospecific, contain antibodies to Ia specificities, and conclusions regarding unexpected specificities must keep these antigens in mind.

CHAIRMAN SMITH: Marianna Cherry and her group (Jackson Laboratory), who kindly supplied the sera used in these studies, share your feeling that there are other specificities.

TERRY: Another point concerns the existence of critical differences between assay systems and possible erroneous conclusions that might be reached if these differences are not appreciated. Antisera exist that detect the antigen β. In addition, β appears to have an important role in stimulation of MLC reactions; that is, it serves as an adequate stimulus for lymphocyte blastogenesis. On the other hand, if an animal is immunized against β (proven by the production of anti-β antiserum), and lymphoid cells from that animal are tested for killer cell activity against β-containing cells, none is found. Either the β-antigen is incapable of inducing cell-mediated immunity, or the β-antigen is inadequate as a target for cell-mediated killing. If we generalize and assume that antigens exist on tumor cells with characteristics similar to β, we must confront the possibility that such antigens may evoke antibody responses only, or may evoke cell-mediated responses that are ineffective because the antigen is not a suitable target for cell-mediated killing. The conclusions to be reached would depend upon whether one was studying this antigen by a serologic technique or for cell-mediated killing.

UHR: With regard to discrepancies between the various assays for tumor immunity, two additional points should be made. The first concerns differences in the repertoire of specificities between serum antibodies and T lymphocytes. Secondly, in a tumor-bearing animal, the tumor will presumably bind selectively cells with the highest affinity for the tumor antigen, as is the case with serum antibody. It is these high-affinity cells which might show the greatest cross reactivity. Therefore a *minimum* of cross reactivity is detected when lymphocytes are examined from a tumor-bearing animal. The extent of cross reactivity might increase if the tumor was removed.

CHAIRMAN SMITH: To answer Uhr's second point pragmatically, not theoretically, after removal of the tumor we observe a much greater degree of specificity toward solubilized antigens from the homologous tumor than toward others; however, not all so-called cross reactions are lost.

UHR: I would think one would expect a higher degree of cross reactivity.

CHAIRMAN SMITH: That is not what actually happened however.

UHR: One should then find cells which have higher avidity for tumor antigens, and these should be able to show greater binding.

CHAIRMAN SMITH: Two elements should be considered in this system. One is avidity at the cellular level, which is a difficult attribute to assess at this point. The other is the relative number of cells comprising the cell subsets responsive to each antigenic structure on the tumor cell surface; i.e., how many cells comprise the principal array versus the cross-reacting array, at various times after tumor inoculation or in varying lymphoid cell masses. When the tumor is amputated, we observe responses that are much more limited to the primary stimulating tumor extract. I must assume that the subsets responding to this multiple antigen complex have given rise to the largest memory population.

COHN: Can we go back to the first point? How do you explain the reaction of an F_1 hybrid against parental cells?

CHAIRMAN SMITH: In F_1 hybrids derived by mating congenic lines, we can identify the genetic locus of the stimulating structure on the target cell as in or linked closely with the MHC locus of the IX linkage group. Since this appears to be a T-cell-mediated response, it seems likely that genetic control of the recognition process is also a function controlled at the locus. In this context, it is construed as an MLC reaction for which we have no known *in vivo* counterpart.

COHN: The response of the F_1 to the parent is dependent on more than the parent acting as an antigen. Is that what you are telling us?

CHAIRMAN SMITH: Yes, it is.

PREHN: I think that is not entirely true. If I understand correctly the work from Michael Feldman's laboratory, one can get the same sort of reaction with the F_1 cell. In other words, true self-to-self, so the phenomenon is probably much more general and does not depend on the F_1 hybrid.

CHAIRMAN SMITH: Yes, a prediction of these data is that F_1 should stimulate F_1. This is borne out in our data but not shown here.

COHN: Since Smith claims that the F_1 reacts against parental as well as F_1 cells, how does he interpret other studies with MLC. Are they spurious reactions, is an antigenic difference being recognized, or are anti-self cells being activated?

CHAIRMAN SMITH: A logical but speculative extrapolation of the data is that all heterozygotes may have self-recognizing subsets. Such subsets might be endogenous in each animal's lymphon, capable of interacting with self structures such as histocompatibility and related alloantigens. Tolerance mechanisms, however, would be necessary to normally prevent possible harmful consequences of expression of this capability. Such a system might regularly function as a built-in mechanism for recognition and disposal of effete, damaged, or unwanted cells. I prefer to cease speculation at this point.

BACH: There is no question, as Smith said, that several investigators have observed proliferative reactions by F_1 cells stimulated with parental cells. The question is, as Cohn says, one of interpretation. There is a very mundane interpretation. If one mixes cells of two individuals or two allogeneic mouse strains, "something" called blastogenic factor is produced. The supernatant of an MLC added to cells of any individual, including lymphocytes from the responding cell donor, will stimulate ^{3}HTdR incorporation, which is the only assay used for "a response." In fact, if both reacting cells are treated with mitomycin-C, even more blastogenic-factor activity is found in the medium. So there may be a trivial explanation for this phenomenon; namely, the parental cells respond to allogeneic antigens of the F_1, produce blastogenic factor, and it is to this factor that the F_1 cells respond.

I personally think this *is* the probable explanation. Smith has just shown us that he has been using Zoschke's BUdR-light techniques for wiping out clones of F_1 cells responding to parental alloantigens. I would fit this in by raising the possibility that stimulating antigens in an MLC, the H-2 or HL-A LD antigens may be clonally distributed. If they are, then Smith is knocking out those cells of the F_1 carrying the specific antigens to which parental cells can respond (and in turn the F_1 cells respond). This would give one the data we have seen. We must also consider that mitomycin-treated parental cells, which recognize foreign alloantigen on F_1 cells, will, by that action, trigger those specific F_1 cells, i.e., the interaction triggers both cells.

COHN: Is it clonally distributed in the F_1 or the parental population?

BACH: It is clonally distributed in the F_1. The only thing I would add is that there are what appear to be one-way reactions which do not stimulate in both directions. For example, mouse strains B10.A(4R) and B10.A(2R), I believe, give a truly one-way reaction.

20

CHAIRMAN SMITH: Bach gives a possible alternative interpretation. As I pointed out, however, we cannot demonstrate the presence of any blastogenic factor in these supernatants, which has the capacity to stimulate other F_1 cells, nor is the clonal character of the response to each parent explained by the operation of a nonspecific blastogenic factor.

ALEXANDER: Regarding Smith's data on the response of the F_1 to parental lymphoid cells, if there are surface antigens which are determined by recessive genes, this would follow logically. I believe that Cudkowicz has shown there are such membrane antigens.

CHAIRMAN SMITH: Cudkowicz's phenomenon is a related one, in overall phenomenology; however, I cannot relate it absolutely to our findings. It seems unlikely that one could demonstrate F_1–parent stimulation with nearly every strain combination if a recessive gene were responsible. If it were true, the postulated recessive genes would code for antigen receptors. Do you agree?

ALEXANDER: Correct.

GOOD: The first experiments Smith presented stimulated much speculation about subsets of immunocompetent cells in F_1 hybrids that can recognize and react to parental cells. I remain confused and resistant. I believe that Smith is duty bound, if he is to move in unconventional directions, to establish that the effects he describes are anything other than the allogeneic influence. He must show formally that what is being observed cannot be the expected allogeneic influence that would account for proliferation of the F_1 cells.

CHAIRMAN SMITH: Would Good define for us what *he* means by allogeneic effect?

GOOD: When I refer to the allogeneic effect, I mean the capacity of immunocompetent allogeneic T cells to provoke nonimmunologic mesenchymal cells to proliferate. This influence has been studied and reported extensively by Lafferty and his colleagues. They observed this influence on chick embryo hematopoietic cells long before the embryos reach immunologic competence. The allogeneic effect could be eliminated by treatment with 50 μg of mitomycin per ml instead of the 20 μg/ml concentration ordinarily used to inhibit division of the putative stimulating cells. Alternatively, one might expect to eliminate the allogeneic influence with very high doses of irradiation to the alleged stimulating cells. In my opinion, until allogeneic influence is ruled out, it is hard for me to take very seriously claims for stimulation of F_1 cells by cells of the parent strain. Perhaps the best way to do this rigorously is to have *no* parental T lymphocytes in the system at all.

CHAIRMAN SMITH: We have accepted the burden of proof, and have gone through a wide range of mitomycin dosage to target cells, up to the point where mitomycin bleeding occurs or it kills the target cells. This point is not far above 50 μg/ml concentration in our hands.

The question Good is raising, it seems to me, concerns whether F_1 proliferation is a function of immunocompetent cells having specific receptors for parental structures or the result of some general noncomplementarity between the membranes of parental and F_1 cells. For several reasons, we have concluded that this is not the case. The recognition reaction differs in no demonstrable characteristic from allogeneic proliferation induced in MLC between mouse lymphoid cells, including proliferation kinetics, time course, T dependency of responding cells, chromosomal identity, and clonal characteristics of responding cells. If this phenomenon does not involve specific T-cell receptors, the same logic must therefore be applied to all MLC between allogeneic cells. There are those here who can argue this point more adequately than I can.

We keep a very open mind about the stimulating structures or structures on parental target cells. Although linked with or located within the MHC locus, we have no direct evidence that these are serologically defined (SD) histocompatibility antigens. It seems quite possible, for example, that the structures could be LD locus determined, or indeed could represent structures under the control of genes within or linked to the MHC locus. For example, the X-1 locus, FMR leukemia viruses antigens or the expression of S-tropic c-particle-type viruses might be involved. It could be more than coincidental that mitomycin is the best blocking agent for target cells in MLC. Although of low order compared to IUdR and BUdR, this compound has a capacity to induce expression of S-tropic viruses in mouse cells. Again, if the membrane structures on target cells prove to be viruses induced in this way, the problem applies to all MLC. It would suggest also that responses to such virus antigens are clonal.

GOOD: That is a real problem.

CHAIRMAN SMITH: It is a fascinating problem.

CHIECO-BIANCHI: Smith's statement involves a very important point. Recent data from Todaro's group at the NIH (Sherr, Lieber, and Todaro, *Cell,* **1,** 55, 1974) indicate that in the mouse MLC, activation of type C RNA virus occurs. The virus shows a peculiar cell tropism since it replicates only in the rabbit SIRC cell line* but not in either N- or B-type mouse cells. Thus, in the MLC a new endogenous virus is produced, possibly by derepression of a virus

---

Editors' note: C-type viruses which proliferate in the SIRC cut line are, by definition, S tropic.

gene present in the cell genome. This might very well determine a change in the antigenic structure of the cell surface.

CHAIRMAN SMITH: I agree with Chieco-Bianchi, but, even if this explanation should be sustained, it does not make the observations uninteresting, just different from the way we have been thinking about them.

BACH: There is one major difficulty, and that is where does the specificity of MLC response come in? You infer a substitution of the C-type virus for the whole LD complex. How can that be in view of all your data regarding specificity of response?

CHAIRMAN SMITH: The clonal elimination experiments appear to stand as a major bulwark against the virus genome expression hypothesis. All one must propose to make it work, however, are the following conditions: (1) there are many S-tropic viruses, (2) that Ir gene–controlled recognition receptors exist for this variety of virus-coded membrane structures, and (3) that these are clonal in distribution on T cells. The Rgv-1 locus represents a possible analogy, in that it is Ir linked, and controls expression of recognition receptors for one type of leukemia virus membrane antigen.

COHN: This is becoming more of a private discussion, and I am not following it. So I would like to put together the points put forward by Smith, Alexander, and by Ceppellini.

It is possible to imagine an F_1 cell population which reacts to antigenic determinants on the parental cell because this parental cell (even though it is mitomycin-treated) stimulates the hybrid F_1 via *abnormal induction* sometimes referred to as *allogeneic induction* (see discussion Session IV, pp 268–276). F_1 stimulation by mitomycin-treated F_1 cells, which Smith and Prehn have referred to, cannot be explained this way. At the moment, I am suspicious of such a finding as not being relevant to the immune reaction, so let us put that aside. What we have to explain is why the F_1 (AB) population behaves, as Smith has put it, "clonally" distributed with respect to its response to the two parental types, P_A and P_B.

The F_1 (AB) antigen-sensitive cell must be recognizing, via its receptor, a determinant which is not expressed or recessive, as Alexander described it, in the F_1 (AB), but is expressed in the parent, P_A or P_B. Immediately, as Ceppellini pointed out, we would think of a Ramseier–Lindenmann type determinant, which is not expressed in the F_1 (AB) because of tolerance. Consider the following situation: An F_1 hybrid AB between parents A and B, expresses *neither* anti-A nor anti-B. In an F_1–P_{AM} mixture, the parent A stimulates, via abnormal induction, the AB hybrid, enabling cells expressing anti-anti-B specificity to respond to anti-B which the parent A expresses. If one now eliminates these stimulated cells with BUdR and light, then assays using P_B, the surviving F_1 hybrid cells with anti-anti-A specificity will be stimulated to respond. This would seem to be a reasonable explanation of the experiment Smith describes.

CHAIRMAN SMITH: This is the only way we can put the Ramseier–Lindenman phenomenon together with the F_1 recognition of parent in MLC.

COHN: It is not the order of magnitude of the response. I would have predicted that very few cells could be responding, and yet from the data on DNA synthesis it appears that many cells respond. So I am a little uncomfortable about interpreting the response unless to the specific component one adds a nonspecific stimulation of DNA synthesis. The clonality and the magnitude of response do not seem to go together.

BACH: Do you want to extrapolate the number of cells responding?

CHAIRMAN SMITH: There is a general correlation, but there are too many factors involved to justify extrapolation.

KLEIN: With respect to differences in cross-reactivity patterns obtained *in vitro* and *in vivo*, I am concerned that our discussion has been restricted to the various ways in which the lymphocyte can look at the same target cell.

MARTIN: We have experiments in mice which indicate that certain tumor antigens are depressed alloantigens. That is, certain components which constitute tumor-specific antigens in a tumor-bearing mouse, may exist as normal tissue components in allogeneic mouse strains. If genetically determined susceptibility to *spontaneous* development of specific types of tumors is related to expression in these mice of particular alloantigens, then the immunology of these spontaneous tumors may differ fundamentally from that of tumors artificially induced by chemical or viral carcinogens in otherwise resistant animals.

The main forms of spontaneous neoplastic disease in mice are mammary carcinoma, leukemia, and alveologenic tumors. These latter tumors occur either as benign or malignant growths. Rice, of the NIH, who has been studying mouse lung tumors for several years, attracted me to the question of why only mice of certain strains develop spontaneous lung tumors. The striking differences in total lung tumor incidence and in the occurrence of malignant lung tumors in various mouse strains are shown in Table 9. Strains C57 and DBA/2 rarely develop lung tumors, whereas strains A, Swiss, and C3Hf develop an appreciable number of lung tumors. An important distinction is that while tumors judged to be malignant by size (3–8 mm diameter or more), and histological features (frequency of mitosis, local invasion or compression of surrounding

TABLE 9

Comparative Susceptibility of Mouse Strains to Spontaneous Lung Tumor Development[a]

Mouse	Mice with tumors %	Tumors/mouse mean	Malignant tumors[b]
A	58	1.3	+
Swiss	49	0.8	+
C3Hf	31	0.4	−
DBA	2.1	0.02	−
C57	5	0.1	−

[a]One-year-old female mice were autopsied. Formalin fixed lungs were sectioned into 2-mm-thick slices and examined under a disecting microscope for lung tumors. Tumors were provisionally classified as malignant on the basis of size (3-5 mm). These tumors, together with representative smaller tumors, were examined histologically to assess frequency of mitosis, compression or invasion of neighboring lung and were then classified as benign or malignant.

[b]Three- to five-millimeter tumors or larger, with malignant cytologic pattern.

TABLE 10

Transplacental Induction of Malignant Lung Tumors in Genetically Resistant Mouse Strains[a]

Strain of mouse	ENU administration (days prior to term)	Average number of tumors/mouse	Malignant tumors observed
A	−5	33.6	+
C57	−5	14.3	+
C3Hf	−5	−[b]	+
A	−2	12.2	+
C57	−2	1.3	−

[a]Data from *Ann. N.Y. Acad. Sci.*, **163**, 813, 1969.

[b]No observation.

normal lung tissue, or mediastinal metastases), occur in strains A and Swiss mice, such tumors rarely develop in C3Hf mice.

Administration of the carcinogens ethyl-nitrosourea (ENU) or urethane to adult mice of a genetically resistant strain greatly increased the incidence of benign tumors. However, this treatment rarely resulted in the development of malignant tumors. Rice showed that genetically determined resistance to the chemical induction of malignant lung tumors may be overcome by administering ENU transplacentally four to five days prior to parturition (Table 10). When the offspring of pregnant C57 or C3Hf mice, treated prenatally with ENU, were examined as adults, multiple lung tumors, macroscopically and histologically resembling the malignant tumors of strain A mice, were detected. Malignant tumors of A-strain mice are usually transplantable to adult syngeneic recipients. In contrast, the tumors induced transplacentally in C3Hf and C57 mice did not transplant to syngeneic mice. Transplantation of two such tumors to (C3Hf × A)F₁ hybrid mice gave progressive tumor growth. These tumors did

TABLE 11

Growth of Transplacentally Induced Lung Tumors of C3Hf
Mice in Syngeneic and in F_1 Hybrid Recipients

Recipient strain	Tumor	Character of tumor growth[a]		
		Negative	Transient	Progressive
C3Hf	38	36/44	6/44[b]	2/44
	85	43/43	0/43	0/43
(C3Hf × A) F_1	38	0/29	0/29	29/29
	85	0/33	0/33	33/33
(C3Hf × Swiss) F_1	38	7/12	4/12[c]	1/12
	85	5/6	1/6	0/6
(C3Hf × DBA) F_1	38	13/13	0/13	0/13
	85	17/17	0/17	0/17
(C3Hf × C57) F_1	38	22/22	0/22	0/22
	85	–	–	–

[a] Mice received 5×10^5 to 10^7 viable lung-tumor cells intradermally from the second to the seventh passage in C3A mice. It was subsequently demonstrated that tumors 38 and 85 would grow progressively in C3H mice.

[b] The transient growth of tumor 38 in C3Hf mice occurred in 6 of 25 mice inoculated with 10^7 lung tumor cells. All but one of these tumors regressed within 20 days after tumor challenge.

[c] (C3Hf × Swiss) F_1 hybrid mice received 6×10^5 or 2×10^6 cells of tumor 38. Transient tumor growth occurred with both doses and, in most instances, persisted for more than 50 days.

not transplant to (C3Hf × DBA/2) or (C3H × C57)F_1 hybrids (Table 11). The resistance of C3Hf mice to syngeneic lung tumor was immunologic by two criteria: depression by treatment with ALS and abolition by sublethal X-irradiation, unless the mice had been preimmunized (Table 12). These lung tumors then express a tumor antigen immunogenic in syngeneic mice.

A possible explanation of why these tumors arise in (C3Hf × A)F_1 mice is that the tumor antigen was, in fact, a normal strain A component inherited

TABLE 12

Lung Tumor "85" in Irradiated C3Hf Mice

Immunization of recipients prior to X-irradiation[a]	X-irradiation[b]	Character of tumor growth[c]		
		Negative	Transient	Progressive
–	–	20/20	0/20	0/20
–	+	2/19	1/19	16/19
+	+	7/19	10/19	2/19

[a] Immunized mice received 2×10^5 lung tumor cells intraperitoneally and 1×10^5 lung tumor cells intradermally 21 and 14 days, respectively, before X-irradiation.

[b] Mice received 400–600 R X-irradiation. All preimmunized mice received 600 R.

[c] Mice were challenged with an intradermal injection of 10^5 lung tumor cells.

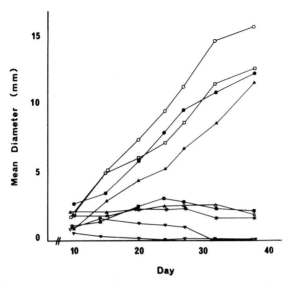

Fig. 7. Mean diameter of tumors developing in mice inoculated intradermally on day 0 with 10^5 "85" lung tumor cells. Progressive tumor growth occurred in normal C3H recipients (○—○), irradiated C3Hf mice, either not preimmunized (Δ—Δ) or preimmunized with normal lung tissue from DBA (□ □), or C57 (○—○) mice. Tumor "38" (▽—▽) or tumor "85" (□—□) did not grow in irradiated C3Hf mice or those preimmunized with normal lung tissue of A (*—*) or C3H (Δ—Δ) mice, or in nonirradiated C3Hf mice (▽—▽). (The results presented in this figure have been pooled from data from 5 separate experiments.) *(Brit. J. Cancer, 28, Supp. I, 48, 1973)*

by the (C3Hf × A)F₁. To test this hypothesis, Rice, Cotton, Esber, and I performed experiments in which sublethally irradiated C3Hf mice were immunized with lung tissue of A mice, then challenged with one of the two lung tumors. The results were that lung of A mice *did* cross react antigenically with the lung tumor antigen. Pooled data from these experiments is depicted in Fig. 7. The antigen was apparently not present in lung of C57 or DBA/2 mice. However, the tumor antigen was present in lung of a related C3H subline.

Lung tumors "38" and "85" grew progressively when transplanted to irradiated or nonirradiated C3H mice. *In vitro* studies have substantiated that this malignant lung tumor of C3Hf mice expresses a tissue antigen of normal A mice. Lymphoid cells from lung tumor–bearing (C3Hf × A)F₁ mice were tested for microcytotoxicity against cultured lung tumor and cultured normal lung. Significant microcytotoxicity was observed against both tumor target cells and normal lung of (C3Hf × A)F₁ and C3H mice, but not against normal lung of C3Hf or C57 mice.

STUTMAN: Since B particles have been found in many of these lung carcinomas, and since both C3H and A lung can immunize, perhaps such effect is related to the presence of mammary tumor virus.

MARTIN: Evidence against this tumor antigen being related to MTV is: (1) DBA/2 mice are positive for MTV, yet lung from these mice does not immunize C3Hf mice against syngeneic lung tumors. (2) The tumors are negative for MTV using MTV antisera. (3) (C3Hf × A)F_1 hybrid mice foster nursed on C57 mothers were still susceptible to tumor challenge as adults.

TERRY: What about other viruses? If other strain-associated viruses were present in normal tissue used for immunization, and the viral antigens were shared by the tumors being studied, the result would be similar.

MARTIN: Of course, I do not know the precise nature of the antigen in normal A and C3H mice. Both strains express the A component in common with the tumor. C3H mice cannot be preimmunized against lung tumor with A tissue. The genetics of expression of the component is consistent with a single dominant genetic locus. The tissue distribution has been studied qualitatively by assessing the capacity of various tissues of A or C3H mice to preimmunize C3Hf mice. Lung, liver, and skin grafts all immunized, suggesting the component is widely distributed. We have not tried infectivity studies, but failure to transfer antigen expression to tissues of C3Hf mice by subcellular extracts of tumor or tissues of A or C3H mice, would not necessarily exclude a virally determined antigen because of a possibly restricted host range of the virus.

KLEIN: How close is the relationship between Martin's C3H and C3Hf strains? Has the latter been derived from the former? Has he tested any C3H × C3Hf F_1 cross? How does it behave?

MARTIN: The C3Hf mice were derived from the C3H mice by foster nursing onto C57 mice in 1956. They have diverged genetically in that reciprocal skin grafts are rejected between day 17 and 28. Both strains type as H-2^k and probably differ at non-H-2 histocompatibility loci. We hope to localize the genetic locus which determines the expression of the lung-tumor antigen.

KLEIN: Are the results in F_1's the same in both reciprocal types, wherever C3H or C3Hf is male and female in the cross?

MARTIN: Progressive lung tumor growth occurs in (C3Hf × C3H)F_1 and (C3H × C3Hf)F_1 hybrids.

GOOD: Just because a single genetic locus is involved, there is no reason to abandon the concept of virus involvement. It is probably not even an argument against a virus if the genetic locus relates to the major histocompatibility region. The new concepts introduced by the work of Dupont and Jersild, and the collaborative work of Dupont and Yunis, and of Ballow and myself, on lacunar immunodeficiency, might be most relevant in this context.

MARTIN: I would not be surprised if a viral genetic locus was involved. In related studies on an ENU-induced brain tumor, similar preferences for growth in the (C3Hf × A)F₁ hybrid mouse over syngeneic C3Hf mice was observed. When C3Hf mice were successful in rejecting an initial inoculum of this tumor, and were rechallenged with an equal or lower number of tumor cells, the tumor grew at a rate similar to that in the (C3Hf × A)F₁. That the loss of tumor resistance is specific for the brain tumor for an immunogenic syngeneic lymphoma is an interpretation that was rejected. We favor an explanation that viruses from the tumor spread to normal tissues, causing an "antigenic conversion" of normal tissues. Virus particles are readily seen by electron microscopy in spleens of tumor-bearing mice. Extracts from both tumor and tumor-bearing spleens are positive for focus-forming activity on embryo fibroblasts. The spleen cells however, express antigenic specificities not present on normal splenocytes. The brain tumor expresses a virus-related tumor antigen, and by analogy the antigen expressed on the ENU-induced lung tumor may be of virus origin.

ALEXANDER: Is Martin's situation formally different from a TL-positive leukemia growing in a syngeneic TL-negative mouse?

MARTIN: Quite possibly it is a similar phenomenon. TL is probably only one of many alloantigens that can be derepressed in malignant lymphoid cells of mice. TL has been reported to be nonimmunogenic in syngeneic hosts and to modulate rapidly when exposed to anti-TL antibody; these are properties which argue that the derepression of TL is immunologically of little significance to the host's defense against lymphoma development. On the other hand, derepression of a lung tumor antigen could explain the rarity of malignant lung tumors in C3Hf mice. The reason we sometimes find an immunogenic lung tumor carrying the depressed alloantigen in C3Hf mice may be that the tumors are induced prenatally, prior to the maturation of the immune system; consequently, the primary host did not reject the tumor.

BACH: Does Martin know anything about the genetic linkage of his locus with any other marker?

MARTIN: Apart from Mendelian segregation as a single locus we have no information as to its linkage group. This information should be available shortly.

COHN: In a cross between a high and low incident strain, is the phenotype that of the high or low incidence?

MARTIN: Sensitivity to tumor development is dominant over resistance. Most F₁ hybrid crosses show a lung tumor incidence near that of the susceptible parent.

COHN: What crosses were done to show that a single locus was involved?

MARTIN: [(C3H × C3Hf) × C3Hf] back-cross mice were challenged with tumor. Progressive growth occurred in 50% of the mice. In (C3H × C3Hf)F$_2$ mice, tumor growth occurred in 75–80% of the mice. Lung tissue of mice which allowed tumor growth induced radio-resistant immunity in C3Hf mice, strongly suggesting that tumor growth occurred because of alloantigen expression in normal tissue.

COHN: Do the spontaneous tumors that arise appear to be clonal?

MARTIN: The tumors are papillary adenocarcinomas. Several lung tumors may occur in the same ENU-treated mouse. The histology does not suggest a tumor of mixed tissue origin.

CEPPELLINI: I would like to put forward an unconventional explanation. Could it be possible that the F$_1$ are resistant because they have an Ir gene which produces a blocking antigen?

MARTIN: In one sense Ceppellini's interpretation is correct. The transplantation studies clearly show that the major tumor antigen is a self-component of (C3Hf × A)F$_1$ hybrid mice. In fact, no evidence suggests resistance to any true tumor-specific antigen when the tumor is inoculated into the F$_1$ mouse. Yet these mice respond immunologically, detected by microcytotoxicity assay, and one can usually detect blocking factors in serum. The question is whether this response is directed against the self-antigen; indeed, this appears to be so. It appears thereby to be a blocked autoimmune response, possibly an extension of the normal homeostatic mechanism preventing self-destruction.

DELLA PORTA: In our laboratory, Parmiani found a slightly different situation with two Balb/c MCA-induced sarcomas, both carrying individual TSTA. They grew in syngeneic animals as well as in two allogeneic strains— C3Hf and C57BL/6. When Balb/c mice were immunized with an allogeneic skin graft, neither tumor grew in Balb/c mice receiving C3Hf skin grafts. One did not grow in mice with C57BL grafts (Table 13). These data suggest that individual tumor-associated antigens of these tumors may be viewed as alien histocompatibility antigens.

MARTIN: Della Porta's data essentially support the notion of derepressed alloantigens; i.e., the MCA-induced Balb/c tumors may express a component present in skin of C57BL/6 mice.

TABLE 13

Effect of Syngeneic or Allogeneic Skin Graft on the Isograft of Balb/c
MCA-Induced Sarcomas Able to Grow in C3Hf and C57BL Mice

Immunizing skin graft	Tumor challenge with 5×10^4 cells s.c.[a] (no. of mice with tumor/no. of mice transplanted)	
	ST-2	ST-5
None	10/10	10/10
Balb/c	10/10	10/10
C3Hf	2/10[b]	1/10[b]
C57BL	9/10	2/9[b]

[a]Seven days after skin grafting.
[b]$P < 0.01$.

DELLA PORTA: Yes. However, absorption with specific antisera shows that the tumors retain the H-2^d of the Balb/c strain.

MARTIN: The derepressed alloantigen is not necessarily related to the H-2 antigen. It is not surprising, therefore, that the Balb/c tumor expresses H-2^d antigens.

DELLA PORTA: Yes, the major difference is that Martin's tumors do not grow in the syngeneic system.

MARTIN: Our lung tumors were induced transplacentally, before the immune system became competent to eliminate strongly immunogenic tumors. Della Porta's data illustrate a point which is also apparent with the lung tumors. After a number of *in vivo* passages tumors "38" and "85" acquired the capacity to grow in syngeneic C3Hf mice. However, these tumors still did not grow in A lung preimmunized irradiated C3Hf mice. The alloantigen was, therefore, apparently present but had lost ability to immunize the host. Loss of immunogenicity of a tumor antigen may be an important escape mechanism for the tumor, but one which can be countered by appropriate allogeneic immunization.

CHAIRMAN SMITH: This discussion has raised several issues concerning embryonic antigens. It is appropriate to focus now upon the biological significance of tumor-borne embryonic or differentiation structures as antigens.

DELLA PORTA: We have demonstrated embryonic antigens on tumor cells, as has been possible in many laboratories. One system involved chemically induced lymphomas. Mouse lymphoma cells induced with urethane were tested with sera raised against 10–14-day-old embryos. These sera killed the target

TABLE 14

Relationship Between Embryonic Antigens and Growth Rate of Balb/c Fibrosarcomas, Spontaneous or Induced by Chemical Agents or Physical State Carcinogenesis

Inducing agent	Growth rate[a] no. of days from injection to a tumor of 10 mm $\emptyset$	Amount of embryonic antigen % of reduction of C57 anti-embryo serum activity after absorption with tumor cells[b]		
		5×10^6	15×10^6	45×10^6
Teflon no. 4	15	88	89	89
DMBA no. 3	15	91	92	90
DMBA no. 1	20	81	87	90
Teflon no. 7	20	32	64	60
Spontaneous no. 3	21	50	62	–
Spontaneous no. 2	25	54	69	73
DMBA no. 2	26	50	81	76
MCA no. 1	28	23	23	64
Teflon no. 3	56	-8	19	27

[a]The growth rate was measured by injection of 10^4 cells in immunodepressed mice.

[b]The serum activity was evaluated on a reference target cell (Ly C57 Ur 24) by ^{51}Cr-release test.

cells by complement-dependent cytotoxicity assayed by ^{51}Cr release (Colnaghi and Della Porta, *J. Natl. Cancer Inst.,* **50,** 173, 1973).

In a second system, DMBA-induced sarcomas were tested *in vitro* for cell-mediated cytotoxicity. In this set of experiments, cross-reacting antigens were found and shown to be closely related to embryonic antigens. After several transplantation passages, individual TSTA were decreased on the tumor cells, with a parallel increase of embryonic antigens (Menard, Colnaghi, and Della Porta, *Cancer Res.,* **33,** 478, 1973).

Some information on the possible biological function of the embryonic antigens was obtained by experiments involving antiembryo immunization, then challenging mice with a series of different tumors induced either by chemicals, or arising by spontaneous *in vitro* transformation. We observed an enhancing effect on tumor growth in antiembryo immune as compared to control mice.

We then tried to correlate the amount of embryonic antigen present on the tumor cells, and some of the biological characteristics of the tumors. We measured (Table 14) the amount of embryonic antigens present on a series of tumors by absorption tests in which we absorbed the antiembryo activity of a standard serum. The tumors which had the larger amount of embryonic antigen grew much faster than the others. Perhaps there is a relationship between the expression of the embryonic antigens and the rate of growth of tumors. This could be an effect of some other biological characteristic of tumors, or perhaps the amount of the embryonic antigen itself is affecting the behavior of the tumor.

BALDWIN: Our point of view is that chemically induced tumors express individually distinct tumor-rejection antigens. This has been extensively analyzed by characterization of the neoantigens expressed on rat hepatomas induced by aminoazo dyes. From these studies, it is clear that hepatomas express individual tumor-rejection antigens since rats immune to their own tumors will not reject challenge with another one, although 10- to 100-fold lower challenge doses of tumor cells are given. In these examples, the individual specificity is also reflected by the specificity of antibody in tumor-immune rats as detected by membrane immunofluorescence or serum cytotoxicity. Similarly, lymph node cell cytotoxicity assayed *in vitro* shows individually distinct specificities.

In contrast, hepatomas induced by 2-acetylaminofluorene (AAF) do not express significant levels of tumor-rejection antigens so that immunity cannot be induced against these tumors even though low challenge doses (10^2 to 10^3) of tumor cells are given. In comparison, the level of immunity elicited against aminoazo dye-induced hepatomas is such that challenge with between 10^5 and 10^6 tumor cells are rejected. Consistent with the data obtained with AAF-induced hepatomas, it has also been established that AAF-induced mammary carcinomas are often deficient in tumor-rejection antigens. There is thus a spectrum of tumor antigenicity ranging from highly immunogenic aminoazo dye-induced hepatomas to essentially inactive AAF-induced hepatomas and mammary carcinomas.

In this context, it has also been shown that many spontaneous tumors, e.g., mammary carcinomas and sarcomas, are deficient in tumor-rejection antigens. It should be stressed, however, that in all of these tumor types where tumor-associated antigens are demonstrable, they show individual specificities. Many of these tumors also express cross-reacting antigens which are reexpressed embryonic components. These antigens are detected by reaction of tumor cells with antibody in sera of multiparous rats either by membrane immunofluorescence reactions or by complement-dependent cytotoxicity. Lymph node cells from multiparous rats are also cytotoxic *in vitro* for tumor cells.

Differentiation between tumor-associated rejection antigens and the embryonic antigens has been made on the grounds of their specificities. Hence, unlike the tumor-rejection antigens, tumor-associated embryonic antigens are common to different tumors. This was initially indicated since a specific multiparous rat serum was shown to be reactive with several individual tumors. Also, absorption of antibody with one tumor removes reactivity with other tumors as well. Further differentiation between tumor-rejection and tumor-associated embryonic antigens is provided by assays of serum blocking of lymph node cell cytotoxicity (Fig. 8). Lymph node cells from multiparous or hepatoma-immune rats are cytotoxic for 15-day-old cultured embryo cells and this can be "blocked" by pretreating plated cells with heat-inactivated multiparous rat serum. Multiparous rat lymph node cells are also cytotoxic for tumor cells, and again this reactivity can be blocked by treating plated tumor cells with multipar-

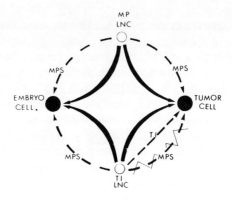

Fig. 8. Diagrammatic representation of serum blocking of lymph node cell (LNC) cytotoxicity for rat tumor and embryo cells. LNC from multiparous rats or tumor-immune rats are cytotoxic for both cultured tumor and embryo cells (solid arrows). Serum from multiparous rats (MPS) has the capacity to block multiparous rat lymph node cell (MP LNC) cytotoxicity for embryo or tumor cells (broken line arrows). MPS also blocks the cytotoxicity of LNC from tumor-immune (TI) rats against embryo cells (broken line arrows) but not against tumor cells (crossed broken line arrows). The cytotoxicity of tumor-immune lymph node cells (TI LNC) for tumor cells is, however, only blocked by sera from tumor-immune rats (broken line arrows). (*Transplantation Reviews,* in press, 1974).

ous rat serum. In contrast, the cytotoxicity of lymph node cells from tumor-immune rats cannot be blocked with multiparous serum, indicating that one population of lymphoid cells is sensitized to tumor-associated antigens which cannot be identified as embryonic antigens.

Utilizing these *in vitro* assays, it has further been established that tumors such as AAF-induced mammary carcinomas, where no significant levels of tumor-rejection antigen can be demonstrated, also express embryonic antigens. Thus, in these examples, lymph node cells from tumor-bearing rats are cytotoxic *in vitro* for the autochthonous tumor. Lymph node cells from a rat bearing a mammary carcinoma are also cytotoxic, however, for other mammary carcinomas, although not for other tumor types, suggesting that an organ-specific neoantigen is being detected. The view that this is an embryonic antigen is supported by studies showing that these lymph node cell cytotoxicities can be blocked by pretreating target cells with multiparous serum. Finally, the available evidence suggests that the expressed cell surface tumor-rejection antigens differ biochemically from the embryonic antigens. In detailed studies with one hepatoma (D_{23}), it has been established that the tumor-specific antigen is intimately associated with plasma membrane and can only be released by a degradative procedure such as extraction with papain or 3M KCl. While this antigen may also be associated with intracellular membrane, it does not occur in the cytoplasmic cell sap. In contrast, the tumor-associated embryonic antigen,

34

which is expressed at the cell surface, can be readily isolated from tumor cell sap and differs biochemically from the tumor-rejection antigen.

PREHN: Della Porta said that tumors which expressed embryonic antigens grew faster than those that did not. Is this true in immunosuppressed animals?

DELLA PORTA: I do not have data on that question.

COHN: In Baldwin's experiments on complement-dependent cytotoxicity, *in vivo* and *in vitro* killing are compared. Is the *in vitro* assay usually carried out with rabbit or with guinea pig complement?

BALDWIN: Guinea pig complement is used in all tests.

COHN: Is there any demonstrable cytotoxicity with rat complement?

BALDWIN: Yes, but rat complement is not very effective.

COHN: Would you say that the rat complement system is not functioning *in vivo* with rat antibody, whereas *in vitro* guinea pig complement is?

BALDWIN: Yes.

CHAIRMAN SMITH: Why is that an important issue?

COHN: We have been discussing the paradox that complement-dependent killing is not operating *in vivo* whereas *in vitro* it is. Why?

BALDWIN: The data I described also showed lymph node cell cytotoxicity.

BACH: When Baldwin speaks of tumors which are not very immunogenic, what is he referring to? What is his *in vivo* assay?

BALDWIN: This is evaluated by the capacity to immunize syngeneic rats either by excision of tumor or by implantation of irradiated tumor cells. So, for example, immunization against an immunogenic tumor, e.g., aminoazo dye-induced hepatoma will permit rejection of 10^5–10^6 challenge tumor cells. In comparison, immunization against AAF-induced hepatomas will *not* induce immunity to challenge with 10^2–10^3 tumor cells. Similarly, immunization with AAF-induced or spontaneous carcinomas will not induce rejection of 10^2–10^3 cells.

SJÖGREN: Is it essential to use multiparous animals in order to obtain potent blocking sera?

BALDWIN: No, it turns out not to be so; we can obtain such sera from animals postpregnancy.

E. KLEIN: What is the nature of the blocking factor in these sera?

BALDWIN: In these sera we think it is antibody, since they contain antibody detectable by membrane-immunofluorescence staining with tumor cells.

E. KLEIN: Can the blocking factor be shown to react to these cells? Is it present on others as well?

BALDWIN: I think that is another question for another day, but we also have blocking factor in immune complexes.

ALEXANDER: There is an interesting difference between the hepatomas with which Baldwin works and the MCA-induced sarcomas in rats. In the latter, the embryonic surface antigen evokes an antibody response, and one gets specific antisera to it in rats after surgical excision of the tumor (Thompson, *et al.*, *Brit. J. Cancer*, **27**,27, 1973). In Baldwin's hepatoma situation, the tumor-bearing host or the host immunized with tumor does not make antibody to the cross-reacting fetal antigen. This onco-fetal antigen in the MCA-induced sarcomas, which we have called OEAI, has been clearly separated from the coexisting TSTA which is unique to each tumor. The respective antigen determinants are on separate molecules with different molecular weights and electrophoretic mobilities.

Also, I think we have to be careful about the term "immunogenicity." As Baldwin knows, there are many tumors against which one cannot immunize in the sense that one can render the animal resistant to a subsequent tumor challenge, and yet one has no difficulty in demonstrating specific cytotoxic factors present in these animals.

BALDWIN: All of these tumor bearers have cytotoxic lymph node cells—that is why I hesitated in using the term immunogenicity—but one needs a simple term to indicate that a tumor does elicit rejection reactions.

ALEXANDER: The last thing we need is a simple term because the capacity to reject the tumor measures at least *two* distinct phenomena. It measures the capacity of the animals to mount an immune reaction, and it measures the capacity of the tumor cells to be attacked successfully by the effector arm *in vivo*.

MANNINO: In this general discussion about embryonic antigens and the specific antigens induced by carcinogens, my concern is whether the various investigators in this complex subject ever exchange products and look for each other's antigens.

BALDWIN: This is part of our trouble—*we* use rats and chemically induced tumors—Della Porta uses tumors in mice. Then, too, we lack the sort of shorthand such as that in the H-2 system which makes for better internal communication.

MANNINO: So what you are finding could just be a general phenomenon of a lot of antigens being exposed.

BALDWIN: Yes.

BACH: I want to come back to this question of a simple term. It could well be that there are highly immunogenic tumors which stimulate that part of the immune response which results in antibody production and thus leads to antigen–antibody complex blocking. Such tumors would then grow well and yet we would say they are not "immunogenic."

BALDWIN: In the tumors we have looked at which do not elicit good tumor-rejection reactions, we cannot detect specific tumor antibody or good cell-mediated immunity.

BACH: But there *are* blocking factors?

BALDWIN: Yes.

CHAIRMAN SMITH: Immunogenicity has the operational definition which Prehn, Old, and Klein gave to it. It is that attribute of transplantable tumors which induce in syngeneic recipients the capacity to reject significantly larger numbers of tumor cells, when challenged after removal or "cure" of the tumor evoking the response. This is still as good a definition as we have.

CEROTTINI: A point of clarification, please. Can Baldwin tell us whether it is correct that lymph node cells from animals bearing a given mammary carcinoma kill *in vitro* different mammary carcinomas, whereas cross reactivity never happens with lymph node cells taken from hepatoma-bearing rats?

BALDWIN: Yes, that is so.

MARTIN: Certain antigens may only find expression during fetal life in some strains, yet may be expressed throughout life in other strains. It may be of interest to determine whether fetal antigens expressed on rat hepatoma cells are also expressed on normal cells of allogeneic rats, or even on xenogeneic animals.
    With respect to Baldwin's contention that fetal antigens cannot be consid-

ered true transplantation antigens, surely tumors which eventually develop in carcinogen-treated rats are selected for ability *not* to evoke effective syngeneic immunity. Appropriate immunization with allogeneic adult or fetal tissue may well reveal that certain of these antigens can still serve as targets for immune destruction *in vivo*.

BALDWIN: I do not suggest that fetal antigens are not immunogenic. Whether they evoke rejection reaction or not probably depends on the stability of the antigens on the cell surface. Probably this accounts for a conflict at the moment between ourselves and Coggin, who has shown that on certain tumor cells fetal antigens function as rejection antigens.

GOOD: How secure are we in talking about tumor antigens as embryonic antigens? For example, has Baldwin taken multiparous sera which interfere with the cytotoxic effect and absorbed them in the male under a variety of conditions of challenge?

BALDWIN: We have looked for these reactivities in adult cells at various times. We have, of course, carried out *in vitro* absorptions. However, the experiment that Good refers to has not yet been performed. We have shown that these antigens appear on fetal cells between day 14 and day 16.

WEISS: On the whole, fetal cells elaborate a variety of soluble factors more actively than do fully differentiated cells, and this is part of the whole business of cell–cell contact which underlies the process of growth, differentiation, and the laying down of organ and tissue systems. Some of these factors undoubtedly are what we call fetal or embryonic antigens. There must be, in all probability, a basic survival mechanism which makes it difficult for such temporarily elaborated substances to be also auto-antigenic. They may lack the biochemical and biophysical attributes which make for effective immunogenicity or they may at least be devoid of intrinsic adjuvanticity, properties which direct immunological responsiveness in cellular directions. In addition, a flooding of the body by such antigens could well affect self-tolerance on the level of effector cell blockade. In any event, the tolerogenicity of fetal antigens may be a necessary condition of development and the expression of such antigens on the surface of neoplastic cells may represent a protective preemption by such cells of a physiological mechanism.

HOWARD: What happens to multiparous females with regard to their resistance to tumor bearing?

BALDWIN: We have not looked at this, but I believe Della Porta has.

DELLA PORTA: We immunized with embryo cells, and in most experiments induced enhancement rather than protection, in the case of sarcomas. However, some recent unpublished data of my colleague Colnaghi show that mice immunized against embryo cells are significantly protected *in vivo* against a challenge of a syngeneic urethan-induced lymphoma previously demonstrated, by serology, to carry embryonic antigens. Also the passive transfer of the antiembryo serum conferred protection to untreated mice. It seems therefore that the *in vivo* outcome of an antiembryo immunization may largely depend on the nature of the target cell.

KLEIN: If embryonic antigens are responsible in Baldwin's system, are all tumors cross reacting at the level of testing for lymphocyte cytotoxicity?

BALDWIN: Yes.

KLEIN: Can Baldwin say that all sera of tumor bearers will cause blocking?

BALDWIN: Yes, that is so.

DELLA PORTA: With antiembryo immunization, however, we also got rejection of lymphomas. Perhaps it depends, in part, on the target cell itself, not only on immunization with embryonic antigen.

HOWARD: In that case, could you say embryonic tissue can be immunogenic in the training sense—can it cause a substantive reaction to the tumor?

DELLA PORTA: When we placed embryonic tissue in intraperitoneal chambers and then challenged the mice s.c. with tumor, we obtained enhancement. Moreover we observed enhancement also when sarcoma cells were implanted in a diffusion chamber and the challenging graft was from the same sarcoma (Table 15). So, perhaps, not only the type of antigen but also the form of its presentation to the immune system is critical in determining the type of the immune response.

KLEIN: Is the resistance that Della Porta induced by immunization with embryonic tissue and the resistance he induced by allogeneic skin graft against the syngeneic transplant of the Balb/c tumor radioresistant in the same sense that the effect shown by Martin was radioresistant?

DELLA PORTA: We have not done that experiment.

KLEIN: I would be worried unless it could be shown that both effects were radioresistant. A number of years ago we found that inoculation of embryonic tissues increased the resistance level of mice to subsequent first inoculations of small cell numbers from syngeneic, MCA-induced tumors. In contrast to true immunization with irradiated cells of the same tumor, this effect was entirely abolished by 400 R whole-body irradiation. We concluded, therefore, that this was not specific immunization, but a boosting of the host's ability to deal with the first challenge of an antigenic MCA-sarcoma isograft.

CHAIRMAN SMITH: Next we shall take up a related set of issues, which concern the production, distribution and characteristics of the antigens produced by growing tumor cells *in vivo* or *in vitro*.

TABLE 15

Effect of Intrachamber Cultivation of Syngeneic Embryo or Sarcoma Cells
on the Growth of a MCA-Induced Sarcoma (ST-2)

Experimental groups (DC's content)	No. of mice with tumor/ No. of mice transplanted with 2×10^3 ST-2 cells s.c.	%	P
Adult tissue fragments (muscle, liver, brain)	7/29	27	
16-day-old embryo fragments (muscle, liver, brain)	21/35	60	< 0.01
ST-2 tumor fragments	12/14	85	< 0.02

Dialysis chambers made with 0.22 μ filters were left for 20 days i.p. and then removed. The challenge was done 7 days later. The ST-2 sarcoma was previously shown, by the standard growth-excision method of immunization, to bear a strong individual TSTA (Permiani, et al., unpublished).

STUTMAN: Antigens on the cell surface of spontaneous mammary adenocarcinomas (MT) of C3H mice as defined by different immunological procedures are presented in Table 16. ML (mammary leukemia) is a cross-reacting antigen, virus dependent, but probably not a part of the mammary tumor virus (MTV) virion. It is also detected in some DBA/2 leukemias, and was defined by Stock, Old, and Boyse, in the 1960s, using serological methods. Another set of cross-reacting antigens is called MTV, for the virus-associated antigens present in the virion. There are at least two or three MTV defined serologically. Some have been associated with the viral envelope proteins. Private, non-cross-reacting antigens are also known, first described by Vaage, which are individual for each tumor and are defined mainly by lymphocyte-dependent reactions. Unexpected is the finding that Thy-1 (θ), defined by complement-dependent cytolysis, is present in MT.

If mammary tumor cell membranes are solubilized in potassium chloride or in similar procedures, ML plus the MTV-associated antigens are readily obtained. The soluble antigen (Table 17) can stimulate specific in vitro responses in immune lymphocytes, measured by blast transformation and thymidine uptake. The antigen is cross reacting (Table 18) and has the characteristic of ML, i.e., ML is probably its main component although MTV antigens are also present (Table 19). The lymphocytes responding to such soluble antigen have characteristics of T lymphocytes (as indicated in Table 20) but B lymphocytes from in vivo immunized mice are stimulated by the antigen rendered insoluble by coupling to sepharose beads.

We now obtain antigen from the supernatants of cells grown in protein-free media or in media with defined proteins which can be easily removed. We observed that both ML and Thy-1 are readily detected in such supernatants.

Without relating details of turnover, we have shown with endogenously labeled antigens, ^{14}C amino acids or sugars, that ML antigen is a glycoprotein

TABLE 16

Surface Determinants in C3H Mammary Adenocarcinoma Cells

Antigens	Characteristics	Techniques for identification	Turnover	"Modulation" by antibody
ML	Cross reacting[a]	SD + LD[b]	Rapid	Yes
MTV (1,2,?)	Cross reactive	SD + LD	?	No
P (Private)	Non-cross-reactive	LD	?	?
Thy-1	—	SD (LD?)	Rapid	Yes ?

[a] Cross reactivity indicates that each of those antigens reacts with other mammary tumors (even from other mouse strains) but not with each other.

[b] SD: antigens defined by serological methods.

LD: antigens defined by lymphocyte-mediated methods.

TABLE 17

In Vitro Response of Lymph Node Cells to Soluble Mammary-Tumor Antigen

Cell type[a]	Antigen[b]	Response (CPM)[c]
C3Hf (nonimmune)	MT	950-2100
C3Hf (immune to MT)	MT	19,950-25,400
C3Hf (immune to MT)	MCS	3000-3800
C3Hf (immune to MSC)	MT	2500-3700
C3Hf (immune to MT)	MCSf	930-1900

[a] 5×10^5 lymph node cells from normal or immune C3Hf adult mice with 20 μg/protein/50×10^6 cells, for 72 hr (last 12 with 3HT).

[b] MT: soluble antigen from C3H mammary tumors.

MCS: soluble antigen from C3H methylcholanthrene sarcomas.

MCSf: soluble antigen from C3Hf MC sarcomas.

All these soluble antigens extracted with $3M$ KC1.

[c] Range of 12 different determinations.

TABLE 18

Cross Reactivity of MT Soluble Antigens

Lymph node lymphocytes immune to MT	Soluble Ag from MT	Net CPM response[a]
1	1	22,000
2	1	15,000
3	1	13,000
4	1	23,000
5	1	13,000
6	1	26,000
7	1	10,000
8	1	7,000
9	1	20,000
10	1	17,500
MCSf	1	600

[a] Expressed as net CPM (background ranged from 800 to 1,300 CPM).

MT: mammary tumors; MCSF: methylcholanthrene sarcoma induced in C3Hf mice.

TABLE 19

Response of DBA/2f Spleen Cells to DBA/2 MT Soluble Ag

Cells	Antigen[a]	Net response
DBA/2 f immune to MT[b]	MT	13,000
DBA/2 f immune to MT	ML[c]	10,500
DBA/2 f immune to ML+L	MT	9,000
DBA/2 f immune to ML+L	ML	11,000
DBA/2 f immune to MT	MC[d]	260
DBA/2 f immune to MT	control	2,300

[a]All the antigens were extracted by $3M$ KCl.
[b]MT: soluble antigen from DBA/2 mammary tumor.
[c]ML: soluble antigen from ML+DBA/2 leukemia.
[d]MC: soluble antigen from DBA/2 methylcholanthrene sarcoma.

TABLE 20

Response of Immune Lymphocytes Depleted of T or B Cells

Type of cells[a]	Antigen	Net response
Whole spleen lymphocytes	soluble	17,000
T-depleted[a] spleen lymphocytes	soluble	600
T-depleted spleen lymphocytes	insoluble	6,000
B-depleted[b] spleen lymphocytes	soluble	13,000
M-depleted[c] spleen lymphocytes	soluble	9,000

[a]T depleted: cells treated by anti-θ 1 and C, dead cells removed by a one step BSA-gradient.
[b]B depleted: cells treated with Anti-Ig and C. Subsequently, CRL are made with sheep red cells + Ab + C, and the lysed cells and rosettes are removed in a BSA-gradient.
[c]M depleted: adherent cells removed by nylon wool columns plus adherence to plastic.

with molecular weight of 60,000, and the antigenic component may be related to galactoside. It is destroyed by β-galactosidase.

Two additional features make this more complicated. At two to six months of age C3H-MTV + mice spontaneously develop MTV antigens in a proportion of their normal lymphocytes. This can be shown by immunofluorescence using a rabbit antidisrupted MTV. Such antigens are readily found in mammary tumor cells and in 20–30% of normal spleen cells, 10% lymph node cells, 10–15% in bone marrow, and 0% in thymus. Thus, at least some antigens are expressed both in the target and in the lymphocyte. The second point is that at approximately the same age, and before detectable tumors are observed, a proportion of the animals have antibodies in serum which react with MTV antigens.

It is clear that the overall immune response in this system is the result of the interplay of such different ingredients. To have expected a simple system was indeed naive.

An important aspect of this system is that some of the reagents are rather well defined: We have "pure" ML and we can produce antibodies in mice and rabbits with it. ML is virus dependent but not present in the virus. We can use either mammary tumor cells or DBA/2 leukemia as target cells for cytotoxicity. Similarly the MTV proteins are well defined. With disrupted virus we can produce a crude anti-MTV antibody in rabbits, or antibodies against external proteins of the virion.

ML is readily modulated by antibodies *in vitro*. The MTV-associated antigens are not. Later I will come back to the effects of soluble antigens on immune lymphocytes and on their ability to kill the mammary tumor target.

CHIECO-BIANCHI: Can Stutman establish these cells as continuous cell lines?

STUTMAN: We may call them "lines," but technically they are not yet established lines. We make a serious effort to have pure carcinoma cells *in vitro*. We achieve this by extensive collagenase treatment and growing the cells in suspension in protein-rich media, thus eliminating the normal cells that will stick under such conditions. We take the floaters, mainly malignant cells, and end up with beautiful epithelial-like monolayers when the cells are transferred to medium with low protein concentration.

CHIECO-BIANCHI: Did you try to modulate these cells?

STUTMAN: We do not have synchronized cells to do that type of thing, but eventually we will try it.

SHELLAM: What of the relative potency of these various antigens, particularly MTV, in inducing immunity?

STUTMAN: To answer Shellam's question I must first define the hosts used for immunization. We have three syngeneic sublines of C3H mice (derived from the Bittner stock) which differ only as to whether they are infected with MTV. C3H is the classic milk-infected strain; it contains MTV-S (Standard) and 100% develop mammary tumors. They are also infected with MTV-L (low, or nodule-inducing virus, of low oncogenic potency) which is transmitted vertically by both male and female parents. We also have a C3Hf that had been derived by Bittner in 1948, which is totally virus free, both MTV-S and MTV-L. The majority of the reported experiments were done with this strain (appears as C3Hf (1) in the tables). The conventional foster-nursed C3Hf strains are only free of MTV-S (i.e., the milk-borne virus).

Of the three antigens present in mammary tumors of C3H origin, C3H responds mainly to ML and P, C3Hf (1) to all three and the conventional C3Hf mice mainly to ML and P and to a lesser degree to MTV antigens. ML is a strong immunogen but it also stimulates antibody production and is readily modulated by antibody. The response to MTV is also strong, but complicating factors in the virus-infected mice are the presence of antigen (i.e., the virus) and also "spontaneous" antibodies, with the possibility of formation of antigen–antibody complexes. I would say that the strongest and most efficient immune response to mammary tumors, measured as *in vitro* cytotoxicity or *in vivo* neutralization of tumor growth, is when the host can recognize all three antigenic types.

CEPPELLINI: Is ML also released from the cell?

STUTMAN: Yes.

CEPPELLINI: I want to point out that there is another antigen, LEA originating on lymphocytes, which sticks on red cells and on lymphocytes, going from lymphocytes to sera and vice versa. In a few hours we are able to change the LEA negative lymphocytes into positive, just by incubating the cells in LEA positive serum and vice versa. It is an extreme case of an antigen which is necessarily endogenous to the cell but is very soluble in cell membrane.

STUTMAN: ML can be endogenously labeled. We digest the surface with enzymes, then measure the regeneration of ML on the surface and its subsequent release in the medium. We produce endogenous labeling with radioactive amino acids. Thy-1 does not label very well, suggesting either a slower rate of turnover or perhaps its "acquired" origin.

VAAGE: Did Stutman say that the C3Hf line is virus free and does not get tumors?

STUTMAN: These are the old Zb mice from Bittner. Hormonal stimulation, multiple pregnancies or multiple pituitary grafting do not produce tumors in this strain.

VAAGE: The C3Hf (Heston) strain which I use, is MTV free although it has the nodule inducing virus, and contrary to what has been reported, the C3Hf mice develop a high incidence of spontaneous mammary carcinomas, if kept alive long enough, and under pathogen-free conditions. The C3Hf mice develop tumors at an average age of 24 months and at the same rate at which the C3H (Heston) mice develop tumors at 8–9 months. The histologic appearance of

44

mammary carcinomas is the same in the two substrains, except that in the C3Hf, appearance is delayed for about 16 months.

STUTMAN: I could not agree more with Vaage. As a matter of fact, in our conventional C3Hf, by 2 years of age about 45% have developed tumors containing viral particles. Incidentally, conventional C3Hf lymphocytes show positive fluorescence for MTV antigens.

MARTIN: I question whether MTV and ML antigens can be called tumor-specific antigens in the autochthonous host. If similar antigens are expressed on nonmalignant cells of the mammary tumor-prone conventional C3H mouse, then these components may not be relevant to tumor rejection.

STUTMAN: ML is not expressed in any normal tissue—only in mammary tumor cells. It is present in some DBA/2 leukemias, but that is a different story.

MARTIN: Is ML expressed in the normal mammary cell of the conventional C3H mouse strain?

STUTMAN: We cannot detect it. With fluorescent rabbit anti-ML we cannot find the antigen in normal mammary gland. It may be detected in nodules, but this is a preliminary observation.

COHN: Stutman says that he had lymphocytes which carry MTV antigens, but the animal is not producing antibody to it. He then inoculates the animal with a tumor which carries MTV and the animal responds to make anti-MTV. Is that correct?

STUTMAN: No. The antibodies against MTV will appear before detectable tumors.

CHAIRMAN SMITH: You have complicated our lives beautifully, Stutman, by presenting these nice data; I presume you also intend to reclarify the situation ultimately. I would like to move to the questions that Stutman raised, dealing particularly with shedding and production of antigen from the cell surface. We will lead off with Cone.

CONE: With Ceppellini in Basel, and Carbonara and Jacot-Guillarmod in Turin, I have been studying the fate of alloantibodies bound to the surface of human peripheral blood lymphocytes when the cells are incubated in cell culture medium. Lymphocytes possessing HL-A specificities 2, 5 and 12 are coated at

4°C with a ^{125}I-labeled IgG fraction of antiserum ToGn which is anti-HL-A 2, 5 and 12. After being washed, the cells are incubated for up to 24 hr in culture medium at either 15°C or 37°C. At intervals during this period, the cells are centrifuged, and the cell pellet and supernatant assessed for radioactivity. In addition, we determine whether the cells can still be killed by added complement.

The gist of the results is that if the cells are incubated at 15°C for 24 hr about 10% of the ^{125}I-labeled antibody is released into the medium. All of the cells are lysed if complement is added, indicating that most of the antibody is still present at the cell surface. Fifty to seventy percent of the released antibody will bind to uncoated lymphocytes. When the cells are incubated at 37°C the picture is quite different. Radioactive antibody is progressively lost from the cell surface so that up to 70% of the antibody is in the culture medium after 24 hr. We also observe a parallel loss in the ability of added complement to kill the cells. Moreover, the antibody released at 37°C will not bind to uncoated lymphocytes. This suggested that the antibody was either destroyed or that the combining sites were blocked by antigen. If the antibody is treated with glycine buffer at pH 2.5, binding activity is restored indicating that at 37°C the antibody is released complexed to antigen.

To determine the nature of the membrane components in the surface antigen-alloantibody complex we labeled the cell surface of lymphocytes with ^{125}I using the lactoperoxidase method. The ^{125}I-labeled cells were coated with ToGn–IgG and the cells were then incubated in culture medium at 37°C for 6 hr. The cells were centrifuged and the released ToGn present in the supernatant precipitated with a rabbit antihuman Ig antiserum. About twice as much ^{125}I-labeled membrane protein is precipitated from the culture fluid of cells coated with ToGn as is precipitated from ^{125}I-labeled uncoated cells incubated for the same period.

The precipitates are dissolved in SDS and the ^{125}I-labeled membrane components are resolved by disc electrophoresis in polyacrylamide-SDS gels. The results are shown in Fig. 9. The upper part of the figure shows membrane components which are precipitated from supernatants containing antibody that has been shed from the cell. These components are not present in control supernatants. The lower part of the figure shows that similar membrane proteins are found when we radiolabel lymphocytes, extract the cells with NP-40 and precipitate the extract with ToGn and rabbit antihuman Ig antiserum. In other words, the shed material complexed to ToGn is similar to what we can actually extract from the cell without shedding.

These results suggest to us that when the alloantibody is released from the cell surface, it is released as a complex with the membrane components to which it binds. Interestingly, if uncoated cells are incubated for 6 hr and ToGn and rabbit antihuman Ig are added to the culture fluid, we cannot detect these

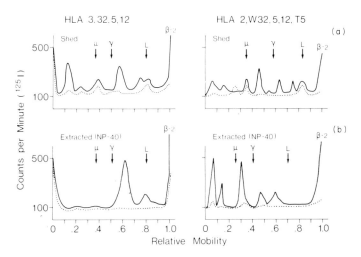

Fig. 9. Polyacrylamide gel electrophoresis of cell surface proteins precipitated from the incubation medium of ToGn-coated ^{125}I-labeled lymphocytes (shed) and detergent extracts of ^{125}I-labeled lymphocytes (extracted). (a) Cell surface proteins precipitated by rabbit antihuman Ig and sheep antirabbit antisera from incubation medium of ^{125}I-labeled lymphocytes coated with ToGn (o——o), uncoated (x——x). (b) Cell surface proteins precipitated from surface Ig depleted NP-40 extracts of ^{125}I-labeled lymphocytes by ToGn and rabbit antihuman Ig antisera (o——o), autologous human serum, and rabbit antihuman Ig antisera (x——x). μ, γ, L, $\beta 2$ refer to the relative mobility of human immunologlobulin μ and γ heavy chains, light chains, and $\beta 2$ microglobulin respectively. ToGn = anti-HLA 2, 5, 12, 4a.

membrane proteins. We interpret this to mean that these membrane antigens are being released from the cell as a result of interaction with antibody.

TERRY: Does the presence of serum in the incubation mixture influence the amount of shedding detected?

CONE: The cells are incubated in RPMI medium which contains 5% autologous serum. We have not tested for what happens in the absence of added protein.

PERNIS: This shedding is not a general phenomenon. It depends on the molecule that adheres to the antibody. Were it a surface immunoglobulin on the lymphocytes, it all goes inside and is chewed up, so there is nothing to shed. So it depends on the antigen. It is very interesting that antigens like HL-A are shed.

CONE: I would qualify Pernis' comment by saying it probably depends not only on the nature of the antigen, but on the nature of the ligand. Under certain conditions complexes of surface immunoglobulin and anti-immunoglobulin antibody *are* shed: It depends on the amounts of antibody used. In the experiments I described, some antigen–antibody complex is also interiorized by the cell.

COHN: Can something be said about the relationship between the number of antigenic specificities and the number of products?

CONE: Yes, this antiserum has a very high titer and may contain antibodies to "non-HL-A" specificities. Therefore, several molecular species are precipitated.

UHR: Since we know that release of tumor antigens into the circulation markedly affects the host response, it is important that we carefully distinguish three possible pathways of release of tumor-associated antigens, namely lysis, shedding and secretion. These forms of release are distinguishable both operationally and mechanistically. The discussions that have just taken place indicate that the terms are not being used correctly.

Let me discuss lysis first. Lysis is accompanied by release of ^{51}Cr, which is not true of shedding or secretion. Shedding should refer to release of molecules which were present on the cell surface. This cannot be ascertained simply by labeling with a precursor. Cell surface iodination, however, can establish that a molecule *was* on the surface before release into the incubation medium.

Figure 10 shows the results of an experiment in which surface iodinated murine splenocytes were incubated for 24 hr. As can be seen, immunoglobulin and other proteins are very rapidly shed during the first 6 hr and then are shed at a very slow rate. The lost immunoglobulin and protein are recovered in the incubation medium, however, no H-2 alloantigens are released during the first 6 hr. They are lost from the cells in small amounts after cells begin to die be-

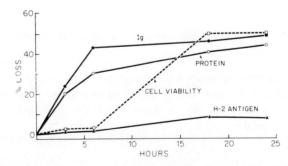

Fig. 10. Release of cell surface molecules from radioiodinated murine splenocytes during incubation.

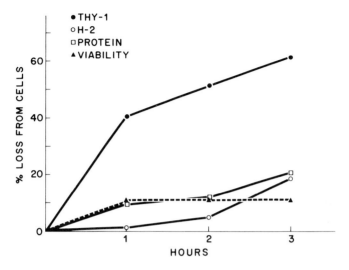

Fig. 11. Loss of Thy-1 and H-2 alloantigens and total protein from radioiodinated murine thymo-cytes during incubation. (Vitetta *et al., Eur. J. Immunol.,* **4,** 276, 1974).

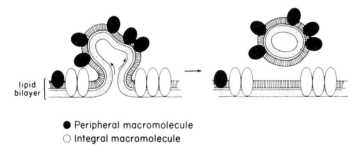

Fig. 12. Model of shedding of peripheral macromolecules from microvilli of lymphoid cells.

tween 6 and 24 hr of culture. In contrast to lysis, therefore, shedding is not associated with cell death.

The antigens released by shedding appear to be released on a fragment of plasma membrane. Thus, the molecular form of the antigen is different from secreted antigen. Figure 11 shows the same experiment in thymocytes. Thy-1 and some other proteins are rapidly released, and H-2 alloantigens are not. Release occurred without significant change in cell viability.

In Fig. 12, I have illustrated a possible model for shedding. I suggest that molecules such as immunoglobulin and Thy-1 are peripheral molecules in the fluid mosaic model. They can migrate into microvilli and are released associated with fragments of plasma membrane when the microvilli pinch off. In contrast,

H-2 alloantigens are integral proteins that penetrate deeply into the membrane and are clustered at the base of microvilli unable to migrate into the villi because of thermodynamic considerations. Thus, the H-2 alloantigens are postulated to have strong protein–protein interactions, and interactions with the hydrocarbon portion of the adjoining lipids which in some way restricts their migration.

Secretion is the active transport of a macromolecule out of the cell and usually occurs *without* a cell surface phase. The criterion of secretion is enrichment, i.e., the proportion of labeled secreted molecules like immunoglobulin to total labeled protein in the incubation medium versus the cell lysate is markedly increased. The ratio is almost unchanged in shedding. For example, after labeling lymphoid cells for 2–3 hr with radioactive amino acids immunoglobulin enrichment is 25- to 50-fold in media versus lysate. Macromolecules like Ig are secreted in their conventional molecular form and not attached to other molecules by membrane. The biology of tumor-associated antigens in the circulation could depend in part on whether they are associated with plasma membrane fragments.

COHN: Consider a third antigen on the surface of Uhr's model cell, is he postulating that it would be shed as a mixed structure?

UHR: Cohn asks if there are other molecules being shed on this fragment. The answer is yes. When incubation media containing shed radioiodinated Ig is immunoprecipitated with anti-Ig without prior detergent treatment, 5- to 10-fold more radioactivity is precipitated than when detergent is used. Detergent by dissolving membrane breaks the link between Ig and other protein molecules. This finding does not occur with secreted Ig.

I want to make the point that it is not a simple matter to differentiate lysis from shedding. Figure 13 shows the results of studies of a Burkitt lymphoma line (Daudi) which was initially isolated by George and Eva Klein. We observed that small amounts of radioactive immunoglobulin could appear in the media of iodinated incubated cells. Did this represent lysis or shedding? To answer this, cells were cultivated at optimal conditions (low density) or suboptimal (stationary growth) and aliquots were labeled with either ^{125}I or ^{51}Cr. Under conditions in which the cells were grown at low density, shown in Fig. 13a, there was much less immunoglobulin released into the medium than when the cells were grown at high density shown in Fig. 13b. Furthermore, the release of immunoglobulin paralleled the release of both total protein and ^{51}Cr. Hence, release is probably by lysis and not by shedding.

The final point I want to make is that in a heterogeneous population of cells, one cell may be secreting a particular molecule, and another cell may have it on its surface either through synthesis or binding of the secreted mole-

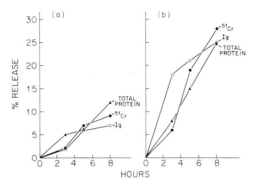

Fig. 13a, b. Kinetics of release of ^{125}I and ^{51}Cr from Burkitt lymphoma cells during incubation. Before iodination, the cells were in (a) log-phase culture and (b) stationary culture (Grundke-Iqbal and Uhr, *Eur J. Immunol.*, **4**, 159, 1974).

cule. For example, we have found that normal thoracic duct cells in mice synthesize and secrete only IgA. Cell surface iodination of this same population reveals only IgM. I believe this dichotomy is because two different cells are involved: IgA is synthesized and secreted by a very small number of plasma cells in the thoracic duct, whereas a much larger number of small B lymphocytes in the lymph have IgM on their surface. Thus, in this population, Ig in the media is not coming from the cells bearing Ig on their surface.

WEISS: By Uhr's discrimination between "shedding" and "secretion," it seems to me that there would be a heuristic appeal to the notion that fetal antigens might on the whole be *secreted* in a soluble, poorly immunogenic form, whereas some of the protective tumor-associated antigens might be shed as fragments with the characteristics, physically and biochemically, of immunogens. This would obviously be subject to testing. Does Uhr have any thoughts on that?

UHR: It is a good idea.

CHAIRMAN SMITH: We must consider another variable in comparing surface membrane behavior of lymphocytes with that of tumor cells. Generally speaking, lymphoblastoid cells shed membrane structures—for example, the MA antigen of Burkitt lymphoma cells or PHA receptor complex on human lymphoblastoid cell lines—whereas small lymphocytes internalize membrane-receptor complex upon encounter with comparable substances.

UHR: That is not true of immunoglobulin which is shed from small lymphocytes.

51

CHAIRMAN SMITH: Yes, but I point out that the fate of immunoglobulin has not been studied on human LCL.

MARTIN: A number of studies show that the type of medium in which cells are incubated determines the rate of release of receptor molecules. Possibly, all *in vitro* culture media cause a degree of nonphysiological shedding and it will be necessary to check one's observations on cells in the *in vivo* environment.

ALEXANDER: My comment relates to Uhr's presentation in that I do not like his terminology. Shedding might also include release of antigens in a monomolecular form. The analogy which Uhr gave us regarding immunoglobulin can be applied directly to tumor-specific antigen. By measuring tumor-specific antigens in the circulation of rats bearing tumors, Thompson made the observation that the concentration slowly built up as the tumor grew. In the case of one tumor he found evidence to the effect that immunologic attack is required to bring about release of tumor antigen into the circulation.* So it looks to me as if the rate of spontaneous release, whether this be shedding or an active process, remains to be resolved. Certainly it can vary considerably from one tumor to another, and it may well correlate with the biological properties of the tumor.

UHR: Shedding should indicate that the antigens were on the cell surface. I do not think it is essential that the shed antigens be on a piece of membrane, but I predict that this will be the case.

TERRY: On how many other tumors has Alexander made this correlation between ease of release of membrane components and the development of metastases?

ALEXANDER: We have studied two other tumors that do not metastasize and did not find high levels of TSTA in the tissue culture supernatant. In addition to the one tumor that metastasizes very readily and where there are very large amounts of TSTA in the tissue culture supernatant, there is an intermediate tumor which metastasizes in about 50% of the animals if the tumor is amputated around day 7. With this tumor one finds significant amounts of the antigen in the supernatant, but nothing like the other.

CEPPELLINI: The main point is that one cannot generalize about all kinds of antigens from this phenomenon, but if I understand Uhr correctly, he said that shedding takes off a piece of membrane. Is that correct?

Editors' note: The phenomenon described by Alexander is reported in *Brit. J. Cancer,* **29,** 72, 1974, and discussed more extensively in Session IV, pp. 235–238.

UHR: I said that in the systems we have studied, shedding involves release of a fragment of membrane.

CEPPELLINI: Just what is a piece of membrane? Each physical unit of membrane antigen engaged by antibody, as Roger Taylor and others have shown, is shed independently; it is not a piece of membrane, but a membrane molecule or a membrane–molecule complex.

UHR: I think the phenomenon which Ceppellini and Cone described is different. They induced release of a membrane protein by adding specific antibody. I discussed what happens in cells *not* treated with exogenous agents.

Regardless, in answer to Ceppellini's question, the evidence that shed immunoglobulin is on a fragment of plasma membrane is indirect but formidable. First, the shed immunoglobulin has the density of a lipoprotein, not a protein. If one pretreats the shed material with detergents, the material bands with protein. Second, if one precipitates shed-iodinated material with anti-Ig, one precipitates 5- to 10-fold more radioactivity than when pretreatment with detergent is used. Third, the immunoprecipitates formed without detergents show many labeled proteins, whereas those formed after detergent treatment essentially reveal IgM only. Therefore, there are many protein molecules along with immunoglobulin on the shed fragment, and these molecules are held together by a structure sensitive to a nonionic detergent.

CONE: I have a comment relevant to Uhr's remarks. Since we observed that HL-A antigens bound by ToGn were not spontaneously shed in six hours, there may be a somewhat different mechanism involved when antibody is added. Therefore we should differentiate between ligand-induced shedding and spontaneous shedding. What we find coming off the surface of the antibody-coated cells is not a large aggregate. The complex appears more likely to be a single molecule of antibody bound to one or two molecules of surface antigen. The interesting thing is that the antigen released in this case is the same size as antigen obtained from detergent lysates. This is somewhat larger than what one would find by papain cleavage. Consequently the antibody is pulling out the hydrophobic portion of the antigen as well, which is normally not removed by papain.

UHR: There is a very simple explanation for Cone and Ceppellini's finding. The interaction of the H-2 alloantigen with specific antibody produces allosteric changes in the H-2 alloantigen, which in turn alters its interaction with adjoining protein and lipid molecules. The affinity of H-2 antigen for the membrane is thereby decreased, and the molecule is released.

HOWARD: Because one gets chromium release is cell lysis actually going on? This is obviously an important issue in the interpretation of what we call spontaneous release and immunological lysis *in vitro* cytotoxic assays. Cells spontaneously release chromium as a consequence of their metabolic activity, and I am unclear in my own mind whether we should necessarily assume that the release of the protein it binds is pathological. Cells release chromium more or less at a constant rate when they first are put *in vitro*, and each cell population releases chromium at a characteristic rate. Perhaps release of chromium bound to intracellular protein may be normal, whether we call it secretion or not, and this may contribute substantially to what we call spontaneous release in cytotoxicity assays. Let me explain why I worry about this. In the next session, we are going to consider specificity and the effects on cells of lymphocytes which are potentially capable of killing them. What is going to be measured is the cytotoxic effect of lymphocytes measured by the release of chromium compared with the spontaneous release.

It occurs to me that if there is a normal process which results in release of intracellular protein, then it is quite possible that its rate may be modulated by nonimmunological means, by the physiological effects of effector cells on targets, irrespective of specificity. If this is so, spontaneous release in the absence of effector cells becomes a completely invalid background for computational purposes.

UHR: I have no argument with Howard's comments, and I think he should continue to worry about the mechanism of chromium release, but it is not particularly relevant to the point I had to make here. I simply was showing data to indicate that it is not a simple matter to differentiate shedding from lysis.

CHAIRMAN SMITH: I would like at this point to recap my interpretation of some of the controversial points we have dealt with thus far.

After having gone through a long period in which I have enjoyed great clarity with respect to the mechanisms involved in modulation, shedding, internalization, and secretion, I found myself hearing these terms used interchangeably as if each involved the same dynamic process. Shedding or internalization, particularly as it concerns whole membrane protein seems to be a one-hit event. By one route or another that protein is lost from the surface membrane, and new membrane structures must be put into the membrane in their stead. Such loss is the first necessary event of modulation.

Modulation, on the other hand, relates to limits placed upon the rate at which replacement of the loss may occur. If the membrane protein is vital to the cell's function or its integrity with respect to its environment, the cell will die unless the structure is rapidly replaced. Histocompatibility structures and structures which bind PHA may be in this category, according to available data.

On the other hand, some structures are clearly lost through interaction with receptor or antigen without any apparent functional effect upon the cell. Examples include the MA complex on human LCL, the TLa system, and judging from Stutman's evidence, antigens demonstrated in the mammary tumor cell system. It is difficult to be certain how the HL-A, anti-HL-A data of Cone fit into this categorization.

CEPPELLINI: I would like to have a definition of modulation. I understand modulation *always* acts in the presence of antibody. It is not true that interaction between antigen and antibody is the essential phase.

Secondly, I agree that capping with the third serologically defined locus of HL-A (SD-3) has been so difficult to recognize, because it is a fantastic supercapper. It caps very easily, even microcapping in spots, and the cell becomes resistant to lysis. It is therefore difficult to recognize a positive reaction.

PERNIS: It is easy to show that capping correlates well with modulation, with respect to a given antigen.

CEPPELLINI: That is a very important point with which I agree. I point out that in protozoa one does not need to have antibody present because modulation continues for generations after the disappearance of the antigen. That does not seem to be the case for mammalian cells.

KLEIN: There must be a fundamental difference between modulation and capping. H-2 antigens cap very well, but they are nevertheless rejection-inducing antigens, whereas TL antigens modulate, and they do not induce rejection responses, obviously because they disappear when they meet antibodies. It is remarkable that TL modulation happens so promptly and so completely. Moreover, the process requires new RNA and protein synthesis. Capping does not require *either* of these and can only be inhibited by reducing the temperature or the energy supply. This is a reason why they are different. To have a complete picture, it will be important to know whether TL caps.

GOOD: If we agree that modulation and capping involve different processes, is shedding fundamentally different from these processes?

UHR: Will Klein discuss the relationship between capping *in vivo* and modulation? For example, as a function of time of exposure to antibody, does the Moloney virus-induced antigen disappear from the surface?

KLEIN: In our experience, the Moloney antigen does not modulate, and it does not cap. It aggregates in dots and spots. I have no other information on the point of capping versus modulation.

UHR: What is the biological significance of capping?

KLEIN: For good reasons I believe that a continuous equilibrium exists between antibody coating *in vivo* and capping (or shedding). When ascites tumor cells, growing in antibody-carrying mice, are harvested and fixed, they have relatively small amounts of immunoglobulin on their surface. When the serum of the same tumor-bearing mouse is reacted *in vitro* with such cells, additional antibody is fixed.* Witz has studied the same phenomenon by radiolabeled antibodies. His findings indicate a dynamic process of immunoglobulin shedding and antigen regeneration.

Another variable concerns the differences in antigen expression on the target cell *in vitro* and *in vivo*. We have evidence of striking changes in the expression of tumor-associated antigens on MCA-induced sarcomas, polyoma tumors, and Moloney lymphomas, even a short time after explantation. Could cross-reactive, perhaps fetal antigens, become expressed *in vitro* but disappear again *in vivo* due to modulation? Herberman has evidence, in a Rauscher leukemia system, that a fetal antigen readily modulates upon antibody contact, whereas the virally determined antigens did not modulate. If cross-reactive, fetal antigens modulate readily, they would not be expressed as rejection-inducing antigens *in vivo*. You will recall the classical TL modulation system; this is a differentiation antigen that cannot serve as a rejection antigen, due to modulation. Perhaps it represents a built-in protective mechanism that prevents the rejection of cells with tissue specific or fetal antigens.

Eitan Yefenoff in our laboratory has been testing the ability of several tumor-associated antigens (Moloney, MCA, polyoma, and H-2) to "cap." They showed interesting differences. The Moloney antigen did not show true capping, only aggregation into large spots and dots. Polyoma- and MCA-induced tumor-associated antigens cap readily, with the exception of one polyoma tumor that did not cap at all; this tumor was refractory to the capping of H-2 antigens as well.

We were interested whether these differences and the capping phenomenon itself were purely *in vitro* phenomena, particularly since they required an indirect (sandwich) type of system, occurring *in vivo* determined by a single antibody technique. We found a way to look at capping *in vivo*. Anticomplement immune fluorescence on fixed cells is a useful method for detecting H-2 and tumor-associated surface antigens on Moloney-polyoma virus and MCA-induced tumors. We sought evidence of *in vivo* capping by passaging various ascites tu-

Editors' note: It was in Klein's own laboratory that the phenomenon of shedding was first elucidated. Whether construed as qualitative or quantitative, it demonstrated that the loss process was energy dependent, reversible and antibody dependent, and that recovery required protein synthesis if not cell division. (Smith, Klein, *et al.*, 1967)

mors in irradiated mice. After four days, a relatively large amount of syngeneic (or, in the case of H-2, allogeneic) antiserum was injected i.p. into the tumor-bearing mice. Two hours later, the cells were harvested; after washing they were exposed to human complement and anticomplement (β 1 C) conjugate and compared with controls not exposed to antibody. Capping did occur *in vivo*, showing essentially the same patterns that Yefenoff found *in vitro*. Its extent is equal to or even more impressive than *in vitro*. This result was obtained with a single antibody, without using a sandwich, in contrast to capping *in vitro* where a sandwich is needed to induce capping at all. It is conceivable, of course, that accessory factors (complement components?) attached to the single antibody *in vivo* promote capping in the same way that the second antibody does *in vitro*. We conclude that it is important to know whether capping has any role in the ability of a tumor cell to free itself from antibody and thereby escape antibody-mediated rejection.

Finally, an important artifact must be considered in all experiments demonstrating cross reactivity between murine tumors *in vitro*, artifacts which do not have a counterpart *in vivo*. Many, perhaps all serially transplanted murine tumors, are contaminated by C-type viruses which can induce specific surface antigens. These cross react *in vitro* but are probably irrelevant *in vivo*. The surface antigens they induce are not universally present on all tumor cells, only on a fraction of the population. Thereby a ''minority escape'' is permitted even in immunized animals. In humoral antibody studies, the C-type viruses can be eliminated by absorbing the antisera with lymphoma cells which share surface antigen specificities with the contaminated target tumor cell.

CEPPELLINI: In our studies on human lymphocytes, modulation is not observed, at least as classically defined. The lymphocyte is a living cell and loses some sensitivity to killing by complement, but with respect to antigens of the LA and Four loci becoming less sensitive, we do not call this modulation. Moreover, when we do capping experiments, we get a beautiful black ring indicating the absence of antigen, as long as everything is at 0°C. In a short time at 37°C there is regeneration of the antigen. If, after capping, antigen regeneration requires a longer time, say 6–7 hr for recovery, we have *de novo* protein synthesis. For some antigens, many hours elapse before reappearance. Therefore, we think that capping is fundamentally different from modulation, but the two phenomena are related.

KLEIN: Ceppellini has just explained very beautifully that capping and modulation *are* different, because modulation requires protein synthesis in order to occur, whereas capping does not require protein synthesis. This shows that there really is a fundamental difference between these two processes.

PERNIS: This problem of capping versus modulation is of interest to me, also. When antigen on the surface combines with specific antibody, it caps and then is shed or endocytosed, and the cell surface becomes relatively free of antigen. By this mechanism, the cell frees itself from the given antigen–antibody complex. But the cell goes on making the antigen at 37°C. If the cell remains in the presence of antiserum, as soon as the newly synthesized molecules appear on the surface, they combine with the antibody, form minor patches, and disappear. If, for instance, rabbit peripheral lymphocytes remain in contact with allotypic antibody, the surface becomes negative for antigen but the cells go on gulping enormous amounts of antibody because of this mechanism. One wonders if something like this may be occurring with tumor cells, in which they become insensitive to the cytotoxic effect of antibody.

Is this modulation? I do not believe that it is. Modulation, in my view, involves permanent loss of an antigen as a consequence of the reaction with antibody. This is what happens with protozoa. They go on capping, and after a given number of cycles of capping, they get bored with that and they *stop* making that antigen and modulate more or less permanently.

CONE: I agree that we cannot equate modulation and capping. One of the striking things about the metabolism of HL-A or H-2 at the cell surface is that the antigen *per se,* without adding an antibody, is stable in the cell membrane. If the antigens are stripped from the surface with papain, the antigens reappear in a period of 6 hr. In a 6-hr period, all these antigens are synthesized and appear in the membrane. In a normal situation, they do not seem to be degraded at the cell surface or shed at any rapid rate. What this suggests to me is that when one removes these antigens from the cell surface, either by stripping them with papain or solubilizing them with an antibody, some sort of synthetic mechanism is activated to replace them rather quickly. An important difference between TL modulation and capping is that modulation requires protein synthesis. When TL is modulated, the site density of H-2 increases. It is conceivable to me that when TL is removed from the surface it is replaced through activation of H-2 antigen synthesis. The actual removal of TL could take place either by capping and endocytosis or by ligand-induced shedding.

GOOD: Does Ceppellini think that the proper experiment to check that might be to put the cells in the demodulating circumstance rather than in the modulating circumstance? The process might require RNA and protein synthesis and its rate could have special relationships depending on whether we have capping, shedding or modulation.

CEPPELLINI: The release of antigens from the cell surface by ligand-induced shedding is a very efficient process. Cone is able to extract by ligand-induced shedding more antigen, than with a detergent, I suppose because the cell is doing the work. The complex shed, as described by Baldwin, is able to block cell proliferation, although we do not know what it does to CML. We can study the antigen without antibody, but we cannot study the antibody without interacting it with antigen. That is why Stutman was very careful to say he was not sure if the antibody alone would block.

Finally, if I may use general transplantation as a model, I want to remind you that when one group of workers, Menner and Van Beckum, transplant kidneys in rats without treatment the kidney is always rejected in five to seven days. When rats are pretreated with passive antibody, perhaps because of *in vivo* shedding, it induces the kidney to stabilize and survive for two years. It means, in my opinion, that an antigen-antibody complex is a better inducer of tolerance than any antigen alone.

UHR: We are all at a very interesting point in the study of cell surface events in lymphoid cells. For the first time, there are techniques available to probe into the biological events of concern at the molecular level. I firmly believe that progress in tumor immunology will be more rapid if these opportunities for biochemical studies are pursued in addition to further descriptive studies of the phenomenology of the tumor–host relationship. Several specific examples come to mind. First, the use of scanning electron microscopy and the discovery of microvilli open a new dimension of lymphocyte and tumor topography. A combination of immunoelectron microscopy at the scanning level and cell labeling techniques should allow mapping of cell surface recognition units and surface antigen from this new three dimensional viewpoint. Second, high resolution biochemistry can be performed on trace amounts of cell surface macromolecules. For example, structural homology between two proteins can be studied by labeling each with different iodine isotopes, mixing the two radioactive proteins, and performing single or two dimensional peptide mapping after proteolysis of the mixture. Such studies should lead to a better understanding of the genetic evolution of the proteins in question. Of course, peptide mapping has significant limitations in this regard, but in several years there may be techniques for performing amino acid sequencing on these small amounts of material. Third, the relationship of cell surface recognition units to each other and to membrane molecules in general can now be approached. I expect that stimulation of lymphocytes by antigen involves a cascade of interactions between ligands, cell surface recognition units, other macromolecules buried more deeply in the plasma membrane, and intracellular structures. To understand the mechanisms underlying stimulation and tolerance it is necessary to elucidate these sequential molecular events by which information is relayed from the antigen-specific receptor across the plasma membrane and eventually into the cell nucleus. In essence, I feel that immunologists will turn more and more to the techniques of molecular and cell biology, and biochemistry to answer fundamental questions concerning the tumor reactivity of lymphoid cells.

CHAIRMAN SMITH: The second major point brought out in our discussions was that embryonic and, perhaps, differentiation antigens show a low degree of genetic polymorphism in defined tumor systems as compared with histocompatibility systems. I would point out that this might be quite necessary if organogenesis and morphogenesis is to be sustained without the potentially damaging interference from large numbers of self-recognition subsets that we postulate may have the capability of interacting with histocompatibility structures. Della Porta's data seem particularly important in this respect.

The last point is that we have heard more than adequate substantiation of the premise that the lymphoid system is presented with a great multiplicity of tumor-borne structures to which it reacts as antigens. This underlines the questions we raised regarding assumption of the existence of unique tumor-specific transplantation antigens. While this fact complicates our experiments and their interpretation, it relieves us of the need for explanations in terms of single tumor-specific antigens or tumor-specific transplantation antigens.

UHR: I am at a loss to fully interpret Smith's comments. I think it would be generally helpful if we could discuss more fully the categories of antigens associated with tumors.

CHAIRMAN SMITH: Perhaps Stutman would care to define the process in terms of his own new model.

STUTMAN: There are antigens expressed only on tumor cells and not on other tissues, and thus could be called "specific." However if Boyse would have studied only TL-positive leukemias appearing in TL-negative mice without studying the antigens of normal thymus, TL would have been a leukemia-"specific" antigen.

UHR: That is not what I meant. Does *every* tumor have a tumor-specific antigen? Have all the ones that have been purified thus far proved to be glycoproteins? How do these antigens relate to the fetal antigens that are present on some tumors. In essence, what can we say about the current concepts of the biochemistry of and relationship among tumor-associated antigens.

KLEIN: In response to the provocation by Uhr, we can start by looking at the way in which that concept has developed. First, there was TSTA, or the tumor-specific transplantation antigens. This simply meant that in contrast to what was previously believed, syngeneic mice could be immunized, under appropriate circumstances, against antigens carried on genetically compatible tumors of certain types, and this induced rejection reactions against small numbers of cells. The word "transplantation" simply reflects the fact that antigens were demonstrated by transplantation experiments.

The term TSTA is still used, but we at least prefer TATA, or tumor-associated transplantation antigen. The reason is simply that TSTA is a rather scholastic concept now, implying that the antigen is truly restricted to the tumor cells and does not occur on *any* normal cells of the same host. As far as the virus-induced rejection antigens are concerned, this is certainly not true, since they are induced by the virus on many normal cells as well that either do not transform at all, or are prevented from growing into frank tumors by host surveillance. TATA is therefore a better term, since we do not have to get hung up every time by the question whether it is really tumor specific or not.

The really important antigens are those responsible for host rejection. It is important to distinguish between antigens that *do* have a rejection potential in a given host and antigens that do *not* have such a potential. TL is a good example of an antigen that does not have a rejection-inducing potential, because it promptly modulates away. I am quite convinced that a number of other antigens, detected by *in vitro* systems, but not by *in vivo* rejection, belong to the same category. We know tumor-associated antigens that do have a rejection potential and are, therefore, expressed as transplantation antigens. These are induced by both RNA and DNA viruses and also appear on the surface of chemically induced tumor cells. This does not necessarily mean, however, that all such rejection antigens are directly related, in some way, to the causative agent. Kobayashi, for example, has shown that very powerful rejection-inducing antigens can be made to appear on the surface of weakly antigenic, chemically induced rat sarcomas by superinfecting them with the Friend virus. This is, in other words, antigenic conversion of an established tumor by a superinfecting virus. Ordinarily, such superinfection experiments do not induce much of a rejection potential, presumably because not enough antigen is induced, or not on a sufficiently large number of cells. Kobayashi has clearly shown that in his system this is as good as or even better than ordinary TATA antigens.

Do all tumors have rejection-inducing antigens? Baldwin's experiments, reported in this session, have clearly shown that there are tumors that do not carry detectable, rejection-inducing antigens. This may be related, however, to the host genetics, particularly whether the host possesses a set of Ir genes that may or may not allow it to mount an efficient rejection response. In fact, we know of Moloney virus-induced lymphomas that do not provoke rejection response in strain A but do induce good rejection responses in F_1 hybrids between A strain and other strains. In one instance, even a congenic-resistant (H-2 substituted) strain gave rise to rejection responses. The most likely interpretation of this finding is that we have introduced into the outcross F_1 hybrid, Ir genes

61

capable of recognizing the relevant antigen. In the congenic cross this indicates that the relevant gene is H-2 linked. I would be greatly surprised if the diverse antigens that can induce rejection reactions in different systems had a common molecular basis. I would rather think that recognition, by host Ir genes, in relation to a number of molecular changes on the surface of cells transformed by a variety of agents, will determine whether a rejection-inducing antigen is recognizable or not. Such antigens, just like other antigens, could vary widely in chemistry and mode of presentation.

BALDWIN: Tumor-associated antigens can now be isolated from tumor cell membranes in relatively defined conditions. For example, specific antigens associated with the plasma membrane of aminoazo-induced rat hepatomas have been isolated by papain digestion; following appropriate purification, these can be resolved as discrete protein fractions (40,000–60,000 M.W.). These procedures are also applicable to other animal tumor systems and to human tumors where antigenic fractions have now been prepared from melanoma and from carcinomas of colon and breast.

ALEXANDER: We have to be rather careful about concluding that the lack of rejection in the host necessarily signifies that there is no immune response to a tumor-specific antigen. Foreign substances can very successfully escape destruction from an existing immune response. Indeed, the infectious diseases illustrate this point as well as tumor biology. Thus, tubercle bacilli grow and kill in the face of a *very active* immune response. It is an important issue to decide whether there are tumors that do not have any TSTA or whether all tumors have them. However, it is essential to recognize that some tumors are exceptionally effective in avoiding destruction by the host, whereas others are less so. The fact that some tumors are not rejected in a suitably immunized animal does *not* mean that they have failed to evoke a reaction. Indeed, one can find specific cytotoxic cells in animals despite their inability to reject a tumor inoculum.

CHAIRMAN SMITH: That is a major point I sought to make. However the term cross reacting carries what I interpret to be an inaccurate connotation—for some reacting cell clones are probably directed toward true self-components, not surrogate ones which share structural configuration. We are impressed with the work of Howard and McKhann, who showed a generally inverse relationship between expression of serologically identified histocompatibility structures representing H-2 specificities and the immunogenicity of MCA-induced tumors. We have reproduced this effect in our own system and expanded it to show that cell proliferation stimulated by solubilized tumor antigens also has a generally inverse relationship to immunogenicity of a wide range of MCA tumors. Perhaps a way to conceptualize this effect is to visualize tumors as having a high proportion of membrane structures being strictly self-structures (those expressed in normal cells) and that these, by virtue of the intensity of their production and release, stimulate proliferation of self-reactive clones. *In vivo,* the tolerant state with respect to these structures is sustained. Those structures which are truly tumor unique, those expressed on tumors but not on normal cells, are immunogenic *de novo* and evoke proliferation of operationally equal clones for which tolerance either does not exist or is too fragile to sustain. In these circumstances, the relative representation of "normal" versus "unique" structures would determine the quality of the target for attack of those clones least likely to evoke effective tolerance. This implies that the more the tumor looks like self, the less the target structures it supplies, and the more possibilities exist for competition with those clones responsive to unique structures.

PREHN: I want to say that I think Alexander has asked us an impossible question, because I think it is formally impossible to ever prove the *absence* of a tumor antigen. Consequently, if we find tumors, as Baldwin has, in which antigens cannot be detected, Alexander would always say that we just did not do it the right way, or that our tests were not sensitive enough. So in this respect, it is utterly impossible to answer the question.

ALEXANDER: In the way Prehn has posed it, one cannot answer the question. However, I would point out that there are other situations where one cannot induce graft rejection by suitable immunization. Yet one can find in animals bearing such a tumor, cytotoxic lymphoid cells, which have all the requisite specificity as judged by *in vivo* tests. So in this situation, one can conclude that we *are* dealing with a tumor which does evoke an immune response, yet for one reason or another is not *effective in vivo* in causing rejection of that tumor.

GOOD: The question raised by Prehn focuses on a most important issue. Baldwin cannot show cellular immunity to a particular tumor but, as I understand it, can show antibody against some of its antigenic constituents. Perhaps in that particular situation, tumor and host relate to one another in a special way that reflects a lacunar immunodeficiency or unresponsiveness of the host to the antigens present on that tumor. To say that the tumor does not have potentially antigenic constituents for this reason may be like saying that the pneumococcus does not have antigenic constituents because it does not stimulate antibody response in an agammaglobulinemic patient, or even more appropriately, that the measles virus is not antigenic because it cannot raise a cell-mediated immune reaction in patients who have multiple sclerosis. Certain multiple sclerosis patients have high levels of antibody to the measles, mumps, and Paramyxo 3 viruses, but do not have demonstrable cell-mediated immunity to the virus. If

63

such patients are given transfer factor, they become able to respond to antigenic configurations on lymphocytes to which they otherwise would not respond, and to the viruses to which they otherwise would not respond. If genetically determined immunological lacunae were responsible for the apparent lack of cellular immunity to Baldwin's tumors, it might be possible to reveal the antigenicity of the tumor after appropriate manipulation of the host, by serological analysis, such as Old and Boyse have used to define the surface antigens on tumors. I conclude that because Baldwin cannot demonstrate antigenicity in a conventional tumor-immunity model does not necessarily mean that the tumor does not have potentially effective antigens at its surface.

BALDWIN: Other examples also illustrate tumors apparently lacking immunogenicity. In this session we have given much attention to MCA-induced sarcomas and other chemically induced tumors, where tumor rejection reactions can be readily demonstrated. On the other hand a considerable number of spontaneous tumors in the rat, e.g., mammary carcinomas and sarcomas, do not elicit immunity in syngeneic hosts. Moreover, where immunity can be demonstrated, the degree of tumor resistance is low as compared to other tumors such as MCA-induced sarcomas. Even so, many of these tumors, which are essentially nonimmunogenic by the criterion of immune rejection, *do* express embryonic antigens, as I pointed out earlier in this session.

ALEXANDER: A possible test is to look at the draining lymph nodes of the tumors. At present I do not know of *any* situation in which the nodes draining a tumor do not show typical characteristic stimulation, even though often one cannot, by immunization, develop a detectable degree of rejection. So, in my view, before we even *begin* to consider that tumors do not have TSTA on their surface, the first and simplest step is to show that the nodes draining such tumors are absolutely normal, i.e., the injected tumor has failed to elicit an immune response.

WEISS: We are bedeviling ourselves by semantics. We know of instances of tumors in which the cell surface antigens strongly expressed are displaced either in time or in place. It is virtually impossible to be certain that an antigen which makes a tumor cell vulnerable to immune attack in the autochthonous host is indeed *unique* to the neoplastic state. And it does not have to provoke immune reactions. Tolerance of self is undoubtedly a quantitative matter, and major displacement of an antigen from its normal time and place of expression in the organism would be quite sufficient to provoke active immunological reactions.

HOWARD: It was not clear throughout the earlier part of this session whether immunogenetic tumor-associated transplantation antigens include proven products of the major histocompatibility complex.

CHAIRMAN SMITH: At least one tumor-associated antigen described by Boyse and his colleagues is clearly linked to the MHC complex, the X-1 locus. The burden of my remarks, however, had to do with the possible roles that other self-responsive clones, directed toward histocompatibility structures determined by the MHC locus and having expression on tumor cells, might have in determining the biologic behavior of a tumor.

HOWARD: Is it true that the chromosomal origin of the proteins which contribute to the very large number of antigens expressed by mouse or rat tumors induced with chemical agents is still completely mysterious?

CHAIRMAN SMITH: As far as I know that is a correct statement.

CEPPELLINI: Howard's question is very important. Up to now we have had no information on the genetic or structural relationship between tumor antigens and histocompatibility antigens. I now think there are two possibilities. First, in that region there is room at least for a number of repressed genes, and it could be that malignancy derepresses these genes and the antigenic molecules appear on the tumor cell surface. Alternatively, "mutation" may change the structure of a *bona fide* histocompatibility antigen. That is an idea that did not surface in these discussions.

CHAIRMAN SMITH: I know of no *bona fide* example of either possibility.

CEPPELLINI: No, but there *is* an approach. For instance, we now know that anti-β-2 microglobulin antibody co-caps with antigens. Will anti-β-2 microglobulin co-cap with tumor antigens? That is a simple experiment.

BACH: But it will not prove that the tumor antigen is a product of the MHC.

CEPPELLINI: It will prove that they are in some way related.

BACH: No, it will prove that β-2 microglobulin is associated with many structural protein components of the surface.

CEPPELLINI: With histocompatibility antibodies, one could try to co-cap a tumor antigen.

BACH: That would be a beautiful experiment.

CHAIRMAN SMITH: Is the β-2 microglobulin present on other than lymphoid cells?

CEPPELLINI: It is present on all cells.

HOWARD: I understood Della Porta to say that he could immunize against a chemically induced tumor by using the tissues of normal animals from another inbred strain as antigen. Furthermore, the inbred strain that supplied the immunizing tissues would be correctly selected on the basis of the growth behavior of the tumor in that strain. Is that correct?

DELLA PORTA: Yes, this was done on two occasions. Howard was referring to the allogeneic skin graft. Although the tumor had the original H-2 antigen, it is rejected in mice previously immunized with a graft of allogeneic skin. But this does not prove definitely that a relationship exists between the chemically induced individual tumor antigens and the histocompatibility antigens. This arose because we observed that a few chemically induced tumors were growing despite a histocompatibility barrier, and one of our students (Invernizzi) wanted to know why.

HOWARD: But it is enormously important that a tumor antigen cross reacts with a transplantation antigen, as in Martin's studies with the spontaneous lung tumors in mice.

PREHN: How would one exclude this phenomenon as being due to some sort of adjuvant effect produced by the grafted skin; there need not be a sharing of antigens.

DELLA PORTA: It does not appear to reflect an allogeneic effect.

KLEIN: The problem of possible linkage between the major transplantation antigen complex and the tumor-associated antigens can be approached in a different way, by using somatic cell hybrids. The following example will illustrate: Wiener and Dalianis in our laboratory have studied the karyotype of an intraspecific mouse hybrid, produced by the fusion of the TA3 mouse ascites carcinoma (derived from strain A) and the MCA-induced sarcoma MSWBS (of strain ASW origin). TA3/Ha has two normal 17-chromosomes, readily detectable by banding analysis. As you know, chromosome-16 carries the H-2 determinants. In ASW, both 17-chromosomes are translocated to two different telocentric chromosomes and can be readily distinguished from each other and, in the somatic hybrids, from the normal 17-chromosomes derived from TA3. There is, thus, the possibility of identifying the H-2^a and H-2^s determinant-carrying chromosomes separately from each other. The hybrid, which is highly malignant and grows in (A × ASW)F₁ hybrid mice, throws off variants that have lost one of the two H-2 complexes. This can be readily selected in the corresponding parental A strain. One A-compatible variant lost the H-2^s complex irreversibly, and, at the same time, it also lost the two translocated 17-chromosomes. Variants compatible with ASW, on the other hand, lost H-2^a and the corresponding two normal 17-chromosomes. It was not possible to select variants that lost all four 17-chromosomes, and one H-2 complex always remains despite strong selection pressures.

One might find out, in this particular system, whether the tumor-associated antigen characteristic of MSWBS is linked to H-2. One could do this by comparing the H-2^s negative with the H-2^a negative variants, for the presence of the tumor-associated antigen derived from MSWBS. Having said this, however, I must also confess that we have not done this experiment. That fact reflects our bias, since frankly, I see no reason why the tumor-associated antigen *should* be linked to H-2. I could be quite wrong, however, and this would be an easy experiment to do.

CEPPELLINI: We know the MLC involves two differences. The MLC locus is associated with initiation of stimulation, and killing the target cell depends upon serologically defined antigens of the SD loci. If one mixes *in vitro* normal lymphoid cells and syngeneic tumor cells, does one obtain stimulation, or does killing occur at the end of the stimulation?

MARTIN: Cytotoxic lymphocytes are generated *in vitro* against EL-4 leukemia cells from spleen cells of C57BL/6 mice. Both EL-4 and C57BL/6 mice express H-2^b major histocompatibility antigens.

CONE: Rollinghoff has shown that a murine, mineral oil–induced plasmacytoma will stimulate the production of cytotoxic T lymphocytes *in vitro* in a syngeneic system. It is a second example.

KOURILSKY: In some systems, no stimulation of nonimmune lymphoid cells is induced by tumor cells. Senik *et al., (Int. J. Cancer,* **12,** 233, 1973) in our laboratory, failed to detect any stimulation of lymphocytes from nonimmune mice in the presence of irradiated tumor cells from various syngeneic MuLV-induced lymphomas, and no killer cells were generated *in vitro* in this system. However, lymphoid cells from mice injected with MSV could be stimulated *in vitro* by syngenic tumor cells sharing common antigenic determinants with MSV-induced sarcoma. Such a stimulation was only detectable using lymphocytes taken 3–7 days following virus inoculation, before the appearance of tumors, and declined to undetectable levels in spleen and lymph nodes of these MSV injected mice.

CHAIRMAN SMITH: Normal syngeneic lymphocytes occasionally give detectable stimulation, when solubilized membranes derived from MCA tumors are added in the system I described earlier. This is not found regularly, however.

BACH: With the exception of certain lymphoid tumors, Rollinghoff's data and the rather weak stimulation demonstrated by Vanky and Stjernswärd, tumor cells are not stimulatory to the nonsensitized individual. Even to lymphocytes of the sensitized individual tumor cells are only weakly stimulatory if assayed in cultures of lymphocytes plus tumor cells.

STUTMAN: There might be a technical problem in the test that Bach describes. Tumor cells in suspension do not give effective stimulation. Cells which have a natural tendency to stick to surfaces give better stimulation and generate killer lymphocytes, provided the target is a monolayer. The time course of these events is completely different from conventional MLC, however.

BACH: In each case I was referring to, we tested tumor cells for their ability to stimulate allogeneic lymphocytes. There is no doubt one can get excellent stimulation and cytotoxicity not only on the allogeneic tumor cells, but also on allogeneic lymphocytes.

SESSION II

IN VITRO ASSAYS FOR TUMOR-SPECIFIC IMMUNITY

Technical problems in assays for cytotoxic lymphocytes—Appropriate controls, kinetic considerations, and interpretation—Comparison of attributes of ^{51}Cr release, prelabeling and microcytotoxicity assays—Selective purification of effector cells—Antibody-dependent lymphocyte cytotoxicity—B-cell-mediated cytotoxicity—Application of lymphocyte cytotoxicity assays to tumor biology—Immunologic memory in tumor systems—Critical importance of target cell sensitivity in assays for cytotoxic lymphocytes—Allogeneic cells as targets.

CHAIRMAN HOWARD: In this session, we shall go, in rather a formal way, through the field of *in vitro* effects of lymphocytes on target cells, starting with descriptions of assays, proceeding to details of the cell populations we know to be involved in mediating these effects, and then branching out into a number of topics which should be easy to follow up with the specialists present.

By studying cytotoxic and cytostatic effects *in vitro,* we examine ways in which lymphocytes or other cell types are potentially involved in effects prejudicial to tumors *in vivo.* It is perfectly clear that accreditation of an *in vitro* mechanism as effective *in vivo* is a far more difficult field in which to establish a foothold. In fact, *in vivo* application is relatively unexplored territory.

Perhaps we should make a rather formal list to work with, to establish the details for both cytostatic and cytotoxic effects *in vitro.* There appear to be three major kinds of cytostatic and cytotoxic assays *in vitro* that are, so to speak, the parents or grandparents of all the other assays. These are colony inhibition, microcytotoxicity, and the ^{51}Cr-release assays. We can deal most comprehensively with the latter two. E. Klein will first describe the microcytotoxicity assay in more or less technical detail, the sort of assay it really is, and the kind of results one gets with it.

E. KLEIN: The microcytotoxicity assay has two important features which distinguish it from the ^{51}Cr-release assay: the use of attached target cells and a test period of 24–48 hr, which makes it a long-term assay. The small plates with wells, charged with a volume of 25 μl, comprise a mini-tissue culture; proper pH and humidity are vital. The target cells are checked for condition throughout each experiment. A ^{51}Cr-release assay in which a high spontaneous release of isotope occurs is not acceptable. Control cells should be in good condition at the end of the assay. A period of 12–24 hr is allowed for attachment of the target cells before lymphocytes are added. The number of lymphocytes added is determined by the number of target cells plated or attached. Appreciable cell growth must occur in controls during the 48 hr of incubation, otherwise, test results are not acceptable. Does using a growing culture as target impair the sensitivity of the assay? We have considered the alternative—that irradiated target cells could be used as static nonreplicating targets. The growth inhibition assay, at times, shows growth stimulation produced by serum or by lymphocytes; this would be missed with static target cells.

It is important to add lymphocytes in varying concentration; we use ratios of 50, 100 or 200 lymphocytes per target cell. Higher ratios tend to give nonspecific cytotoxicity. A 200:1 ratio involves about 40,000 lymphocytes per well, or over one million cells per ml. This is a high concentration for ordinary cultures. If one works with cells that are capable of growing well in culture, growth also occurs in the microplate. Granulocytes are detrimental to this assay; the effector cell population should, therefore, be purified. The fast Ficoll–

Isopaque separation procedure does not, in our hands, yield a cell population with specific effects. In mouse and rat systems, the assay performs well in the detection of lymphocyte-mediated, antibody-dependent cytotoxicity. Growth stimulation does occur in this assay. We often found that serum dilution to the point that the cytotoxic effect subsides may give a stimulatory effect.

CHAIRMAN HOWARD: So that we can compare the assays directly, Cerottini will now give a description of the ^{51}Cr-release assay.

CEROTTINI: What kind of target cells can be used in the ^{51}Cr-release assay? Most cells grown in suspension have been used. Macrophages, fibroblasts and sarcoma cells also work; one is not limited by the availability of cell suspensions. The choice of target cells is chiefly limited by their rate of spontaneous ^{51}Cr release. ^{51}Cr as sodium chromate is incorporated into the cytoplasm of the target cells where it binds to ill-defined proteins.

Spontaneous release of the isotope into the supernate always occurs following incubation of the target cells in culture medium. For unknown reasons, spontaneous ^{51}Cr-release rates are quite different from one target to another. Uhr pointed out in the preceding session that spontaneous release will decrease or increase depending upon culture conditions used. Also, the manipulation of the target cells after labeling must be gentle, as we found that resuspending the labeled cells by pipetting increases spontaneous ^{51}Cr release.

Several groups use Petri dishes which are placed on a rocking platform. We prefer round bottom tubes, of a small diameter, in which lymphoid cells and target cells tend to concentrate in the bottom. To increase the initial rate of interaction between the effector cells and the target cells, the cell mixtures are best spun down at $200 \times g$ for a few seconds at the onset of the incubation period. This procedure seems to shorten the latent period necessary to detect specific ^{51}Cr release. In fact, in very sensitive systems, no latent period can be demonstrated in contrast to what was described some years ago.

Another point is that chromium release into the supernate is a relatively late event. A delay occurs between the time the target cell is lethally hit and the time the target cell releases its isotope; this is because the mechanism of lysis involves at least two steps. The first step is dependent upon the presence of the effector cells and is probably related to permeability changes. The second step is independent of the presence of effector cells and is related to osmotic lysis which ends in release of cytoplasmic proteins, including those which have bound isotope. In model systems, this delay varies from a few minutes to several hours.

A possible limitation of the ^{51}Cr assay is a requirement for relatively large numbers of target cells, and hence for lymphoid cells. With the specific activity of ^{51}Cr presently available, a minimal number of 10^4 labeled target cells per individual tube is required. In exceptional systems, this can be reduced to as little as 100 cells. The optimal duration of the assay depends very much on the target cells being used. If spontaneous ^{51}Cr release is low—that is, it does not exceed 25%—it is possible to run 24 hr tests. Usually, however, the optimal incubation period is 3 to 6 hr.

CHAIRMAN HOWARD: What about terminal labeling of microcytotoxic assays, since this modification is the closest relative of the original visual cytotoxicity (e.g., trypan blue) test. Is it possible to estimate the number of cells remaining by using a post-label?

WEISS: We have taken E. Klein's assay, with one major and some minor changes, and employed it to study CMI. We use Miwa's medium (Miwa, *Acta Med. Okayama,* **23,**393, 1969) throughout, and find it to be a more satisfactory medium for a variety of mouse tumors and for mouse lymphoid cells than any other we have tested. At the end of incubation, we wash the attached cells repeatedly in order to remove most, if not all, of the lymphoid cells. The last washing is with 0.3 *M* sucrose. Then we terminally label the remaining attached targets with ^{51}Cr, cut the plate with a thermal cutting device, and count each well. The correlation between label uptake and direct microscopic counts is very good; it is linear over a large range of cell numbers and proportions including those used by Klein. We also avoid the labor and inherent error of counting the cells by simply estimating their numbers by their radioactivity and comparing the values with controls.

MARTIN: The use of ^{51}Cr to postlabel might lead to a false negative result since any lymphoid cells remaining in the wells could incorporate the label. It is possible that immune lymphoid cells are more adherent than normal control lymphoid cells, because of their specific interaction with target cells, or because of increased numbers of macrophages.

The problem with ^{125}IUdR incorporation as a postlabel is that it reflects division rate as well as cell number. If cell lysis occurs, increased cell proliferation by the remaining cells may sometimes result in more ^{125}IUdR uptake than in control; thus giving a false negative result.

TERRY: Our experience with the ^{51}Cr-release cytotoxicity test relates in part to the issue Martin has raised. Specifically, immunized animals yielded large numbers of lymphoid cells incorporating label, which paradoxically gave high residual counts. In our hands, a major problem was lymphocytes sticking to the wells. The problem was particularly severe with lymphoid cells from immunized animals, where it appeared that we were seeing immunoadherence. Has Weiss had any difficulty with this?

WEISS: We obtain a clear difference between sensitized lymphoid cells and normal ones, despite any artifacts of increased label uptake by adhering immune effector cells strengthening the results. We have, of course, examined our reaction wells visually, in order to make the initial correlations between cell counts and terminal ^{51}Cr uptake. We find no morphological evidence of significant lymphoid cell retention. Perhaps such retention is reduced by use of Miwa's medium or by the fact that we wash our effector cells six or more times before adding them to the targets. Addition of labeled serum to the attached cells, specifically directed at the effector cells, revealed very little lymphoid cell residuum.

Our impression is that any error of lymphoid cell retention is small. To the extent that it actually exists, it increases the significance of comparisons between the cytotoxic capacity of normal and immune effector cells. The correlations we have seen between our method and the direct evaluation of cell numbers has been so good with all the tumors that we have used, that we feel we can rely on it.

ALEXANDER: If specific increase in ^{51}Cr over the spontaneous release level is relatively small, how can one tell whether this is due to actual cell lysis, or due to an increased export of protein from the cells after some pathological process?

Another question is what happens if the cell number goes below that inoculated, meaning there must have been some cell detachment. Does one know whether such cell detachment invariably means that such detached cells cannot grow?

E. KLEIN: Alexander asks whether the growth inhibition or cytotoxicity is primarily due to detachment of the target cells. It is not possible to say with any degree of certainty that this is a mechanism by which effector cells or their products function. Essentially, detachment leads to cell death because most cells which grow in monolayers do not survive unless attached to a surface.

CHAIRMAN HOWARD: Does growth inhibition operate at mitosis and do the cells become grossly detached at that point?

E. KLEIN: I do not know.

CEROTTINI: I agree that Alexander raises an important question. It is very difficult to make any valid interpretation when ^{51}Cr release in the presence of immune cells is close to the level of spontaneous release, even if the difference is significant by statistical analysis. One way of getting around this problem is to select, by various procedures, cell subpopulations which are enriched in effector cells and, hence, are able to produce much higher cytotoxicity on a cell for cell basis.

ALEXANDER: When the kinetics are linear everything is fine. How do you react to reports of new phenomena based solely on getting an extra 10–15% ^{51}Cr release over spontaneous levels? This is often the only measurement which has been made, and the conclusion is that cytotoxic cells have been produced *in vitro* or something of that sort.

CHAIRMAN HOWARD: I have seen reports where we are asked to accept a calculated 3% excess label release as being significant. Even appreciating the very small difference that can be significant if the numbers are good enough, it is worth remembering that the minimum variance for any radioactivity estimation is the Poisson variance, obtained if all samples contain precisely the same amount of label. In a Poisson distribution the standard deviation is equal to the square root of the mean, or 32 on a mean of 1000. Thus, for the usual 3 replicate values in an assay, a 3% release value cannot achieve statistical significance. Yet this is the kind of figure that some claim as a significant result.

DELLA PORTA: How does Klein interpret her assay if she has a 25% difference between the medium alone and the control lymphocytes?

E. KLEIN: I adjust the number of test lymphocytes to the population density of the target culture.

DELLA PORTA: Not to the number of control lymphocytes?

E. KLEIN: I estimate the effect of the control lymphocytes and compare it with the performance of the test lymphocytes. Calculations are made in relation to the control lymphocytes. If control lymphocytes also cause a decrease in target cell numbers, the experimental lymphocyte effect will be larger. I prefer to compare the effect of the control situation with that of the experimental, and not in regard to the untreated control. When the control lymphocytes cause no effect there is no problem. When they have an effect it cannot be disregarded.

DELLA PORTA: The control lymphocytes may have stimulatory effects.

E. KLEIN: A raised "minus" cytotoxicity compared to the experimental makes for an even higher quantative effect for the test lymphocytes. Therefore a dose-response curve is very useful, both in the case of control and experimental lymphocytes. If we take the values for control lymphocytes as base line we introduce bias.

CHAIRMAN HOWARD: The question of what are the right controls is a very important one. What are the right comparisons to demonstrate a specific effect? Let us consider the following parameters available for use in assessing the chromium-release assay, with representative values:

Total available label $T = 100$
Freeze-thaw release ("releasable label") $FT = 75$
Spontaneous release (medium control) $SR = 30$
Control release (in presence of "control" population) $CR = 45$
Specific release (in presence of experimental population)
   $ER = 60$

All these parameters except the freeze-thaw release have clear analogies in the microtoxicity assay. There are a number of ways these numbers can be juggled to estimate the magnitude of the specific effect, and by using different calculations one can get amazingly different results. For example, to minimize the apparent effect, use the following calculation:

$$\frac{ER - CR}{T} = 15\%$$

for intermediate values use either:

$$\frac{ER - CR}{T - CR} = 45\%$$

or:

$$\frac{ER - CR}{FT - CR} = 60\%$$

and to maximize the apparent effect use:

$$\frac{ER - SR}{FT - SR} = 75\%$$

Now it is not immediately clear which of these is "right," but it is evident that a rather mediocre increase in chromium release can be expanded by the appropriate calculation to a highly impressive effect. My inclination would always be to use the most conservative figure on general methodological grounds. It is nearest to the raw data and requires the minimum number of assumptions. It is easiest to calculate a true significance for the difference, for example, between the specific and control releases. I am unhappy about the validity of subtracting the control release from the experimental release to obtain a single, "corrected," specific release value. Usually, different "control" populations give different control release values; some may even be lower than the spontaneous release. How can one be sure that the particular control population used is the "right" control? If one uses as control an immune population as similar to the experimental population as possible, but directed towards irrelevant specificities, how can one be sure whether some or all the control release do not have a specific immune component through an unsuspected cross reaction? If such a component does exist, does it invalidate the control subtraction? Does this consideration thereby prevent one from *ever* using the "best" control population, corresponding most nearly to the experimental population, in case such a cross reaction occurs? I do not have answers to these questions; I raise them to emphasize the serious difficulties that arise in the handling of chromium-release cytotoxicity data. It is usually possible to say definitely whether some specific activity is present in a population. It is usually very difficult to give a sensible answer to the question—How much?

BACH: I would simply like to warn you that statistical evaluation of this type of data is difficult since one is dealing with three values, each with a standard deviation. Either this must be taken into account in a parametric evaluation, or nonparametric tests should be done.

KOURILSKY: The ^{51}Cr release in the presence of control lymphocytes may well be higher or lower than the spontaneous release, depending upon the lymphocyte–target-cell systems used. In the latter case, analysis of chromium release by test lymphocytes based on the comparison with the spontaneous release, may lead to negative values, even if the test lymphocytes are clearly cytotoxic as compared to the control lymphocytes.

CHAIRMAN HOWARD: I agree with that. One of the most serious problems with introducing control release at all, in estimating the magnitude of an effect, is the fact that control release varies in unpredictable fashion. In view of this, it seems to me that control release has a questionable value as a correction in estimating the "true" magnitude of experimental release.

PERLMANN: In the microcytotoxicity test the control lymphocytes are definitely the best control because the cell numbers are most comparable with those in the experimental sample. In comparison with medium controls, there may be different numbers of target cells surviving, but if one then makes the comparison with the experimental sample, one gets essentially the same specific result. However, it is extremely important to have well-standardized preparations of purified lymphocytes. This is particularly important when one works with lymphocytes from patients, as they may contain a large fraction of nonlymphocytic cells. Such cells used as controls may give poor target cell survival. This is actually the reason why some have difficulty detecting tumor-associated cytotoxic reactions in certain patients. Likewise, effector cell preparations from tumor patients contaminated with nonlymphocytic cells may destroy unrelated target cells as well.

CHAIRMAN HOWARD: I do not mean that control cells should not be run in cytotoxic assays. They must be run, because how else may one know whether one is dealing with an effect at all? In dealing with the statistics of the effect, one has to decide what is an appropriate control population, as well as being very sure what one is going to do about control effects when they differ from medium controls.

GOOD: There is something wrong here. What Cerottini says is well and good for some tumors, but I am certain the ^{51}Cr release presents problems with other tumor systems. Could he clarify this for us? Is the problem one of chromium release after damage, or is it one of reutilization of chromium or what? Just what are the restrictions that make it impossible to apply chromium release to *all* tumors? If we could use it more widely it would give us a most precise and quantifiable method for studying cytotoxicity for all tumors. I know this is not the case.

CEROTTINI: There are two major limitations: (1) The choice of target cells is restricted to those which show a low spontaneous ^{51}Cr release and (2) the number of lymphoid cells required to reach levels in excess of that killing target cells is relatively high. This is because the number of labeled target cells necessary to get enough radioactivity per individual tube is high for many tumors. There is no evidence or reincorporation of the ^{51}Cr label released from damaged target cells into the supernatant fluid.

CHAIRMAN HOWARD: Stutman uses a prelabeling microcytotoxicity assay. Would he briefly describe it and say whether he thinks that it is basically like the Cerottini assay or the Klein assay?

STUTMAN: It is like neither. It measures cytotoxicity. It is the assay described by Bean and collaborators *(Nat. Cancer Inst. Monograph,* **37,** 41, 1973). Briefly, it consists of taking the target cells, growing them in proline-free media (the majority of the conventional media are proline free), and then labeling them with ^{3}H-proline. This produces 100% labeled cells. We had been labeling with ^{3}HTdR, but this was inconvenient because of the tolerated doses required for adequate labeling, and the resultant assays were not really "micro"; 5000 cells had to be seeded to get adequate counts. The same problems existed with IUdR. It is also toxic for a wide variety of tumors at doses that give good labeling. Proline has the advantage that it is well tolerated by the target cells, not reutilized, and after labeling the cells are grown in media with available cold proline. What is measured is the cells that stay attached to the plastic dish. This is an indirect measure of the number of cells that are lost—either dead or floating. Obviously one cannot detect any form of stimulation. The number of cells that can be plated in the proline assay is 200 to 500, so it is really a microcytotoxicity assay. One can use either cells or antibody and complement to induce cytotoxicity, but it is basically a measure of the remaining attached target cells.

CHAIRMAN HOWARD: Clearly there is a complex of cytotoxic and cytostatic assays in common use which grade into one another. At opposite poles are the pure Brunner–Cerottini cytotoxic assay and the pure Klein microcytotoxicity assay. The Cerottini assay is short (4–6 hr) and measures only target cell lysis. The Klein assay is long (24–48 hr) and measures target cell detachment from a surface and/or growth inhibition. In its pure form, the Klein assay can also measure immunostimulatory effects on targets caused by specific effector cell populations. The prelabeling modifications of the Klein assay, described by Weiss and by Stutman, differ considerably from the parent assay in that neither growth-inhibitory nor immunostimulatory effects can be recorded, only target cell lysis or detachment. In this sense the assays approach the Brunner–Cerottini cytotoxicity assay, while still being distinguished from it in duration. A microcytotoxicity assay, where a postlabel is used to count the remaining target, is a much closer replica of the original Klein assay in being sensitive to the same target cell effects, but, as Weiss will tell us later, inhibition of DNA synthesis is among the specific effects of immune cells on a target. While this is recorded in a postlabel assay, it is not necessarily seen (at least to the same extent) by direct cell counting.

Somewhat out on a limb is the true colony inhibition assay, commonly confused in name with the microcytotoxicity assay of Klein, and usually measured as a decrease in the plating efficiency of a target cell population as a result of contact with effector cells. Here direct cytotoxicity and growth inhibition could both be involved, though they are hard to separate. It seems to bear the closest resemblance to the Klein assay, based on the assumption that all cells remaining in such an assay are potentially the progenitors of new "colonies." If this is not so, then colony inhibition measures yet another dimension in which cytopathic effects can be induced in target cells by specifically immune effector cell populations.

As we shall discuss later on, these different assays can yield substantially different results with a given immune effector cell population. Clearly it is important to understand these assays properly before generalizing about the manifestations of a state of cellular immunity.

We should now consider the quantitative aspects of the various assays, the extent to which we can estimate by titration the cytotoxic activity of a cell population. In other words, can one deal with immune cell populations in cytotoxicity assays, as one titrates antibody, both with a view to comparing the magnitude of different states of immunity and to purifying the cytotoxic cells? Here I suspect there is something of a great divide between chromium-release cytotoxicity (at least with the P-815 mastocytoma system) and the microcytotoxicity assay. Would Cerottini develop these issues for us?

CEROTTINI: I have discussed this issue extensively in a recent review (Cerottini and Brunner, *Adv. Immunol.* **18**, 67, 1974). In brief, it is possible under appropriate conditions to get an estimate of the relative frequency of effector cells, or at least of the relative activity of these cells, in different cell populations. Such an estimate is based on the existence of a quantitative relationship between the number of target cells lysed and the concentration of effector cells. In well-defined systems, in which a constant number of labeled target cells has been exposed to increasing amounts of immune lymphoid cells for a constant period of time, it has been found that specific cytotoxicity varied linearly with the logarithm of the number of lymphoid cells. Moreover, it was observed that dose-response curves obtained with different lymphoid cell populations resulted in parallel lines. It is, therefore, possible to get some estimate of the relative frequency or the relative activity of the effector cells in different cell populations by comparing the number of cells required to achieve a fixed value of ^{51}Cr-release; for example, 50% of the releasable isotope.

CHAIRMAN HOWARD: Would Wigzell comment on the microcytotoxicity assay? His recent data have troubled me.

WIGZELL: They not only troubled Howard, but they troubled us as well. They should trouble everyone working with this procedure. In essence, we found no simple linear dose-response relationship in the Moloney leukemia microplate assays.

CHAIRMAN HOWARD: Is this the system described by Klein?

WIGZELL: Klein is a coauthor of the papers you are referring to; the name of the principal investigator is Lamon *(Int. J. Cancer*, **13,** 91, 1974).

In contrast to the ^{51}Cr-release assay where one has a simple dose-response curve, in the Moloney microplate technique this is frequently not the case. When one adds increasing numbers of "control" lymphocytes, a growth stimulating effect on the target cells is frequently produced. At too high concentrations of lymphocytes, "nonspecific" inhibition is frequently encountered. Superimposed on these effects is a specific inhibitory effect when using proper immune lymphocytes. Due to these complicated processes, differences between normal and immune cells do not titer out in a simple linear manner. Thus, statistical comparisons were made between control and immune lymphocytes at the same effector: target cell ratios. Significant differences could be observed, but no simple quantitative relationship was found in this system. The microplate technique looks more promising in other systems.

CEPPELLINI: I am not sure that it is clear to everyone that we are talking about cell-mediated lysis, but that some of these tests could also be applied to antibody-mediated lysis.

CHAIRMAN HOWARD: We have been dealing with cell-mediated effects; all the techniques that have been described have been used to study cell-mediated, target cell damage. Nevertheless, it is likely that all these effects could also have been mediated by antibodies in conjunction with cells (LALI, LDA, etc.) though I doubt whether the quantitative results would be identical.

BACH: Cerottini has shown *(Adv. Immunol.,* **18,** 67, 1974) a very good linear relationship between the percent killing and the log of the number of effector cells. They use a very sensitive target cell. In the cell-mediated lympholysis (CML) assay, using PHA blast cells as target cells, we do not always find a simple linear relationship. The difference may be related to the fact that the PHA blast is a less sensitive target cell than the lymphoma cell, or that the target cell population is heterogeneous.

Peck has studied MLC activation using a PHA-stimulated target cell in a mouse system. At low ratios of the effector to target cells, a linear relationship to cytotoxicity is seen. High ratios of effector to target cells give a higher percentage of cytotoxicity than that predicted by linear extrapolation. This finding questions the reliability of simply using the number of effector cells needed to get 50% lysis as a quantitative expression. In some systems matters seem to be more complicated.

E. KLEIN: Titration curves were a subject of discussion among our group, even while the work was being carried out. The fact that we did not obtain a titration effect in the MSV system, using one particular target cell, does not mean that one does not generally get dose-response curves in the microcytotoxicity assay. In studies that included the H-2 system, the MSV-rat system, and human bladder carcinoma, MSV was the only system in which we had problems with dose response. A slight effect could be seen at a 25:1 ratio. Above a 200:1 ratio, the controls also gave effects. Within that range a nice titration curve was obtained.

CHAIRMAN HOWARD: Then you can get linear titration curves?

E. KLEIN: Yes. I would like to emphasize that the assay is amenable to titration, and one generally gets a good dose response. It should be remembered that the assay is used with many different kinds of target cells. Not all cells are suitable, due to peculiarities of growth behavior, lack of attachment to surfaces, etc. Not all cells can be used in the ^{51}Cr assay either, as some show a high spontaneous release of isotope.

TERRY: The probability of obtaining interpretable dose-response curves in any of these *in vitro* assays may well be determined by the duration of the assay. With assays of short duration (2–6 hr), dose-response curves should be readily interpretable. With longer assays, all of the effects already discussed come into play. Cells are dividing, differentiating, dying; membranes are turning over and shedding; responsive cells are being "educated" and releasing blastogenic factors, toxins and so on. All of these factors may play a role in the outcome of the assay, and any dose-response curve must be interpreted in the light of a complex series of interactions.

CHAIRMAN HOWARD: Then let us say that both assays are titratable but in some circumstances one gets curious results with microcytotoxicity. Terry's reservations are very important here; there is room for an enormous number of secondary effects in microcytotoxicity. If a linear titration is observed that would seem to be a fortunate outcome.

MARTIN: Using a constant number of effector lymphocytes and varying the number of target cells one observes that, over a wide range, the absolute number of target cells lysed varies directly with the number of target cells added. If one uses too few target cells, however, a false negative result may be obtained. If one uses too many target cells the actual percent lysis, in contrast to the absolute number of cells lysed, falls below significant levels. Thus with low levels of activity, especially in syngeneic systems, one may have to use a range of target cell numbers for its detection.

CHAIRMAN HOWARD: Cerottini would have reservations about cytotoxicity titrations in very weakly active populations. I agree that the results of such a reverse titration are relevant and interesting. By electronic analogy, increasing the size of the target increases the gain in the amplifier. Nevertheless, a stronger signal in the form of a more active effector population yields a proportionally greater output for any gain, giving a Cerottini titration. As I understand it, Cerottini has described a method for increasing the sensitivity of the system for assaying weakly active populations. He does this by enriching the effector compartment before assay.

GOOD: There is absolutely no question about the extraordinary usefulness of the Brunner–Cerottini system vis-a-vis certain kinds of target cells. It is the most useful method we have for quantifying T-cell-mediated cytotoxicity. The admonitions Terry imposes, concerning changes that can take place during the analysis, are not limited to long term analysis. Boyse and Komura and their associates induce, in a period of 90–120 minutes, the expression of the products of some 11 genes at the surface of T lymphocyte precursors by exposure to nanogram or even picogram quantities of G. Goldstein's thymin. Similar changes in cell surface can occur in microcytotoxicity systems as well. This could be one of the problems when we use different tumor systems and different tumor–target-cell ratios, or systems that involve complex mixtures, which contain substances that might themselves influence surface characteristics of the cells.

WEISS: We touch here on the general question of the titratability of all assays of cell-mediated cytotoxicity, including those based on terminal labeling. If one compares the fate of target cells exposed to different ratios of sensitized lymphoid cells, to normal lymphoid cells, and to no cells at all, it becomes obvious that there are two competing effects exerted by the lymphoid cells, at least with regard to some tumor targets. There is both a cytotoxic effect where the lymphoid cells are cytotoxic, and a stimulatory effect on the growth and/or survival of the target cells which can be exerted by *any* lymphoid population. This is much more pronounced with regard to some tumor cells than with others. Thus, if one picks up cytotoxicity and can titrate it only over a limited range of cell ratios, it may be a reflection of a cancelling out of two opposite actions by the effector cells. If this is taken into account, then the narrowness of titratability often observed is not all that surprising.

CHAIRMAN HOWARD: I am glad Weiss raised this very important point. I was hoping we could have some discussion of immunostimulatory or feeder effects in microcytotoxicity assays, as they clearly could have exactly the influence Weiss mentions: cancelling out and making invisible a concomitant cytotoxic or cytostatic effect. This problem, if it is real, clearly only affects the results of the microcytotoxic assay when it is recorded visually or by terminal labeling. Prelabeling techniques almost certainly record only cytotoxicity.

WEISS: If the degree of sensitization of the effector cells is limited, and the target cells do not do very well in culture and require a sort of feeder effect, then cytotoxic potential could be largely obscured by the positive feeder effect, especially at crucial levels of total cell numbers in the system.

CHAIRMAN HOWARD: It is worth pointing out something that came up earlier regarding the comparability of the chromium-release and microcytotoxicity assays. The best of the chromium-release assays, using mastocytoma or lymphoma cells in suspension as target, are now usually used to analyse either the mechanism of a particular well-defined type of killing, or the mechanism by which specifically immune populations (usually of T cells) are generated *in vivo* or *in vitro*. These assays are essentially effector mechanism oriented rather than target oriented.

This is rather different from the normal use of the microcytotoxicity assay, which is a more general purpose assay for assessing immunity to any tumor that may occur either spontaneously or experimentally. It is almost always used in situations where the potential immunogen is the tumor itself, while in the chromium-release assays the immunogen is often normal allogeneic tissue. It is only very recently that the mechanism of microcytotoxic effects has begun to be studied. More often it is the existence of the effect in a particular "clinical" situation that has been the subject of interest. I get the impression that we have put these two assays in opposition to each other. I suspect this distinction is artificial and that they have quite different uses operationally.

It is now appropriate to consider the cells involved in killing. Wigzell will deal first with evidence that T cells are involved in the killing mechanisms.

WIGZELL: We have been trying, during the last few years, to develop techniques that permit us to purify and characterize subpopulations of cells by the use of their surface markers, and to assess the immune capacity of such cells. I would like to mention some work done together with Golstein, in which we used the classical system involving spleen cells taken after primary immunization of mice across an H-2 barrier. If these cells are passed through a column coated with anti-Ig, the cells carrying surface markers of B-lymphocyte-type are eliminated. Simultaneously a significant increase is observed in the capacity of the effluent cells to function as cytolytic effector cells in the ^{51}Cr-release assay. Removal of T lymphocytes by anti-T-cell serum and complement (or by passing the cells through anti-T-cell column as designed by Andersson) removed the cytolytic capacity. From this we can say that the cytotoxicity of spleen cells after primary *in vivo* immunization across an H-2 barrier, without addition of antibody, is due to the T lymphocytes in the cell population. With Svedmyr, we have analyzed which cells in the MLC will become cytolytic against the specific target cells. So far, in human and in mouse systems, and testing for cytolytic cells in ^{51}Cr assays, we have shown that the dominant cytolytic effector cells carry the surface markers of T lymphocytes.

The problem of cytophilic antibody functioning as effector molecules in such systems will be discussed later. However, I want to emphasize that spleen cells taken from double-immunized animals are absorbed on a given allogeneic monolayer in such a way as to remove only the relevant killer cells. In other words, we find no evidence that T cells can generate antibody-like molecules which can then bind to another T cell and make that T cell into a killer cell.

UHR: Do these columns remove monocytes as well as B cells?

WIGZELL: Yes.

CHAIRMAN HOWARD: It is very unfortunate that the chicken has not been one of the species in which cells responsible for killing has been defined; so far as I know, this species can be made into the most B-cell-deficient animal of all.

CEROTTINI: With the ^{51}Cr-release assay such as used in our system, the effector cells involved are *only* T cells, throughout the immune response. With the microcytotoxicity assay one finds, at the beginning of the immune response, a mixture of T and non-T effector cells. However, later on, starting at about day 30, 40 or 50 of the immune response, I believe that only non-T effector cells are detected. It appears that the two assays measure two different types of effector cells. This is the problem we face.

CHAIRMAN HOWARD: Would Perlmann now describe for us non-T killing?

PERLMANN: Let me briefly emphasize again that cell-mediated killing induced by humoral antibodies *in vitro* has been seen in a large variety of immune systems. Tissue culture cells including tumor cells as well as erythrocytes (except from human) are very good target cells for this type of assay. More recently, lymphoid cells have also been shown to be excellent target cells. The antibodies may be heteroantibodies as well as alloantibodies, including anti-H-2 or anti-HL-A, or even autoantibodies. Effector cells may be normal peripheral lymphocytes, or lymphocytes from the spleen of animals immunized against the target. In the latter case, it has been shown that target cells are killed without addition of antibody. With certain foreign antigens, such as erythrocytes or haptens, target cell killing by immune spleen cells has been shown to be mediated by antibodies released during the incubation period.

I will briefly summarize some of the important facts which have been established in several laboratories during the past few years. What I am going to say is based on the results of chromium-release experiments in which labeled target cells have been incubated in suspension with purified lymphocytes from normal donors, in the presence of antibodies against surface antigens of the target cells. It has been shown that the antibody doing the job is of the IgG class. Antibodies of IgM class or of any of the other major immunoglobulin classes (e.g., IgA and IgE in man) are inactive. Under optimal conditions only a few hundred antibody molecules/target cell are sufficient to induce a reaction. With optimal antibody concentrations and effector cell, target cell mixtures incubated in small volumes, the reaction may be completed within a few hours and has kinetics similar to those seen in T cell killer systems. The cytotoxic reaction requires contact between effector cells and target cell, and destruction of the latter is by a non-phagocytic mechanism.

The points I would like to make are as follows:

1. Effector cells kill antibody-carrying target cells, *or* antibody-free target cells by utilizing antibody from adsorbed complexes.

2. Cytotoxicity inhibited by antigen/antibody complexes (third party antigen).

3. Cytotoxicity inhibited by large amounts of IgG (including human IgG subclasses 1, 2, 3, 4 ?).

4. Cytotoxicity inhibited by antibodies to donor type immunoglobulin but *not* by F(ab')₂ anti-Ig.

5. Effector cells retained on columns charged with antigen/antibody complexes *or* activated C3.

6. Removal of T cells increases cytotoxicity of effector cell preparation.

The inducing antibody is not cytophilic in the sense that it is easily absorbed to the effector cells when it is present in a monomeric form. However, when aggregated or present in the form of a complex with antigen, it is much more firmly absorbed. The reaction can therefore be induced by adding free antibody to a mixture of effector cells and target cells or by pretreating the target cells with antibody. The reaction can also be induced by adding antibody complexed with antigen. When effector cells which have taken up such complexes are washed and added to fresh target cells (not coated with antibody), the antibody will be utilized in a cytotoxic reaction. It has also been shown that the effector cells can pick up such complexes from the surface of antibody-coated target cells and can thus acquire a specific killing reactivity. While antigen–antibody complexes containing the relevant antibodies can induce a reaction, complexes containing antibodies against unrelated antigens have been shown to have blocking effects. Actually, depending on the quantitative balance between the different components, the same antibody can be shown either to induce or to inhibit the cytotoxic reaction.

From these results, it can be concluded that the event which triggers the cytotoxic reaction is the interaction of the Fc receptor on the effector cells with the Fc part of the antibody on the target cells. That the Fc fragment of the antibody is a prerequisite for the reaction and that the effector cells must have Fc receptors has also been shown in direct experiments.

When human blood lymphocytes have been used as effector cells with rabbit IgG antibodies as the inducer, the reaction can be inhibited by addition of large amounts of normal IgG. Rabbit and human IgG have been seen to be equally inhibitory. When the inhibitory effects of the different human IgG subclasses have been compared, IgG1, 2 and 3 have been found to be equally inhibitory. For IgG4, different results have been reported but it seems also to have certain inhibitory effects. In any event, these results would seem to distinguish the Fc receptor of the effector cells from that on monocytes which only interacts with IgG1 or IgG3.

In a system consisting of human lymphocytes and rabbit antitarget cell antibodies, addition of rabbit antihuman immunoglobulin inhibits the cytotoxic reaction, However, when the antihuman immunoglobulin is added as the Fc-free F(ab')$_2$, there is no inhibition. This indicates that inhibition by the unfragmented antibody against the Ig of the effector cell donor is due to the formation of complexes which block the Fc receptor of the effector cells. While the possession of an Fc receptor is typical for B lymphocytes, the effector cells do not seem to have surface bound immunoglobulin because they are not retained on columns charged with the F(ab')$_2$ fragments of antibodies against effector cell immunoglobulin. As indicated by immunofluorescence, this procedure removes the lymphocytes with surface immunoglobulin. It has also been seen that the effector cells have complement receptors. When purified lymphocytes are passed through columns charged with human C3b, effector cells active in antibody-mediated cytotoxicity are retained. They can also be removed from a preparation by centrifuging off the cells which form rosettes with complement-carrying sheep erythrocytes. This raises the question of the possible importance of the complement receptor for the triggering of the cytotoxic reaction. When purified human blood lymphocytes are mixed with chicken erythrocytes carrying a few antibody molecules of IgG type, a cytotoxic reaction is very easily induced. However, when the erythrocytes are coated with much larger amounts of complement (human C3b) in the absence of IgG antibody, no cytolytic reaction is triggered in spite of rosette formation. This suggests that the Fc–Fc-receptor interaction may constitute the important triggering event for the chain of reactions leading to the destruction of the target cells.

Now I would like to return to the question of the nature of the effector cells. Good evidence exists for both mouse and man that nonactivated T cells are inactive in this system. Because several types of mononuclear cells possess the Fc receptor, which is needed for the acquisition of the recognition factor, the humoral antibody, it can be assumed that there exist several types of antibody-dependent cytotoxic effector cells. Available evidence suggests that this is so. For example, Holm in Stockholm has recently shown that human RBC coated with hyperimmune human anti–blood group A are easily lysed by the monocytes from human blood but are not affected by the lymphocytes taken from the same blood. In contrast, the latter cells efficiently lysed antibody-coated human tissue culture cells, while the monocytes did not lyse these target cells. Susceptibility of different target cells to the various kinds of potential effector cells also has to be considered in this connection.

We have recently gone through serious efforts to characterize lymphocytic effector cells (from human blood), lysing chicken erythrocytes in the presence of rabbit anti–chicken erythrocyte antibody. This is a very efficient lytic system at low effector cell: target cell ratios even with very highly purified lymphocytes. Morphologically, as judged from both light and electron-microscopic studies, the cytotoxic effector cells have a lymphocytic appearance but morphology may not be very helpful in resolving the question. Some of the criteria typical for these cells have been listed in Table 21. For comparison the corresponding properties of mature human blood monocytes analyzed at the same time are also given. Both monocytes and the monocyte-depleted lymphocytic fraction do lyse chicken erythrocytes in the antibody-dependent chromium-release assay.

As can be seen, the lymphocyte effector cells are distinct from monocytes in several respects but seem to lack easily detectable surface Ig, characteristic of mature B lymphocytes. Lack of adherence and phagocytic potential may, perhaps, also be found in very immature monocytes, although the occurrence of such cells in human blood is not well established. The inhibition of the cytotox-

TABLE 21
Antibody-Dependent Effector Cells

| | Cell type involved | |
Property	Lymphocyte-like	Monocytes
Adherence to plastic dishes at high serum concentrations	−	+
Phagocytic potential	−	+
Surface Ig	−	not tested
Inhibition of interaction with antitarget antibody	Human IgG1, 2, 3, possibly 4	Human IgG1, 3
Complement receptor	C3b, C3d	C3b

88

ic reaction by three or possibly all four subclasses of human IgG has already been mentioned. This is clearly different from the monocytes which in parallel experiments with the same inhibitors are only inhibited by IgG 1 and 3. An additional difference is seen in the interaction with C3. It has recently been shown by others that human B lymphocytes have two distinct complement receptors, one for C3b and another for enzymatically inactivated C3b (= C3bi or C3d). This also seems to be the case with these lymphocytic effector cells, since removal from the preparation of cells forming rosettes with sheep erythrocytes carrying either C3b or C3bi (= C3d?) efficiently abolishes its cytotoxic capacity. In contrast, mature monocytes (like granulocytes) only seem to possess the C3b receptor.

In summary, then, it would appear that the antibody-dependent effector cells which I have discussed do not belong to the monocytic series, but further work is needed to establish this. It should also be stressed that antibody-dependent effector cells from mouse spleen have, at least by some, been assigned properties which would appear to be more on the monocytic side. Since we have so many cell types with Fc receptors, it is not surprising to find several types of antibody-dependent effector cells.

GOOD: The cells Perlmann describes are so much like B lymphocytes in every respect except for the absence of the immunoglobulin on the surface. Can he give us some idea of how many there are in normal blood as compared to the number in some pathological states?

PERLMANN: It is difficult to be precise, because we always start from purified cell preparations before we make our counts. In normal blood, the proportion of purified cells which have no T cell markers and do not carry immunoglobulin but which have complement receptors may be from 2–7 percent. At least such a fraction contains the effector cells.

In patients, the situation may be very different. For instance, in the blood of certain myeloma patients, Mellstedt and Holm have found increased numbers of effector cells, even after removal of phagocytic and adherent cells. I would be inclined to believe that the antibody-dependent effector cells which I discussed belong to the lymphocytic series or represent an independent lineage. They could be immature B cells or B cells which have lost their surface Ig.

GOOD: Has Perlmann carried out experiments in which he incubates these cells *in vitro* to see whether immunoglobulin appears on the surface?

PERLMANN: No. We have looked for antibody-dependent cytotoxicity of lymphoblastoid cell lines, together with Klein. These are all B cell lines but any cytotoxicity observed was very weak.

CHAIRMAN HOWARD: Perlmann has now described a rather well-defined cell in human blood with a collection of properties which certainly makes it distinct from what have previously been called T cells and what we have been calling B cells. The question struck me, during his presentation, whether the properties of this lymphocyte-like cell in human peripheral blood are the same properties as the Stobo, Rosenthal, and Paul, non-B, non-T cells (*J. Exp. Med.,* **138,** 71, 1973). Can anyone comment on those cells?

GOOD: These cells are strikingly similar to the cells that Siegal, Wernet, and Kunkel have described in a patient with immunodeficiency. This patient had agammaglobulinemia and thymoma. She had in her circulation many cells that did not synthesize immunoglobulins but which had the other markers of B lymphocytes. When these cells were cultured, in the fluids or in plasma from normal individuals, or even calf serum, the cells developed into typical B lymphocytes with surface immunoglobulin. It may be that killer cells in cell-mediated antibody-dependent cytotoxicity are B lymphocytes in an early stage of differentiation. Such incompletely developed B lymphocytes have also been seen in circulation in quite large numbers in some patients with X-linked infantile agammaglobulinemia according to Buckley *et al.* and Kersey *et al.* Also, we always see a small number of these cells in the circulation of normal, healthy individuals. But in many diseases, the accounting gap between fully differentiated B lymphocytes plus fully differentiated T lymphocytes and all other lymphoid cells becomes very large. Such gaps may be made up, in part at least, by cells with the characteristics Perlmann describes. I wonder whether the functional aspects he has now ascribed to this small population of B lymphocytes in normal persons is present in the large population of lymphocytes found in the circulation in disease states.

CHAIRMAN HOWARD: In these cases we want to know whether these populations are also rich in Perlmann-type cells.

PERLMANN: I do not know that.

CHAIRMAN HOWARD: It may be that immunodeficiency patients provide a means of getting a pure, or nearly pure, population of Perlmann-type cells.

ALEXANDER: A physiological way of attempting to define these cells is by their behavior *in vivo*. The point is, should one call a cell a lymphocyte if it is found in the blood but is not present in lymph, or is there only in very small numbers.

CHAIRMAN HOWARD: That seems to me an interesting, but pedantic, point. I say it is interesting because on the whole I agree with the stricture, and because Parish, working in Oxford, found rare lymphocytes in the rat thoracic duct that have the right surface properties for the Perlmann cells. They are Ig-negative C3 and Fc positive, and yet, McClennan found that they are inert in an antibody-dependent cytotoxicity system which is almost certainly identical to the system described by Perlmann (McClennan, *Transpl. Rev.*, **13,** 67, 1972). This case may simply represent a concentration problem since pure populations of these cells have not been analysed. It should be emphasized that there may be other cells with the right combination of morphological and surface properties, lymphocyte-like cells, which are not potential killer cells. The cells involved in the antibody-mediated killing may also be in fact quite heterogeneous.

WIGZELL: It may be appropriate here to describe briefly our studies of immune cell populations, in which we find that immune non-T cells are effective in the absence of added antibody. The systems are not formally Perlmann systems, because we do not intentionally add antibody. Our final conclusion from the study of two systems in mice is that the effector cell is functioning through antibody that the cells have synthesized *in vitro*.

The original starting population is immune spleen cells, deprived of most macrophages and monocytes prior to other *in vitro* fractionation procedures. The first system examined in collaboration with Lamon involves mouse anti-Moloney leukemia antigens, and microplate cytotoxicity. Comparatively pure subpopulations of either T or B cells were obtained by passing cell populations through specific anti-Ig or anti-T columns or by treating the cells with anti-Ig or anti-T serum plus complement followed by proteolytic enzymes, to remove possible antigen-antibody complexes and allowing the lymphocytes to recover *in vitro*. Providing the test assay was carried out 50 days or longer, after virus introduction, inhibitory activity of cells was present only in the B-enriched population, not in the T-enriched population. Earlier assay disclosed activity in both populations. Since the B and T subpopulations were produced by methods identical in principle, this suggested that the inhibitory activity observed was truly B cell dependent.

This result does not mean, however, that the cytolytic cells in this 48 hr assay, are the B lymphocytes. Other precursor cells such as monocytes or the like, surely could differentiate during the time of the assay to become effector cells in an antibody-induced, cell-mediated-type lysis. Favoring this interpretation, in fact are results obtained in the second system. We used chemically defined antigens coupled covalently to target cells. Haptens or proteins were coupled to chicken erythrocytes and spleen cells were taken for *in vitro* ^{51}Cr cytolytic capacity against relevant target cells. To our surprise purified specific immune T or B lymphocytes did not give specific lysis of antigen-coated CRBC, despite the fact that such cells were perfectly capable of transferring reactivity *in vivo* as measured by delayed hypersensitivity helper cell activity or humoral antibody production.

To my knowledge, no one has shown that *specific* immune T lymphocytes can lyse erythrocytes. In this CRBC system we found that cytolytic effector spleen cells, contrary to Greenberg, were adherent; they are removed by passage through any kind of column, unless the separation is performed in the cold and with EDTA. The characteristics of lysis in this system are summarized as follows: If antibody produced by the immune cell donor is added to normal spleen cells, lysis starts immediately. If immune spleen cells, but not extra antibody were added, a 3-hr delay occurred before lysis started. This was inhibited by puromycin, in contrast to the lysis induced by antibody plus normal cells, as described by MacLennon and coworkers. These data suggested that active protein synthesis by the immune cell system was required for lysis. In fact, we isolated IgG antibodies from the immune B cells after 3 hr. Such antibodies transferred to normal spleen cells made these cells aggressive.

Furthermore, when we assessed the affinity of immune cell-mediated lysis by adding the specific hapten or protein as inhibitor, we found that the molar concentration required to inhibit the killing capacity of the immune spleen cells was identical to that required to inhibit the serum IgG of the cell donor from agglutinating target cells. In this defined system, we found no evidence of cytophilic antibody. Antibody must be produced *in vitro*, and the antibody will then retain another cell type to become the effector cell. Whether this is always the case when one uses immune cells and finds non-T cell lysis, remains to be established.

TERRY: In the experiment where cells are passed through anti-IgG columns, I would assume that the anti-IgG itself is aggregated. This sets up the possibility that cells with receptors for aggregated IgG would be removed. In the next experiment anti-IgG plus complement was used and there is the possibility that aggregates could be created and bind to cells with aggregate receptors and block their activity. Were aggregates clearly removed from that situation? I raise the possibility that during the incubation of cells and anti-IgG, IgG is released by the cells, formed into complexes with the anti-IgG and that these complexes would then abolish the killing effect of aggregate-binding cells. The question is whether or not the experiments yielded cells selected for IgG or for aggregate receptors.

WIGZELL: Terry's question is valid. However, we have been unable to find any evidence to support it.

CHAIRMAN HOWARD: If one gets non-T-cell killing by cells from immunized animals, can one assume that it is mediated by the Perlmann mechanism?

The experiment just described by Wigzell is slightly different from Perlmann's, but they both seem to involve similar events at the target cell level.

WIGZELL: I must stress that the two systems reported involve mice. There is no evidence of a lymphocyte-like cell in the mouse, analogous to those in human peripheral blood, effectuating cell-mediated antibody-induced lysis. No one, to my knowledge, has analyzed mouse peripheral blood lymphocytes in this test assay. They always use spleen cells.

PERLMANN: When Wigzell shows no killing of erythrocytes in his system this may reflect a failure in the induction of a specific killer cell. This does not mean that erythrocytes are not susceptible to T cell killing. PHA-activated T cells of mouse or human origin lyse sheep and chicken erythrocytes efficiently. The mechanism of this lytic reaction is probably similar to that of killing by *specific* T cells.

STUTMAN: All adult Balb/C nude homozygous mice (nu/nu) injected with Moloney sarcoma virus develop tumors, but no regression of such tumors occurs such as in normal heterozygote nudes (nu/+) within a week or so after tumor development. If the *in vitro* studies in any way reflect *in vivo* effects, this suggests that T cells are required to generate either killer lymphocytes or antibody-forming cells mediating tumor regression *in vivo*.

WIGZELL: We agree. It is well known that the production of IgG antibodies which induce antibody-dependent, cell-mediated immunity is highly thymus dependent. These experiments do not tell us at what level the system is thymus dependent.

GOOD: Wigzell's studies show the killer effect of T cells, and a clearly defined killer B cell population in tumor immunity. In these experiments there seemed to be a sharp dissociation between the period killer B cells were present and the period the killer T cells were present. I am referring to the experiments of Lamon. Could Wigzell straighten out this issue?

WIGZELL: I should stress a point that will be made later by Kourilsky, that is, we employ an oversimplified concept when we talk about T cells. First, we know that there are several subclasses of T cells, and it is also evident that what is called T cell lysis might very well be a multistep process. Secondly, T cell-dependent target cell lysis, as revealed by chromium release in our first system and by T cell lysis in our second system, may involve different mechanisms. The third variable is the susceptibility of target cells to T cell lysis. Specific immune T lymphocytes, in our hands, do not lyse red cells. However, Perlmann showed that nonspecific PHA-activated T lymphocytes, as well as non-T lymphocytes, are capable of lysing certain red cells. This may be a question of induction rather than of target cell fragility; different effector T cells may be involved in different situations.

GOOD: To try to clarify this issue, can red cells coated by antigens stimulate the T lymphocytes to divide or is this model just not suitable for addressing the T lymphocytes? Specifically, will T lymphocytes proliferate after stimulation with chicken red blood cells coated by antigen?

WIGZELL: We have not done that experiment.

CHAIRMAN HOWARD: It is quite possible that antibody-mediated cytotoxicity is more efficient against red cells than is T cell-mediated cytotoxicity simply because of structural conditions on the red cell or haptenated red cell surface. Possibly the avidity of binding achieved by free antibody, followed by secondary lymphocyte attachment through Fc receptors, is greater than that achieved by a T cell with only its intrinsic receptor molecules available.

GOOD: The beauty of the fact that only B cells appear to act as killer cells in this model may be that only B cells can be stimulated by antigens in the form in which they are displayed on the RBC.

UHR: Can Perlmann tell us whether, in the system of PHA-induced cytotoxicity in which red cells are killed by lymphoblasts, rosette formation accompanies or precedes killing?

PERLMANN: Uhr's question is difficult to answer, because PHA causes strong mixed aggregates between lymphocytes and red cells. However, there is good evidence that the essential trigger of the lytic reaction is the activation of surface-bound processes in the effector cells. Although effector cell, red cell, contact is needed for the lytic reaction to start, and this might be facilitated by the gluing effect of PHA, when the mixed agglutination is strong, the cytotoxic reaction may actually become inhibited. It should be noted that nonagglutinating mitogens may also cause this type of cytotoxicity, the mechanism of which in regard to lytic events very much resembles that produced by specifically activated T cells.

MARTIN: I would like to know how mouse systems compare to human systems with respect to ease of detecting lymphocyte-dependent antibodies (LDA). Our experience is that in mice it is rather difficult to detect LDA using the standard ^{51}Cr release or dye-exclusion test for cytotoxic antibodies. One of the controls used in these assays is antibody incubated with lymphoid cells in the absence of complement. I cannot recall finding greater lysis in the control group than in the control group containing lymphoid cells plus medium. Possibly, since all the lymphoid cells are coated with antibody, the effector cells would be inhibited, but this concern should not apply to anti-theta-treated spleen. In these assays the antibody goes onto the T-cell population, presumably leaving the B-cell population available as effector cells for LDA. Again in my experience, I do not find lysis occurring, specific for anti-θ-treated spleen cells, in the absence of additional complement. My question is whether some special technique is required to demonstrate LDA in the mouse.

CEPPELLINI: We have had some experience in trying to block the Perlmann phenomenon only to find that we had effected lysis. Why should there be such a difference between mouse and man? To obtain information on this point we screened lymphoid cells from a number of animals with varying doses of cells. Our findings showed that human cells with either human or animal antibodies are the best effector cells in this system. Rabbit cells are much less efficient and those from the rat and the mouse are the poorest we have tested. Thus, from our experience, I would say it is important that those working with mice, who use murine antibodies, should always include in this test human lymphocytes as effector cells.

PERLMANN: Let me add to this list recent experiments made in Boston by Carpenter and collaborators. They show that rats also are excellent producers of antibody-dependent cytotoxic lymphocytes. These lyse histoincompatible rat thymocytes with the proper alloantibodies within a few hours.

CHAIRMAN HOWARD: We should next discuss briefly the selectivity of assays with respect to the effective killing mechanisms. In fact, Perlmann's original description was of chromium release by erythrocytes, but we know, independently of his telling us, that immune T cells are not able to lyse erythrocytes. Is this because different assays reveal the activities of different effector mechanisms? Because Kourilsky's laboratory has made such comparisons perhaps he can tell us whether the microcytotoxicity assay favors non-T cell effector mechanisms while the ^{51}Cr-release assay favors T-cell-mediated cytotoxicity, respectively?

KOURILSKY: The nature of the target cell in microcytotoxicity assays and in chromium-release tests undoubtedly influences the detection of the various effector mechanisms. This was recently demonstrated by Plata *et al.* (*J. Immunol.*, **112**, 1477, 1974) in comparative *in vitro* studies on effector cell diversity in cell-mediated immune responses to MSV-induced tumors in mice, as already mentioned by Cerottini. The test systems were the following: C57BL/6 mice received one injection of MSV under conditions in which regressive local tumors are induced, and the time evolution of cell-mediated cytotoxicity against tumor cells was determined in spleen lymphoid cells by two assays: (1) the chromium-release test, using syngeneic target lymphoma cells (EL-4) bearing antigens common to MSV tumors, and (2) a microcytotoxicity assay using monolayer cultures of recently explanted MSV tumor cells as targets, with the proper controls. Only T cells (purified on anti-Ig-coated columns) were efficient as cytotoxic cells in the chromium-release test with the lymphoma target, whereas both T and non-T cells (obtained following treatment with anti-θ and C') were active in the microcytotoxicity assay with the MSV tumor cell target. The macrophages were apparently not involved in either assay, as shown by carbonyl-iron treatment of effector cells.

The time evolution of the T-cell-mediated cytolytic activity of spleen cells in the chromium-release test was monophasic, starting at the time of tumor growth (7 days) with maximum values around day 12–15, at the peak of tumor size; it declined progressively thereafter. Comparative studies of the same lymphoid cell suspensions in the microcytotoxicity assay showed a somewhat different pattern. Non-T effector cells became detectable at the same time as in the chromium-release assay and persisted for several weeks, but T effector cells in the microcytotoxicity assay, which became detectable at the same time as the non-T effectors, were not found after day 25.

The first point relevant to our discussion is that, at the time of maximum tumor size, a transitory drop of cytotoxic T or non-T cells was found by microcytotoxicity, whereas , in the same spleen cell suspensions, the cytolytic activity of T cells in the chromium-release assay was at its peak value. How, then, can one explain why the same T cells, cytolytic for ^{51}Cr-labeled lymphoma cells, have no effect on monolayers of MSV tumor cells, in the microcytotoxicity assay, although both target cells have antigens in common?

Our proposed explanation is that MSV tumor cells are relatively insensitive to the direct membrane attack of cytolytic T cells, whereas lymphoma cells are highly sensitive. This was demonstrated by labeling MSV tumor cells with ^{51}Cr. These cells, in fact, appear to be almost "unbreakable" in the chromium-release assay by either syngeneic anti-MSV or allogeneic anti-H-2^b immune T cells, whereas lymphoma cells are highly susceptible to the lytic effect of the same effector cells.

A second comment follows from the previous observation. The chromium-release assay measures a direct membrane lesion, whereas microcytotoxicity detects a long term effect which effector cells produce on the growth of target cells. What is the effect of a cytolytic T cell on a target cell which is resistant to T-cell-mediated immune lysis? We suggest that, in this situation, perhaps other mechanisms of cell damage by immune T cells may be evidenced, and one of them may be responsible for T-cell-mediated growth inhibition in the microcytotoxicity assay. Additional support for this concept has come from blocking experiments to be discussed later.

CHAIRMAN HOWARD: I am afraid that the main points are not clear to me. Perhaps I could ask Kourilsky to give us a brief resume.

KOURILSKY: Only T cells were demonstrated to be responsible for the specific chromium release in this syngeneic tumor system, as already published (Leclerc *et al.*, *Int. J. Cancer*, **11**, 426, 1973; Plata *et al.*, *J. Immunol.* **111**, 667, 1973), but both T and B cells were found operative in microcytotoxicity.

The point is that, while the lymphocyte suspensions are the same in both assays, the target cells are different, even though they bear some of the same antigens. Target cells used in the microcytotoxic assay are resistant to direct immune cytolysis by T cells. This suggests that the mechanism of cell damage induced by T cells is different for growth inhibition and short term cytolysis, and, perhaps, the T effector cells are not the same. It is conceivable that the growth inhibition effector pathway can be blocked independently of the cytolytic effector pathway, as will be discussed later on.

MARTIN: There are a number of situations in which immune activity is detected by microcytotoxicity or colony inhibition but not in ^{51}Cr-release assays. For example, I have tested lymphoid cells of mice bearing a variety of tumors on ^{51}Cr-labeled tumor target cells. Cytotoxicity was not demonstrated in any of these assays. Similarly, lymphoid cells of mice pregnant to an allogeneic mouse are not directly lytic in ^{51}Cr assays for cells bearing the alloantigen of the fraternal strain, even though activity in the colony inhibition assay can be demonstrated.

Esber and I have studied both ^{51}Cr release and microcytotoxicity or colony inhibition by the same lymphoid cell population in the following four specific situations:

1. Balb/c mice immunized with EL-4 leukemia cells: Allogeneic tumor challenge is rejected and lymphoid cells are active against EL-4 in both ^{51}Cr release and colony inhibition.

2. C57BL/6 mice immunized with irradiated EL-4 leukemia cells: No anti-EL-4 activity can be demonstrated in the ^{51}Cr-release assay yet their lymphocytes are active in the colony inhibition assay. However, when spleen cells from these mice are cultured with EL-4, high levels of activity develop as measured in the ^{51}Cr-release assay.

3. C3Hf mice immunized with the transplacentally induced lung tumors bearing the strain A alloantigen as a tumor antigen (see elsewhere), are resistant to tumor challenge; yet their lymphoid cells are inactive as tested in ^{51}Cr-

release assays against ^{51}Cr-labeled lung tumor cells. These cells are active against tumor, however, in the microcytotoxicity assay.

4. (C3Hf × A) F₁ hybrid mice bearing the same lung tumor show no evidence of effective *in vivo* immunity, presumably because tumor-specific antigens evoke no response. Yet their lymphoid cells are active against the tumor in the microcytotoxicity assay. No activity can be detected by ^{51}Cr-release assay. It is, therefore, not possible to distinguish *in vitro* the reactivity pattern of cells from these tumor-susceptible mice from those of tumor-immune C3Hf mice.

These discordant findings suggest to us the following:

1. A positive result in the microcytotoxicity assay does not distinguish cell populations containing cells active in ^{51}Cr-release assays from those not containing such cells.

2. The presence of cells active in ^{51}Cr-release is usually associated with *in vivo* resistance. The same cannot be concluded from a positive microcytotoxicity assay.

3. The *in vivo* production of cytotoxic lymphoid cells is suppressed in C57BL/6 mice immunized with EL-4; this may indicate that lymphoid cells whose activity is detected in the colony inhibition assay may function *in vivo*, not as potential "effector" cells, but rather as "regulator" cells responsible for the arrested maturation of cytotoxic cells.

4. The findings of microcytotoxicity in a situation in which no tumor antigen seems to be present, i.e., in the (C3Hf × A) F₁ hybrid bearing a lung tumor, suggests that the reaction is against self-antigen. Indeed, as discussed earlier, reactivity of lymphoid cells of these mice against cultured lung cells obtained from (C3Hf × A) F₁ mice has been observed. This finding again suggests that in some circumstances the cells effecting microcytotoxicity *in vitro* may be involved in the regulation of potentially destructive autoimmune processes. These considerations have been explored recently (Martin, Esber, and Wunderlich, *Fed. Proc.*, **32,** 173, 1973; Martin *et al.*, *Brit. J. Cancer*, **28,** Suppl. I, 48, 1973).

ALEXANDER: The situation Martin has outlined is better understood than he has indicated. It is known that macrophage cytotoxicity is, by and large, cytostatic and that it is frequently difficult to detect ^{51}Cr release following attack by specific immune macrophages unless they are contact-activated, achieving cytotoxic potential. Unless spontaneous release of ^{51}Cr is very low, their cytotoxic activity cannot be detected in a short-term test. Therefore, at least two types of immunologically-specific effector cells exist, the cytotoxicity of which cannot be easily detected by ^{51}Cr release but which is readily demonstrable by growth inhibition. The contact-activated memory-type cells can be easily distinguished from the immediate lytic cells, because the latter are more radioresistant. There is one more point related to Kourilsky's data. The dip in Kourilsky's curve is not unique. The same situation has been found in mice immunized with allogeneic cells. The growth inhibitory activity of their spleen cells shows a dip at about ten days.

WEISS: Responding to Martin's remarks, we have studied several tumor systems in which cytotoxic activity by lymphoid cells could not be demonstrated, but in which repeated washing of the effector cells revealed them to be highly effective. Washing less than six times was often ineffective. We have seen this with regard to both mammary tumors and MCA-induced sarcomas in Balb/c mice. An inhibitory factor, which at least in terms of specificity—and we have made no other characterization—behaves as if it were antigen, appears to come off in the washing. When instead of washing a crucial six to ten or more times, we simply let the effector cells stand at room temperature at 37°C for 24–48 hr, they also regained some of their cytotoxic reactivity. When one combines the procedures of incubation and washing, potential but masked lymphoid cytotoxic capacity may be best revealed.

It is remarkable that even lymphoid cells obtained from animals carrying very large tumors, lymphoid cells which seemed at first to be totally nonreactive *in vitro*, and coming from hosts which showed no evidence of resistance to tumor growth, nonetheless showed remarkably good cytotoxic activity after such repeated washings. Workers in several other laboratories have made similar observations.

CHAIRMAN HOWARD: That is a very important idea that failure in a cytotoxic test might be due to blocking, providing demonstrable activity is present in another assay. It is possible that blocking is responsible for the dip in activity in Kourilsky's data at the time of peak tumor size. Martin makes a good point that direct cytotoxic activity is associated with resistance, while microcytotoxic activity can be found in nonresistant individuals. It should be pointed out, in addition, that resistance may occur in the absence of direct cytotoxic activity— for example, in Martin's own case of the tranplacentally induced lung tumor in C3Hf mice.

TERRY: I would like to introduce an additional aspect of this problem as it relates to the evolution of the immune response to tumors. This derives from Glaser and Herberman's work in an experimental system involving Gross virus-induced lymphomas in rats. The system is artificial, in the sense that it involves tumor transplantation and the observations may be different if one follows the evolution of a spontaneous tumor. Two assays are used to evaluate the evolution of the immune response. Cell-mediated cytotoxicity is assessed with a 4 hr chromium-release assay at different times after tumor inoculation. The chromium release caused by spleen cells is detectable before day 5, peaks at day 10 and is undetectable again by day 20. The other assay used is stimulation of ^{3}HTdR incorporation occurring when spleen cells are stimulated by tumor cells. The stimulation assay does not become positive until after day 10, peaks at about day 40, drops markedly by day 60, and then remains positive at a low level for quite some time.

The point is that during the evolution of a tumor and the immune response to a tumor, different assays will give positive results at different times, and it is not possible to make generalizations about the absence of immunologic responsiveness without using a multiplicity of assays.

Finally, in agreement with Weiss, Herberman reported several years ago that, in some tumor systems, cell-mediated immunity assays (for anti-tumor-cell activity giving negative results) could be converted into ones giving positive results if lymphoid cells were removed from the animal and held in tissue culture medium overnight. It does not work with all tumor systems.

STUTMAN: Another important factor determining the type of response is the class of antigen involved and the capacity of the host to respond to such antigens. Using only one test in the C3H mammary tumor system and selecting for individual antigens of the array that I showed in the preceding session, we find every possibility, and we can actually push the responses in any direction we desire. A virus-free animal immunized with a mammary tumor will recognize ML, MTV and private antigens. Such an animal will produce T lymphocytes that kill target cells *in vitro*. We also detect conventional complement-dependent cytotoxic antibodies. If we add that cytotoxic antibody to the mixture of lymphocytes and target, it usually potentiates target cell killing. If different dilutions are employed something akin to blocking is revealed. No complement is added to this system. So in this system, T lymphocytes kill target cells specifically, and conventional cytotoxic antibody is demonstrable early after immunization.

After six periodic injections of irradiated cells, peak cytotoxic T-cell activity in regional lymph nodes becomes less and less, and antibody-dependent lymphocyte cytotoxicity, using non-T lymphocytes, is then easily detected. On the other hand, the virus-infected animals react mainly to ML and private antigens, not because of tolerance to the MTV antigens, but because that antigen is already present in excess. Early after immunization, in this case, little peaks of T cell killing are observed, then lymphocyte-dependent antibody cytotoxicity catches up. In this system we never find conventional cytotoxic complement-dependent antibodies directed against tumor target cells.

Therefore, depending on the antigens involved, the type of responses elicited, and manipulations of the host, different answers can be obtained using different tests, different target cell types, and different syngeneic systems.

CHAIRMAN HOWARD: Cerottini has been working on the evolution of the cellular response to target antigen in immunized animals. What kind of mechanisms occur with what tempo? What kinds of cell populations are produced during immunization? The nature of immunological memory in these cellular immune phenomena is of great interest. It takes one back to the old observation by Medawar that second-set skin grafts reject more rapidly than first skin grafts, something which has never been satisfactorily explained in terms of cell populations, although it was used by him as evidence that an immune response is involved in graft rejection. Despite the multiplicity of experiments now being done on cytotoxic phenomena, there is actually no explanation for second-set graft rejection.

CEROTTINI: The question of memory has often been raised in transplantation immunology. To study this question, Brunner and I have tried to use a model system of allograft immunity in which the formation of cytotoxic thymus-derived lymphocytes (CTL) can be easily quantified by the method I described earlier. It was, thus, possible to demonstrate that mice injected twice with the same irradiated allogeneic tumor cells developed a secondary response characterized by earlier appearance and higher peak of cytotoxic activity than was found after a single injection of allogeneic cells (Brunner and Cerottini, *Progress in Immunology*, B. Amos, ed., p. 385, Acad. Press, N.Y., 1971). More recently, we have tried to confirm this finding by using *in vitro* systems. As you know, CTL can be generated in MLC. Using quantitative methods, we have studied the formation of CTL in MLC, using irradiated DBA/2 spleen cells as stimulating cells and C57BL/6 spleen from either normal or primed mice as the source of responding cells. Primed mice had been immunized with DBA/2 tumor cells 2–4 months earlier, in such a way that little residual cytotoxicity was detectable in their spleens at the time of the onset of MLC. Quantitative analysis of the formation of CTL revealed an earlier appearance and a higher peak of effector cells in secondary versus primary MLC (Cerottini, Engers, MacDonald, and Brunner, submitted for publication).

Since a secondary antibody response is quantitatively and qualitatively different from a primary response, we looked for qualitative differences in the antigenic stimulus leading to CTL generation *in vitro*. Thomas, in our laboratory, was fortunate enough to find that allogeneic membrane fractions, in contrast to irradiated lymphoid cells, were able to stimulate the formation of CTL *in vitro* in primed spleen cell populations but did it very poorly in normal cells. The results of a representative experiment are shown in Table 22.

It can be seen that the membrane preparation, used at an optimal dose, was over 30 times less efficient than the irradiated lymphoid cells in inducing the formation of CTL in primary MLC, whereas the same preparation was almost as efficient as irradiated cells in secondary MLC. Altogether, these studies suggested that primed mice possessed long-lived progenitor cells which were in

TABLE 22

In Vitro Generation of CTL: Immunogenicity of Allogeneic Irradiated Cells or Cell Extracts[a]

Responding spleen cells	Alloantigen stimulus	% Specific ^{51}Cr release 0.3 at L:TC[b] ratio of					LU/culture[c]
		0.3	1	3	10	30	
Normal	Whole cells	6	20	55	90	99	59
	Cell extract	N.D.	N.D.	4	12	30	3
Primed[d]	Whole cells	20	58	95	99	100	312
	Cell extract	10	30	78	98	100	122

[a]Spleen cells from either normal or primed C57BL/6 mice were incubated with either 1000 R-treated DBA/2 spleen cells or particulate membrane extracts prepared by sonication of DBA/2 spleen cells. On day 5, each cell population was assayed for cytotoxicity *in vitro* using ^{51}Cr-labeled P-815 (DBA/2) target cells.
[b]Lymphocyte: target cell ratio in the assay system (number of target cells: 10^4; incubation time: 3 hr).
[c]Lytic units calculated as mentioned in *Adv. Immunol.*, **18**, 67, 1974.
[d]C57BL/6 mice injected with 30×10^6 P-815 (DBA/2) tumor cells 2 months previously.

higher numbers and perhaps qualitatively different—in terms of the antigenic requirement for triggering—than in unprimed mice.

In order to get further insights into this phenomenon, we tried to repeat these experiments in a completely *in vitro* system. MacDonald thus investigated the formation of CTL in long-term MLC following repeated antigenic stimulation over periods of time of more than 2 months. Normal C57BL/6 spleen cells were incubated with irradiated DBA/2 spleen cells for 2–3 weeks. By that time, about 1/5 to 1/10 of the original cell number was recovered, and this cell population showed little cytotoxic activity. However, it was observed that the readdition of irradiated DBA/2 spleen cells resulted in a return to peak level of cytotoxic activity when measured 4 days later. When the kinetics of the reappearance of cytotoxic activity in MLC populations after restimulation was studied more closely, it was found that greatly enhanced cytotoxicity was already demonstrable 24 hours after stimulation. Viable cell counts for the same cultures revealed no increase in cell number during these 24 hours, but a constant increase from that time until the fourth day. Indeed, the absolute number of cells increased 5- to 8-fold after restimulation, and the cytotoxic activity reached a level more than 3 times higher than that observed at the peak of the primary response on day 5. Further studies established the specificity of the cytotoxicity of CTL obtained after secondary stimulation.

Using this system, it was possible to perform 4 successive stimulations of the same MLC cell population at 3 week intervals. As shown in Fig. 14, each restimulation resulted in the reappearance of cytotoxic activity which reached peak levels as high (if not higher) than those observed after the first stimulation (MacDonald, Engers, Cerottini, and Brunner, manuscript submitted for publication). In addition, the following points could be established: (1) The effector cells in long-term MLC repeatedly stimulated with antigen belonged to the T

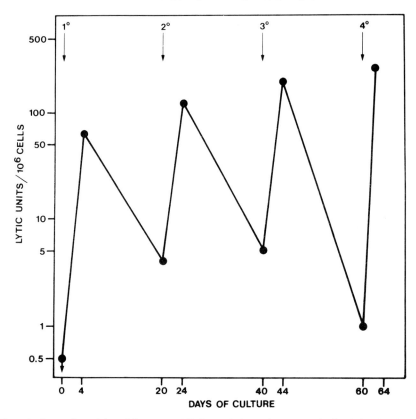

Fig. 14. Cytotoxic activity of long-term MLC populations after repeated stimulation *in vitro*. Spleen cells from C57BL/6 mice were incubated with heavily irradiated DBA/2 spleen cells for 20 days. The remaining cell population was then transferred into new culture tubes together with freshly prepared heavily irradiated DBA/2 spleen cells. Twenty days after the secondary stimulation, the same procedure was repeated. A quaternary stimulation was performed 20 days after the tertiary stimulation. On day 4 after each stimulation, cell aliquots were assayed for cytotoxicity using ^{51}Cr-labeled P-815 (DBA/2) target cells. Lytic units per 10^6 cells were calculated as in *Adv. Immunol.*, **18**, 67, 1974.

cell class; (2) the cells which become cytotoxic after secondary stimulation belong to the small lymphocyte series; (3) these cells, however, derived from the large lymphocyte population which appeared on day 4 after primary stimulation; (4) the appearance of cytotoxic activity within 24 hours after restimulation of day 14–20 MLC populations did not require cell proliferation as shown by the lack of effect of cytosine arabinoside, a DNA synthesis inhibitor. After the first 24 hr, however, the increase in cytotoxicity was closely related to cell proliferation. These results thus suggest the following differentiation pathway in MLC populations: CTL progenitors, which are small lymphocytes, respond to alloantigenic stimulus by proliferation and differentiation into medium and large lymphocytes which are highly cytotoxic. (Whether or not this process involved T–T-cell cooperation will not be discussed here.) These cells are unable to further proliferate following alloantigenic stimulation until they revert in size to small lymphocytes. Then, these small lymphocytes, which are poorly cytotoxic, become highly cytotoxic within 24 hr after secondary stimulation and then proliferate during the following days. Although these results are highly suggestive of such a lymphocyte differentiation pathway, it is as yet impossible to prove or disprove that the cells which become cytotoxic after secondary stimulation derive from precursor cells which are cytotoxic after stimulation. A specific marker for CTL is needed before such a question can be answered.

CHAIRMAN HOWARD: For a long time many of us have been puzzling over why explicit cytotoxic effector cell activity was long gone from primed animals while second-set rejection function was absolutely unimpaired for many, many months. These experiments of Cerottini provide an elegant explanation for this paradox, and I would imagine it is as true for tumor systems as for grafts. There is no reason to doubt that what has been described here is in fact a primed effector cell precursor which has no intrinsic cytotoxic effect or functions, which can be reactivated to effector function in the absence of DNA synthesis, and which is also potentially a dividing cell, so it amplifies its function by mitosis.

I should like to know about the persistence of this new cell type *in vivo,* for if it does persist *in vivo,* an explanation of the persistance of secondary functions *in vivo,* and of second-set graft rejection may be available. From the Sprent and Miller experiments concerning persistence of cells derived from primary allogeneic immunization and transferred *in vivo,* it appears that thymidine-labeled transferred cells have essentially vanished a week to ten days later. Do cells in Cerottini's experiments, obtained after one or two cycles of *in vitro* immunization, confer long term secondary responsiveness to unprimed animals? If such cells do persist *in vivo* for a long period, conferring second-set capabilities on the unprimed recipient, then the explanatory cycle will be complete, and we will have an explanation for the secondary T cell rejection phenomenon.

The importance of this for studies of tumor immunity must be emphasized. The standard technique for demonstrating immunization by a tumor is to allow a tumor to grow, to remove the tumor, and then subsequently re-challenge the animal with living tumor cells. This is analogous to Cerottini's experiment or to any experiment dealing with first- and second-set skin grafts. A primary stimulus is applied, a long period passes, and immunity is demonstrated by the outcome of a second stimulus. Can we postulate that tumor immunity measured by this kind of application, ligation, and second application, expresses the activity of cells of the type Cerottini has described—secondary reactivatable cells? That is a very important question.

There are two further questions. First, do the cells that Cerottini recovers from his multiple immunized cultures have any GVH activity measured as F_1 hybrid spleen enlargement in the Simonsen assay? I should predict that they would be inactive on the grounds that immunity to transplantation antigens, though marked and persistent by skin graft rejection, is never seen as a increase in the GVH activity of the lymphocyte populations of the immunized animal (Ford and Simonsen, *J. Exp. Med.*, **133,** 938, 1971).

Second, if the cells from Cerottini's cultures can be shown to persist *in vivo*, what is their distribution? Are they recirculating cells in the sense that they migrate continually from blood to lymph, or are they restricted to the blood vascular system; are they localized in the solid lymphoid tissues or in extravascular sites such as the serous spaces? And are they persistent *in vivo* because of a long life span or by repeated division?

ALEXANDER: Howard felt little was known about memory cells in graft rejection but this is not so. The fact is Gowans and Uhr *(J. Exp. Med.,* **124,** 1017, 1966) clearly showed that small lymphocytes carried memory in a second-set response. More recently, but still 4 years ago, Denham *et al. (Transplantation,* **9,** 366, 1970), using tumor allografts showed that after suitable immunization of mice and rats, there were lymphoid cells present which were very sensitive to all types of inhibitors of DNA synthesis (such as X-ray, and cytotoxic chemical agents) which, after contact with the specific target cell, become cytotoxic *in vitro*. These cells persist in the animal for more than 30 days and their presence coincides with the capacity of the animals to reject an allograft in a second-set fashion. These cells were found in the spleen but not in the thoracic duct. Again, compare the experiments of Gowans which point invariably in the same direction.

CHAIRMAN HOWARD: Surely effector cell activity does not persist in allogeneically immunized animals as long as second-set graft rejection. The normal figure for the recovery of cytotoxic cells from primarily immunized donors is about five weeks, while second graft rejection lasts for many months or years. I can imagine that different antigen systems vary in duration of cytotoxic-cell persistence, but we are still left with the paradox that grafting immunity outlasts the presence of cytotoxic cells.

ALEXANDER: No, I said *memory* cells. The persistence and distribution of the immediate killer cell is different. Howard poses the question of the persistence of memory cells. These can easily be recognized by the fact that they require contact activation before they become killers and by their susceptibility to all kinds of inhibitors of DNA synthesis. After they have been contact-activated by specific antigen, they are no longer nearly as susceptible to radiation. The memory cell found *in vivo* is characterized by the fact that it has seen antigen and is very susceptible to all forms of DNA inhibitors. Within 12–24 hr after contact with the antigen it becomes relatively resistant. Transformation is required for these cells to turn from memory to effector cells, and this requires some form of nucleic acid biosynthesis.

CHAIRMAN HOWARD: If that is so, we have yet another cell to be concerned with, for that requirement is explicitly absent from Cerottini's cytotoxic cells. In his work, transformation from nonactivity to activity occurred in the first 24 hr, and was specifically insensitive to DNA synthesis inhibitors.

CEROTTINI: That is the main point. There was no difference in the appearance of cytotoxicity during the first 24 hr after restimulation, whether or not the inhibitor of DNA synthesis was added to the culture.

ALEXANDER: I see, that is interesting.

COHN: I interpret the Cerottini experiment, in which a primed population in the presence of cytosine arabinoside responds to induction in a limited way, to mean that an antigen-sensitive cell can be induced to differentiate to an effector T killer cell without division. This also seems to be true for the induction of B cells to plasmacytes.

CHAIRMAN HOWARD: A similar difference exists in the antigen requirement for secondary responses, which again has a pleasantly old-fashioned sound about it. It is as if these cells are more avid or something.

COHN: We should remember that in order to induce differentiation to T killer cells, cooperating activity (associative antibody) is required. If a primary antigenic stimulation raises the level of associative antibody (cooperating activity), then the secondary induction of T killer cells would require either a much lower concentration of antigen or one of lower affinity. Consequently, as Cerottini finds, a comparison of the capacity of an antigen or intact cells to induce, with that of membrane components, would show a much greater difference in a primary than in a secondary response.

GOOD: I may have missed the point of Cerottini's experiment. The crucial experiments relate to Alexander's evaluation of the sensitized animal (to know whether any memory cells are present before starting the *in vitro* system). Can one, by prior treatment with DNA inhibitors like Ara-C, irradiation, or alkylating agents *in vivo,* eliminate this cell population capable of resisting Ara-C and producing killer effects *in vitro?* It appears as though Cerottini has duplicated for T lymphocytes what has long been known for B cells.

CHAIRMAN HOWARD: Another point which relates to this is that as long as immunity is demonstrable by rapid graft rejection "Cerottini cells" should be found. There are some problems about describing these two functions, but it would be interesting to correlate second-set graft rejection with the presence of a cell evolving into an effector cell and not requiring DNA synthesis.

ALEXANDER: Fifteen to twenty days after allogeneic stimulation, the cytotoxic activity of lymphoid cells can be totally obliterated by radiation with 300–500 R.

CEROTTINI: In experiments done by Brunner, it was evident that cytotoxic lymphocytes taken from mice immunized 3–6 weeks earlier were not affected by 500 R. It was necessary to use a dose higher than 1000 R before the activity of the effector cells decreased.

STUTMAN: After immunization of C3Hf mice (by progressive tumor growth followed by amputation) it is easy to detect cytotoxic lymphocytes in regional nodes and other lymphoid compartments as early as day 5 after amputation (Fig. 15). This response peaks by day 7 and then progressively returns to background levels. The magnitude of the response is variable depending on the type of lymphoid cells tested (Fig. 15) but the peaks usually have the same timing.

After the second inoculation, peak is again rapidly detected (Fig. 16). After a third inoculation, the results are variable depending on the timing. When the third inoculation is given during the peak of the second response, cytotoxic lymphocytes in regional nodes actually decrease (Fig. 16). This is probably due to migration of lymphocytes to the subcutaneous site of tumor injection. This phenomenon is comparable to results described by Mackaness in immunity to bacteria. If the third stimulation is given during the decrease of the secondary response, a sharp peak of rapidly dividing cells is observed (Fig. 16). Similar sharp peaks after fourth and fifth immunization are observed (Fig. 17). The main difference being that as hyperimmunization *in vivo* proceeds the magnitude of the peaks progressively diminish (Fig. 17).

Apparently progressive decay occurs in the ability of regional lymph node cells to kill target cells. These *in vivo* results are somewhat different from those of Cerottini in an *in vitro* system. It may also be of interest that sera from these animals give readily detectable lymphocyte-dependent antibody cytotoxicity.

BACH: I want to question the extrapolation which Howard made earlier, to the effect that memory cells detected *in vitro* are cells which are likely to account for second-set graft rejection. Cerottini himself pointed out that there may be

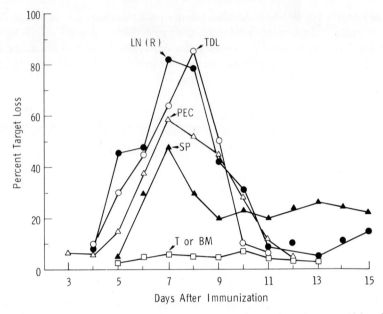

Fig. 15. Generation of cytotoxic lymphocytes *in vivo*. Lymphocyte-dependent cytotoxicity of syngeneic C3H mammary tumor cells (prelabeled with ^{3}HTdR and adherent at 500:1 lymphocyte-target ratios) is expressed as % target cell loss after 36 hours incubation and as a function of time after immunization (animals were C3Hf injected with 5×10^5 tumor cells in the right foot pad and amputated 10 days later; "days after immunization" equals days after amputation). LN(R): regional lymph node, TDL: thoracic duct lymphocytes, PEC: peritoneal cells, SP: spleen, T: thymus, BM: bone marrow.

a selection as the culture continues, with certain cells dying. The somewhat greater responses seen in secondary, tertiary and quarternary stimulation, which he showed us, could be due to stimulation of selected cells without a particular change in these cells. After *in vivo* sensitization, he could use membrane fragments to stimulate, getting almost the same results as with lymphocytes, whereas after *in vitro* sensitization he was unable to do this. I am not convinced that the cells examined are memory cells. They may be cells which can respond—stay around in culture and respond exactly the same way the second time.

CEROTTINI: To answer Bach's question, MacDonald has done only a few experiments in which he tried to use a membrane fraction to restimulate primary MLC cells kept in culture for 20 days. So far the results have been negative. There is, however, a problem which might explain these negative results. As shown by Wagner and others, including Bach, adherent cells apparently are required for the proliferation and formation of CTL in MLC. Long-term MLC populations are probably devoid of such cells. When they are restimulated with

108

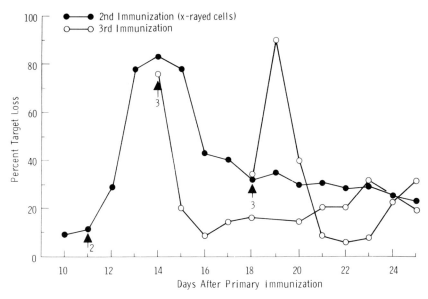

Fig. 16. Effect of second and third immunizations on generation of cytotoxic lymphocytes, primary immunization, as in Fig. 15, and other immunizations by injection of 1×10^6 X-irradiated (2000 R) tumor cells, subcutaneously.

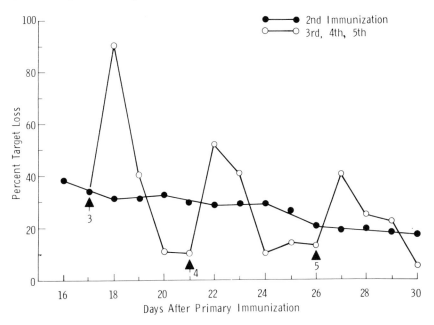

Fig. 17. Effect of second, third and fourth immunization on the generation of cytotoxic lympho-cytes *in vivo* (see text of Figs. 15 and 16 for details).

109

irradiated cell populations there are enough adherent cells provided to substitute for those missing in the responding cell populations. Obviously, this is not the case when membrane fractions are used for stimulation. Further experiments using an extra source of adherent cells are thus needed to clearly establish this point.

CHAIRMAN HOWARD: Bach has an important point—that the stimulability with antigenic membrane fragments is separable from other properties of these immune cells. Nevertheless, I think Cerottini's caveat is valid, and we must simply await the outcome of the experiments.

GOOD: To bring Cerottini's experiments into perspective with *in vivo* data presents a problem. One can understand, from earlier data, how memory cells may effect second-set graft rejection. After all, memory cells last a long time and can be rapidly expanded by proliferation to large numbers of effector cells. It is not difficult to understand, then, how a skin allograft can be rejected in 6–7 days rather than in 10–11. I wonder if the model Perey and I described a few years ago is not explained by the findings Cerottini presented. Agamma-globulinemic chickens unable to make antibody, were repeatedly immunized with allogeneic cells. This brought them to a point of rejecting a skin allograft as a white graft. With Cerottini's findings it would be possible to explain this model, which was difficult with Alexander's prior data.

VAAGE: As a counterpoint to the present emphasis on *in vitro* systems and on the cellular factors in tumor immunity, I offer the following observation. In a system of MCA-induced fibrosarcomas in mice, conditions can be achieved where a proportion of tumors will spontaneously reject after implantation. This is done by sensitizing the mice with one subcutaneous injection of killed tumor cells in saline plus one intraperitoneal injection of killed tumor cells in Freund's adjuvant. Live tumor cell pieces are then implanted subcutaneously. In about 2–3 weeks, about 10% of the implants grow slowly and regress, and about 90% grow progressively and kill the hosts. Histological study of tumors during the process of regression, even very small ones, shows insignificant or no lympho-cytic infiltration.

In further experiments, the effect of passively transferred tumor antiserum was found to increase the number of rejections, compared to normal serum-treated animals, and growth was delayed in those tumors which grew progres-sively. It would be difficult to ascribe a role for cells in these instances of anti-tumor immune protection.

CHAIRMAN HOWARD: Perhaps with that early reminder of how complex *in vivo* effects usually are, we should move on to some of the most confusing aspects of the cytotoxic phenomena that have been described.

The first point is that when cytotoxic assays are attempted *in vitro*, the result is very much dependent on the target cell. It is necessary for the target cell to be susceptible to the effects that one is attempting to document; in fact, one will fail to find the effects if the target cell is inappropriate. The general rule is to assume that the effects are absolute, so to speak, and that the target is merely a passive illuminator of the effect, just as a piece of film will passively reveal the image on it as long as it is properly exposed. I am quite convinced that this is not so and that there are very significant differences in target sensitivity, differences so great that they can create a negative result, implying that a particular effector-cell population does not exist. If the assays are negative, one is obliged to say that effector cells are absent.

We have heard enough experiments which convey loudly and clearly that responsibility for a negative can sometimes be laid on the target. The first clear observation on this was undoubtedly by Cerottini and Brunner and colleagues. They showed in their early experiments that certain differences exist in the ease with which different targets are killed by cytotoxic cells from allogeneically immunized donors. The P-815×-2 mastocytoma was a very special target in that it was much more easily killed than other targets. We know now that other target cells used for chromium-release cytotoxicity are essentially as sensitive as P-815, i.e., EL-4, and at least two lymphomas in rats. But many other cells are not as easy to kill.

Why is this so? Several points have come up in discussion which either illustrate the target cell susceptibility issue in a new way, or provide what might be mechanisms to explain it.

Weiss will describe some work concerning the ability of immunized cells to bind to target cells and the failure of the target to show a cytotoxic effect.

WEISS: Doljanski, Ben-Sasson, Wainberg, and I have been studying interactions between chick-embryo fibroblasts transformed by the Rous sarcoma virus *in vitro*, or whole tumor cells taken from autochthonous or allogeneic tumor-bearing chickens, and lymphoid cells derived from chickens with actively growing or regressing Rous sarcomas. We found that lymphoid cells from tumor-bearing chickens attached specifically to autochthonous or allogeneic tumor cells, with a clear preference for the former. In this binding assay, we employ ^{51}Cr as a label on the lymphoid cells and so can obtain a rapid and simple indication of attachment to the targets. In parallel, we found that such sensitized lymphoid cells also bind macromolecular substances released *in vitro* from chicken embryo cells transformed by RSV and from tumor cells, with a high degree of specificity. To quantitate the binding of materials "shed" by these cells, we introduced labeled choline and glucosamine into the transformed cell growth medium and followed the uptake by lymphoid cells of the labeled cell surface material released by transformed cells into the medium.

111

In parallel cytotoxicity studies (i.e., liberation of ^{51}Cr from the neoplastic target cells), we found cytotoxic effector cell activity in a limited number of instances, in the same population of sensitized lymphoid cells which were positive in the binding tests. Where cytotoxic action was demonstrable, there was again a clearly greater activity towards autochthonous than toward the allogeneic targets. These observations also suggest to us the presence of individual antigenic components on the surface of Rous sarcoma cells, in addition to common RSV-associated or other antigens.

It then occurred to us that those instances in which cytotoxic activity was not demonstrated, the failure to kill might be due to the presence on the surface of these lymphoid cells of free blocking antigens, shed by the tumor and attaching to the lymphoid cells *in vivo*. However, when we attempted to block the activity of those cells which could kill, by exposing them to the macromolecular cell surface material peeled off *in vitro* from RSV-transformed chicken fibroblasts, we failed to neutralize the cytotoxic activity. When we removed by repeated washing from lymphoid cells that could not kill, material which seemingly was applied to these cells *in vivo*, the eluted material could neutralize cytotoxic activity of other, active effector cells. It also appeared from further experiments that the bond between tumor target cells and lymphocytes not capable of cytotoxic action is less firm than the bond between such targets and lymphocytes capable of killing.

It might be argued from these observations that there is a critical degree of affinity of binding, or of density and complementarity of the target cell surface antigenic determinants for specific effector cell receptors, or of some other factor making for strength of attachment, which is necessary to bring about that intimacy of union necessary for severe cell damage. A considerably lesser degree of binding avidity may still give a positive attachment test with no subsequent destruction of the target. Similarly, what peels off the transformed cell surface *in vitro* and can attach specifically to sensitized lymphocytes does not necessarily block their ability to kill, whereas the material which the cells shed which attaches to effector cells *in vivo* seems better able to block cytotoxicity. It could be that the constituents coming off the surface of the transformed cells *in vitro* lack some of the properties which make for a firmness of interaction with the sensitized effector cells which is requisite for interference with their cytotoxic capacity. These observations are becoming fairly clear; their interpretation may be questionable.

PREHN: I want to be clear whether the variation in killing effect was due to variation in the target cells or the lymphoid cells.

WEISS: This is due to variation in the lymphoid cell populations, because we can have in a series of experiments identical target cells, coming either from the same tumor or from the same chicken embryo transformed *in vitro* by Rous sarcoma virus; one can really rule out target cell variation. To repeat, we find almost 100% lymphoid cell-binding, but a lesser frequency of killing in this system.

CHAIRMAN HOWARD: I am afraid I misunderstood the implications of these experiments at first. I now realize that we are indeed dealing here with an interesting variation in lymphocyte performance rather than of target susceptibility. It is unclear whether binding and killing, and binding and failing to kill, represent two poles of a statistical distribution of binding avidity or some more fundamental qualitative difference between two classes of binding cell.

STUTMAN: For those who use adherent cells, additional factors must be considered. Appreciation of one of them caused us to abandon the study of MCA-induced sarcomas *in vitro*. This factor is the ability of certain tumors to produce collagen *in vitro*. If they synthesize collagen, they grow in rather organized structures which are virtually impossible to kill. It was very tempting, obviously, to select tumors that were easy to kill and tumors that were very difficult to kill and manipulate the results in any direction.

KLEIN: The variation in the sensitivity of different cells to immune effector mechanisms is a very important point. It is also a difficult point, and it is obviously easiest to study the antibody-complement mediated cytotoxicity.

Probably the first experiment involving the selection of immunoresistant variants was done by E. Möller and my wife in 1965. They exposed a chemically-induced sarcoma to the selective pressure of H-2 incompatible recipients and found that "nonspecific" sublines appeared, readily transplantable to H-2 incompatible hosts. When the H-2 antigen expression was compared to the original strain-specific lines from which they were derived, a ten fold reduction was found. Later, Fenyo *et al.* in our laboratory, exposed a Moloney virus-induced lymphoma, YAC, to selection in syngeneic , Moloney virus-immunized mice. Again, an immunoresistant subline arose (YACIR) that had a tenfold reduced concentration of the Moloney virus-induced surface antigen, without any change in H-2 antigen concentration. All this has led to the conclusion that immunosensitivity is essentially a function of surface antigen concentration. I might also mention that we recently succeeded in showing that the YACIR subline actually contains a Moloney virus variant, defective in its ability to induce membrane antigen in susceptible indicator cells (JLSV-9) compared to the virus derived from the original, wild type-YAC line.

Recently, the somatic hybridization technique gave some very interesting new information. Friberg has analyzed the behavior of the immunoresistant TA3/Hauschka line, in comparison with the immunosensitive TA3/St mammary carcinoma, of strain A origin. Both sublines grow as ascites tumors and express H-2[a] antigen, but there is an approximately 30- to 50-fold difference in expression, with TA3/St as the high and TA3/Ha as the low antigenic line. In parallel, TA3/St is exquisitely specific for the original A strain, whereas TA3/Ha grows indiscriminately in foreign strains. Again, the first conclusion was that difference in sensitivity to rejection and to cytotoxic isoantibody (and, incidentally, also to lymphocytotoxicity *in vitro*) is exclusively dependent on antigen concentration. When, however, the low-antigenic TA3/Ha line was fused with normal ACA fibroblasts, and high malignant ascites tumors were re-selected, first in (A × ACA) F₁ hybrids and then also in the parental A strain, 12 independently selected hybrid-derived segregants all showed a high H-2[a] antigen concentration, quite comparable to the original TA3/St tumor. Only 4 of the 12 regained the original, high cytotoxic sensitivity characteristic for TA3/St, however, whereas the remaining 8 were moderately or even completely resistant to cytotoxicity. This, therefore, shows that high antigen expression, although it may be necessary for high cytotoxic sensitivity, is not sufficient by itself and that there are obviously other membrane properties, perhaps membrane repair, that can counteract antibody and complement-mediated killing. This work has been recently published (Klein, Friberg, Wiener, and Harris, *J. Nat. Cancer Inst.*, **50**, 1259, 1973; Friberg, Klein, Wiener, and Harris, *J. Nat. Cancer Inst.*, **50**, 1269, 1973).

CHAIRMAN HOWARD: If Klein were to make a list of targets in order of their known susceptibility to lysis by one method, for example, antibody-complement dependent lysis, would he arrive at the same order if he were then to test the target cells for susceptibility to either T-mediated direct cytotoxicity or to lymphocyte-dependent, antibody-mediated cytotoxicity?

KLEIN: This has not been studied very well. The only results I am aware of are the findings of Friberg, who found a direct parallel between the antibody and complement-dependent cytotoxic sensitivity of the immunosensitive and immunoresistant TA3/St and TA3/Ha lines (in relation to anti-H-2[a] antibodies) and their sensitivity to lymphocytotoxicity, in short-term isotope-release tests.

TERRY: Are these cells equally lysed through some other antigen?

KLEIN: Yes, there is no difference between the lines with regard to their sensitivity to xenogeneic antibodies, directed against species antigens.

COHN: The same type of result has been found for the theta (Thy-1.2) antigen by my colleague Hyman. (*J. Nat. Cancer Inst.*, **50**, 415, 1973).

If one is going to try to select a complement-resistant line, it seems to me one would put a double selection pressure on the cells, i.e., selecting simultaneously with anti-H-2 and anti-viral antigen. In that case the possibility of escaping both lytic processes would be small and selection would favor a line intrinsically resistant to complement lysis. Such a case might be very revealing.

I would like to ask how Klein interprets the stable loss of an antigen and its return to a high level on hybridization.

KLEIN: We already have two models. In the TA3/Ha model, low antigen expression is "recessive" in the hybrid. This means that upon fusion with a normal fibroblast, e.g., of the ACA strain which does not carry genetic information for the H-2 complex that is suppressed in TA3/Ha (H-2^a), full expression of the H-2^a complex reappears (Klein, Friberg, and Harris, *J. Exp. Med.*, **135**, 839, 1972). This means that the immunoresistant, low antigenic variant is missing something required for antigen expression or assembly. It is interesting, however, that Friberg found that the 30- to 50-fold difference between TA3/St and TA3/Ha narrows down to 3-fold when lyophilized materials or isolated plasma membranes are compared (Molnar, Friberg, and Klein, *Transplanation*, **16**, 93, 1973). This suggests that some steric feature of the living cell membrane prevents full expression of the antigen that is there, cryptic, but in relatively high quantities, in the TA3/Ha cell.

COHN: Has Klein ever tried to fuse two independently derived negative lines to see whether he can get a positive expression of H-2 by complementation?

KLEIN: No, we have not explored that possibility.

ALEXANDER: I would suggest that fragility and ease of lysis is an entertaining test tube phenomenon which may be irrelevant to the *in vivo* situation.

For tumor control the tumor cells must be "sterilized" (i.e., prevented from dividing). How quickly they actually break up and disappear is irrelevant. This comes out very clearly in radiotherapy where some tumor cells, like lymphomas, break up and lyse within hours after receiving a sterilizing dose of radiation while most sarcoma cells may stay intact, i.e., remain physiologically alive, but are incapable of dividing (i.e., reproductively dead). It is quite wrong to refer to the former as radiosensitive and to the latter as radioresistant. Radiosensitivity is related to the dose needed to sterilize the tumor. Fragility is not the important end point.

COHN: Alexander is worried that castration is synonymous with death. When a cell is irradiated, it does not know that it is dead until it divides.

This question of sensitivity to killing is terribly important to any immune surveillance hypothesis, in which a cell when transformed to neoplastic is eliminated by the immune response, but, as a result of some variation to resistance, it escapes the immune system. We have to look at all the ways in which cells escape the immune system, and loss of expression of tumor-specific antigen is obviously one of the escape mechanisms.

ALEXANDER: In terms of the tumor cells, the important difference is reproductive death. How long a nondividing tumor cell hangs about, whether it succumbs in 4 hr, 24 hr, or 24 days is relatively unimportant. So my query really is, in connection with these variations in fragility, what constitutes physiological death. Is this also reflected in the same variation in reproductive integrity, and especially in reproductive death, which is, after all, the important end point?

KLEIN: I agree with Alexander about the utter irrelevance of radioresistance. As far as radioresistance is concerned, the basic definition of all the variants I have referred to was made *in vivo*. This means that the same immunized mice that could reject the immunosensitive variants of a given tumor were more or less completely unable to deal with the immunoresistant variants. Obviously, immunoresistance is relative, but it can be seen in relation to the threshold effect, typical for all immune killing, and basically different from radiation sensitivity that proceeds by a single hit mechanism. One can also express this by saying that a tumor cell variant that reaches immunoresistant (i.e., nonrejectable) colony size at a lower cell number will be more resistant to the various immune effector mechanisms than a tumor that has a higher threshold.

ALEXANDER: I want to point out ·that Klein's experiments involve complement-dependent lysis *in vitro*.

KLEIN: Perhaps one could rephrase the question by asking whether the immunoresistance development, demonstrated by *in vivo* experiments involving serial transplantation of tumor lines in the presence of immune response, is also relevant for the growth or recurrence of spontaneous tumors. Here, there is no solid evidence. In Burkitt's lymphoma, we have a strong suspicion that immunoresistance may play a role. Virtually all tumors are highly sensitive to chemotherapy but some recur whereas others go to long lasting total tumor regression, probably cure. The recurring tumors often accumulate IgG on their surface, suggesting some kind of blocking or self-enhancement mechanism operating with cells that are more resistant to antibody-mediated killing than the primary tumor that virtually never shows a similar accumulation of IgG. At least two of the recurring tumors were found to be tetraploid, incidentally, and this has considerable interest when considered against the background of the experimental work that has shown that tetraploid variants are often more immunoresistant than the diploid tumors from which they are derived. All other Burkitt lymphomas that have been examined cytologically were diploid or near diploid.

CHAIRMAN HOWARD: This discussion began with a concern whether the concentration of antigen on target cells was a relevant consideration in determining the susceptibility of the cells to any killing mechanism. The evidence makes it quite clear that antigen concentration may be relevant, but is not the whole answer.

Cone mentioned a phenomenon earlier, while talking about the antigenic products of the HL-A region, which could conceivably influence the susceptibility of a cell to lysis whether antibody or cell mediated, i.e., that the antigenic products of the recently described third locus in HL-A were much more rapidly shed *in vitro* than were antigenic products of the LA and Four loci. In other words, three different antigenic determinants on the cell surface, which are products of three different loci, may have quite different potential as targets for cytotoxicity. If one of them is shed rapidly, then it may be an insufficient target by dilution from the cell surface, or it may be an insufficient target by producing blocking of some kind.

CONE: These experiments were done with Bernoco in Ceppellini's laboratory. In these experiments protein synthesis by human peripheral blood lymphocytes was blocked by cyclohexamide and changes in the amount of HL-A of the first, second and third segregant series were determined. Bernoco found that antigens of the first HL-A locus did not decrease appreciably for 24 hr after inhibition of protein synthesis, antigens of the second HL-A locus decreased about 50% in 24 hr and antigens of the third HL-A locus were no longer detectable 12 hr after inhibition of protein synthesis. These results suggest that if a tumor-specific antigen is turning over rapidly, chemotherapeutic drugs which block protein synthesis could cause the loss of this antigen, thus rendering surviving tumor cells nonimmunogenic.

UHR: May I ask why this phenomenon is described as shedding, when basically what was detailed was turnover?

CHAIRMAN HOWARD: Because I remembered that the antigen had been recovered in a soluble form, after radioiodination of the cell surface.

CONE: No, there is loss of detectable antigen from the cell surface.

CEPPELLINI: I think that Cone is wrong on this point. In fact, it is a kind of exhaustion phenomenon. The third locus product is exhausted before the product of the first and second loci.

117

UHR: The biochemists use the term "turnover" to describe the rate of degradation and replacement of particular molecules. It is a misuse of the term, because in the case of the cell surface they have never looked for release into the culture medium. An appropriate use of the term turnover would be to describe loss from the cell compartment in question without implication as to mechanism. Incidentally, shedding has only been described *in vitro,* and we do not know its physiological significance.

CHAIRMAN HOWARD: There is one particular class of cell surface determinant in the mouse which is rather interesting, because it shows a really quite special resistance to being a target for lysis. The antigens which I have in mind are those of the central region of the MHC complex, the antigens which have been called lymphocyte-defined or LD antigen and the presumably homologous antigens which lie outside the serologically defined loci in the human HL-A chromosome. I bring up these antigens, because they have been used to generate some very important insights into the way cytotoxic lymphocytes in general are produced.

First let us consider these so-called lymphocyte-defined antigens in terms of target cell fragility.

TERRY: The Chairman raised the question earlier as to whether antigens can be detected on cell surfaces which do not serve as appropriate targets for cell killing. I would like to present an example of one such system, which comes from the work of Sachs, Shearer, Simpson, and their collaborators.

The serologic system is that which defines Ia antigens, which are cell surface antigens controlled by genes that map in or near the Ir-1 region. The specific system is one in which B10.A animals are immunized with lymphoid cells from B10.D2 animals. These two strains differ at H-2.31, and, as a consequence of this immunization, the B10.A animals make anti-31 antibodies. When this antiserum is tested against spleen cells from B10 animals (which lack H-2.31) lysis is again observed.

This observation is unusual in two respects: First, it should not have been found according to the H-2 specificity charts, and second, because only about 45% of the spleen cells were lysed. Subsequent experiments showed that the cells being lysed were predominantly B cells. Genetic studies made it possible to map the genetic control of these antigens in the Ir-1 region. A number of antigens have been defined and it appears that there is a locus containing a series of allelic genes which control products detected on the surface of B cells. Neither direct studies nor absorption studies have revealed expression of these products on the surface of T cells, but the possibility remains that they may also be there but at a very low density. Because of the location of the genes, it has been agreed to refer to this locus as the Ia (Ir-associated) locus.

118

The next observation was that the MLC reactions detected after mixing B10.A and B10.D2 spleen cells required Ia antigens in order to produce stimulation. B10.D2 stimulator cells were found to stimulate B10.A responder cells to a significantly greater extent than they stimulate (B10 × B10.A) F₁ responder cells. Both responders differ from B10.D2 by the same H-2 specificity (H-2.31), but only the B10.A also differs by the Ia antigen described above (since B10 also shares this antigen). Furthermore, spleen cells were separated on nylon wool columns into adherent and nonadherent cell populations. In both directions, one way MLC's showed that the adherent (B cell) population caused the majority of stimulation. Thus by both criteria the Ia antigens appear to be important in stimulating the MLC.

As I have indicated, B10.A animals immunized with B10.D2 cells make antibodies against H-2.31 and the Ia antigen designated "β" by Sachs. This antiserum will lyse B10 cells, which lack H-2.31 but contain β. When cell-mediated killing is assayed, it is clear that although B10.A spleen cells are cytotoxic for spleen cells carrying H-2.31, they are incapable of killing spleen cells that contain only the β-antigen, for example, B10 spleen cells. Separate experiments show that B10 cells are susceptible to cell-mediated killing, since spleen cells from B10.A animals immunized against B10 are cytotoxic for B10 cells.

It is not clear from these experiments whether no appropriately sensitized killer T cells are formed, or whether they are formed but cannot kill β-bearing cells because of some property of the Ia-cell-surface antigens. In either case, one can conclude that these antigens can stimulate an MLC and can serve as adequate targets for antibody and complement but are not capable of leading to effective killing by cell-mediated mechanisms. The implications for tumor immunology of either of these interpretations is quite obvious.

CHAIRMAN HOWARD: The experiments Terry describes illustrate an example of fragility differences.

MEO: The question is what sort of target was Terry using. Was it a PHA blast?

TERRY: No, either T cells or B cells.

MARTIN: What is the evidence that Terry has generated an anti-B cytotoxic lymphocyte?

TERRY: There is no way one can say that it is directed against theta, that is generally impossible. That being the case, it would reflect another example of the same thing we are talking about, namely an antigen which will induce anti-body but which will not induce cell-mediated immunity.

CHAIRMAN HOWARD: This makes target cell fragility worth talking about. But we do not know whether these antigens are inadequate targets for cell-mediated cytotoxicity because they do not elicit effector cell activity or because the antigens are inadequate as targets for a cytotoxic effect. We cannot know the answer to this question at present. The conditions, which lead to the appearance of effector cells *in vitro,* may have something to do with the generation of effector cells in general. Could Bach give us, briefly, evidence that he thinks would support cell collaboration?

BACH: The mouse H-2 complex, or MHC, is divided into four regions, K, I, S, and D, as shown schematically in Fig. 18. Each region has one marker locus. The K and D regions contain the H-2K and H-2D loci respectively, alleles of which determine the classically defined H-2 antigens. I will refer to these as the SD regions, loci, or antigens. The I region contains immune response or Ir loci, which control the animals response to a variety of antigens and the S region marked by the Ss locus. In addition to the SD, there are loci in the I region, which, if different in two animals, lead to MLC reactions, GVH responses, and skin graft rejection. This locus is now called Hld-2; the locus and antigen are referred to as LD. A separate, weaker LD locus, Hld-1, maps between the S and the D region. SD region differences lead to relatively much weaker MLC stimulation and GVH responses than LD differences.

Several years ago, Häyry and Defendi described in the mouse, and Solliday and Bach in man, that, after several days of MLC incubation, cytotoxic

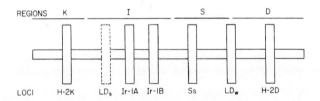

Fig. 18. Scheme for the mouse major histocompatibility complex (MHC). The mouse H-2 complex is divided into four regions—K,I,S, and D—each designated by a marker locus, H-2K, Ir-1A, Ss, and H-2D. The alleles of the H-2K and H-2D loci determine the classical serologically defined H-2 antigens. The Ir-1A and Ir-1B loci determine the immune response of the animal, and the Ss locus controls the quantitative levels of a serum protein. Differences between the two LD loci result in activation of lymphocytes in MLC and are associated with GVH reactions *in vivo;* the alleles of the LD-s locus are relatively stronger, in this regard, than alleles of the LD-w locus. The LD-s locus has not been formally separated from the Ir-1A locus. Differences in the LD-s locus are also associated with skin graft rejection without concommitant H2K or H-2D disparity.

cells develop which are capable of causing ^{51}Cr release from target cells taken from the same strain or individual whose stimulation, or sensitizing, cells were used in MLC. This reaction was made generally applicable by the introduction, by Ceppellini, Lightbody, and coworkers, of PHA-stimulated lymphocytes as target cells. The cytotoxic test is referred to as CML. Since H-2/LD differences lead to MLC activation, we tested whether, in such cases, CML also occurred towards the LD target. In the first combination tested by Alter in our laboratory, excellent CML took place. This was the C57BL/6-H(21) combination of Bailey. In two subsequent H-2/LD different but SD identical combinations, however, there was no detectable CML against the LD target despite good MLC activation, confirming the finding of Eisjvoogel in a family in man.

Schendel and Alter showed that in order to get CML in the mouse, the sensitizing cell in MLC had to differ from the responding, or eventual effector cell, by both LD and SD components and that the target cell required the SD region difference present on the sensitizing cell in MLC. Under these conditions, CML was positive. In fact, there was equally good killing on a target cell carrying only the specific SD region differences, which had been on the sensitizing cell in MLC, as on a target cell carrying both the SD and LD differences in question. Studies by Ceppellini and Eisjvoogel, and their colleagues also suggested that the SD antigens are the target.

These same results are obtained in another manner in a "three-cell experiment" defined by Schendel and shown in the following tabulation:

Cell combination in MLC	^{3}HTdR incorporation in MLC	CML on C target cells
AB$_m$	+++	—
AC$_m$	±	—
AB$_m$C$_m$	+++	+++

The responding cell is from donor A. Strain B differs from A by H-2/LD differences. Strain C differs from A by H-2/SD differences. I use the same reference system of A, B and C having these relationships with respect to LD and SD throughout. The results obtained in early experiments are illustrated. There was no CML on B target cells under any conditions; in order to generate cytotoxic cells against C, both the LD and SD differences were needed during *in vitro* sensitization.

As we developed more sensitive culture conditions for MLC sensitization, we did see positive MLC activity in AC$_m$ mixtures and positive CML on C target cells. In every case, however, the three cell combination, AB_mC_m increased the percent CML on C targets. Our colleague, Widmer, working with MacDonald in Brunner's and Cerottini's laboratory, was able to obtain essentially maximum lysis with AC_m mixtures alone. The question thus arose whether the SD antigen could stimulate a maximal response alone under some conditions, or whether there were LD loci in the SD region.

Schendel has recently obtained some preliminary evidence that is consistent with the latter possibility. She has used heat treatment of MLC-stimulating cells, similar to the protocol used by Eisjvoogel, to abrogate the ability of the cells to stimulate thymidine incorporation. The results she gets are illustrated in Table 23. The tests were performed in a more sensitive MLC system where AC_m mixtures do stimulate and lead to CML as discussed. We interpret these data to mean that there is some physiological cooperation between LD and SD. The LD response makes possible or enables the development of CML activity. We do not know whether the CML attack is on the SD antigens themselves or on a phenotypic product of genes closely linked to those determining the SD antigen. Further, we must hold open the possibility that CML can be demonstrated on LD targets. The lack of cytotoxicity demonstrated here could be explained in many ways. First, LD may be clonally distributed, and as such is present on too few cells to show up in CML, even if those few cells are killed. Second, LD may not be expressed on PHA blasts. Third, LD may be shed or modulate so rapidly that it cannot allow the cell interactions needed for cytotoxicity. Of course, many other explanations are possible.

Likewise, several mechanisms can be proposed for LD-SD cooperation. One or two separate populations or lymphocytes of A exist—a proliferating helper cell, or PHC, responding to LD, and a cytotoxic lymphocyte, or CL. A response to LD would then either allow or make possible the CL response à la T–B-cell collaboration. In this case, it would be T–T-cell collaboration in all probability. There is, of course, an analogy to the hapten-carrier system.

TABLE 23

Heat Lability of MLC-Stimulatory Cells

Cells in MLC mixture	^{3}HTdR incorporation in MLC	CML in C target cells
AB_m	++++	−
AC_m	++	++
AB_mC_m	++++	++++
$AB_\Delta C_\Delta{}^a$	±	±
AB_mC_Δ	++++	++++
$AB_\Delta C_m$	++	++

[a] Δ = heated cells.

122

The fact that we can separate LD and SD onto different stimulating cells, under these *in vitro* conditions, in the "three-cell experiment" does not, in my mind, argue against this postulate. The degree of cell crowding that pertains in culture might bring the PHC and CL together very easily, especially given the high frequency of LD responsive cells. We cannot measure the relative efficiency of the LD–SD collaboration in the "three-cell experiment." Thus, one may not need the theoretical bridge required by the hapten-carrier complex as in the T–B-cell collaboration that leads to antibody production.

Secondly, the B mitomycin-C treated cell may actually recognize the foreign LD antigens on the A cell and thereby activate A, which then allows the A cells to respond to the CML target antigens on the cells of C. If LD differences on A, which are recognized by mitomycin-C treated cells of B, are not clonally distributed, but present on all A cells, then this is a reasonable mechanism. In fact, it can be tested.

Third, A cells, as single cells, may recognize both LD and SD differences, even though the ability to respond to either stimulus is clonally distributed. I do not favor this mechanism but certainly have no way of ruling it out.

COHN: If we are trying to convince the *"in vivo* people" not to be afraid of an *in vitro* system, like that just described by Bach, we will have to give them better information on how to interpret it.

CHAIRMAN HOWARD: In closing this session on mechanisms of cell-mediated cytotoxicity, I should explain why I brought up the issues of target cell-specific influences in *in vitro* assays and cell collaboration in the induction of *in vitro* effector cell activity. These issues are currently relevant only in highly refined systems using inbred mouse strains and individual humans of known HL-A phenotype. The reason I raised them is that they illustrate effects, which any proposed cytoxic immune mechanism involved in tumor rejection must explain.

There are many ways of finding out whether any given antigen is present on a cell. I assume, that as immunologists, we all believe that it is through cell surface antigens that immunosurveillance and tumor rejection must be mediated. What we have learned here is that our assays for antigen are all highly selective. The examples that have been discussed are probably the most dramatic illustrations of this target cell selectivity. Some antigens are vigorous stimulators of lymphocyte proliferation but are apparently undetectable by cell-mediated lysis. Other antigens are excellent targets for cell-mediated lysis but induce little or no proliferation. Still other antigens are beautiful targets for antibody-mediated lysis but are undetectable by cell-mediated lysis. Under some conditions cell-surface antigens are apparently accessible to cell-mediated cytostatic mechanisms but undetectable by cell-mediated cytotoxic mechanisms. No doubt direct binding of fluoresceinated or radiolabeled antibodies can detect further antigens.

Since we do not have any clear idea which immune mechanisms serve to cause rejection of tissues *in vivo* we must be prepared to use all the *in vitro* assays available in a systematic approach to elucidating the role of the immune system in natural or induced control of cancer. In the present state of knowledge, no single *in vitro* assay suffices to mirror the *in vivo* phenomena that accompany tumor or tissue rejection. We must use them all and understand the value and limitations of each one of them.

A second effect of interest is cell collaboration. It has been easy to think of an immune response as simply due to an antigen causing a precursor cell to differentiate through to an effector stage: B cell—blast cell—plasma cell, or, T cell—blast cell—effector cell. This simplistic view, if not totally wrong, is clearly incomplete. We now know that B cells will only differentiate to plasma cells under very special circumstances, and the evidence can no longer be ignored. That similar complications exist for the differentiation of the T cell is now becoming apparent.

The experiments described by Bach, showing apparent collaboration between the cells responding to "LD" and "SD" determinants of the H-2 complex in mice, based on a precisely analogous finding by Eijsvoogel and colleagues in man (*Transpl. Proc.*, **5**, 1301, 1973), showed that antigens not detected by cell-mediated cytotoxicity may nevertheless induce a proliferative reaction that in some way promotes a cytotoxic response to other antigens. These findings may be of general interest in predicting the fate of an antigenic cell *in vivo*, and especially of a tumor cell. As has already been pointed out, there is really no such thing as a tumor antigen. "Tumor antigen" is really a bundle of things; the changes in the tumor cell surface are many and varied. It may well be that, because of the extreme complexity of the tumor cell surface, conditions may be created which resemble the degree of complexity presented to the immune system by an allogeneic cell, which bears antigens derived from the large number of known polymorphic histocompatibility loci. Antigens like LD on tumors may induce only a proliferative response, and others, like SD determinants, may present adequate targets for cell-mediated cytotoxicity so long as LD-like differences are also present. If either form of antigen is present alone on the cell, no effective carcinostatic mechanisms may be available, though *in vitro* antigenicity may still be demonstrable by one means or another.

Finally those who are particularly interested in the *in vivo* actions of the immune system in cancer must not be afraid of, irritated by, or overwhelmed by seemingly abstract and overcomplicated *in vitro* experiments. They are enormously informative, and provide the only methods we have as yet to determine the range of immune phenomena available to influence the fate of tumor cells *in vivo*.

124

SESSION III

ECOLOGY AND RELATIVE CONTRIBUTIONS OF VARIOUS LYMPHORETICULAR CELLS TO TUMOR RESISTANCE

Destruction of tumor cells *in vitro* by activated macrophages—Arming versus nonspecific activation of macrophages—Nonimmune character of target recognition by activated macrophages—Macrophages and tumor-virus infection—Lectins as probes for membrane changes associated with transformation—Capacity of activated macrophages to discriminate between transformed and normal cells—Development of cytotoxic macrophages in the tumor-immunized animal—Immunologic factors in metastatic spread—Characteristics of dormant tumor cells—Ecological basis of apparent immunodeficiency in tumor bearing—Macrophage sequestration in tumors with consequent depression of DTH—Immune suppression in virus infections.

CHAIRMAN UHR: Many variables affect a given *in vitro* assay for tumor immunity. It is, therefore, difficult to assemble a picture of the total immune response to a particular tumor by comparing the results of the many *in vitro* assays. The "gut" question of this conference is what components of the immune response are critical to the *in vivo* tumor–host relationship. We could have reached this point without having performed a single experiment in tumor immunology. Look at the consequences of over a half century of experimentation in immunity to infectious diseases. Take as an example, antibody-mediated immunity to bacterial infection. Our understanding of the mechanisms of this type of immunity and our capacity to develop appropriate vaccines to the relevant infectious agents are still imperfect. In fact, aside from the toxin-producing organisms, the gaps in our understanding here are awesome. In the case of antitoxic immunity to *C. diphtheriae* or *Cl. tetani*, a small amount of immunogen given several times at appropriate intervals results in long-lasting primary immunity and life-long anamnestic responsiveness. But the problem of *V. cholerae* is another story. Whether the antibody response should be aimed at toxin or at the bacterial cell is not at all clear. Current immunization practices for cholera are certainly not satisfactory. It is difficult to get any anamnestic response to a cholera antigen.

Plague immunization is also unsatisfactory, requiring repeated booster injections. After years of experience, immunity to typhoid is difficult to produce—in fact, the protective effect of any vaccine is controversial. Streptococcal immunity and streptococcal vaccines have been studied for a half century, and I am sure they will continue to be studied far into the future, perhaps without the ultimate resolution of a safe and completely effective vaccine.

Microorganisms are probably more heterogeneous than tumors but the same principles apply. We should expect that tumor antigens will be quite heterogeneous with respect to their biochemistry, immunogenicity, density, and topography on the cell surface. Their presence on microvilli, whether or not the antigens are peripheral or integral membrane components, and whether they modulate or are shed, are all important variables. By analogy to infectious diseases such variables will affect the impact of tumor antigens on the immune system with respect to the type of immunity that is stimulated by any particular tumor and, conversely, the response of such tumors to various immune components.

For these reasons, it will be well for tumor immunologists to look back over their shoulders every once in a while at our rich past experience with immunity to microorganisms. There are important lessons to be learned.

The cell class on which we shall concentrate first is the mononuclear phagocyte or macrophage. The lymphocyte has received much attention during the last decade and notably during the preceding sessions here. It is fair that the macrophage now has its share of the limelight. To start our discussion of macrophages there are clear indications of parallelisms between their established role in host resistance to infectious diseases and a relatively recent implied role in tumor immunity. One of the first questions to be asked is what happens when normal macrophages interact with syngeneic tumor cells *in vitro*.

KELLER: Recognition of a role for normal, nonimmune macrophages in dealing with tumor cells is a rather recent development. As far as I know, four groups have contributed to this knowledge: they are Hibbs, Remington, and collaborators at Stanford, Alexander and colleagues at the Chester Beatty Institute, Holtermann and Klein at the Roswell Park Institute, and our group at the University of Zurich. I will refer from time to time to the work by Hibbs and Remington and by Edmund Klein, and Alexander will himself report his findings.

Our investigations started with the observation that the growth of Walker carcino-sarcoma was entirely suppressed or greatly enhanced in rats infected with the nematode, *Nippostrongylus brasiliensis*, depending on the timing of the tumor-cell inoculum in relation to the parasite infection. Early in the immune response to the parasite, the tumor did not grow; once the immune response had developed, tumor growth was enhanced (Keller, Ogilvie, and Simpson, *Lance*, **1,** 678, 1971). Further studies showed that inhibition of the growth of Walker carcino-sarcoma in rats was also achieved by passive transfer of activated macrophages (AM) from rats pretreated with peptone or infected with the nematode parasite. Moreover, *in vitro* culture of tumor cells with peptone-induced peritoneal macrophages for only a few hours led to a marked decrease in the number of targets (Keller and Jones, *Lancet,* **2,** 847, 1971; Keller, *Schweiz. Med. Wschr.,* **102,** 1148, 1972). These and other studies (Keller and Hess, *Brit. J. Exp. Path.,* **53,** 570, 1972) indicated that AM contribute effectively to tumor resistance but a more appropriate *in vitro* model system was needed to explore the cellular interaction.

Normal resting macrophages (NM) and AM are most conveniently available from the peritoneum where rodents have a relatively large resident population of these cells. This population is increased in number and in activity by the i.p. administration of various "inflammatory" agents, such as peptone, starch, glycogen, BCG, endotoxin, double-stranded RNA, etc. (Alexander and Evans, *Nature New Biol.,* **232,** 76, 1971; Keller and Hess, *Brit. J. Exp. Path.,* **53,** 570, 1972; Parr, Wheeler, and Alexander, *Brit. J. Cancer,* **27,** 370, 1973). Such treatment not only "activates" resident peritoneal macrophages but also leads to emigration of blood monocytes. Recent observations (Daems and Brederoo, *Zschr. Zellforschg.,* **144,** 247, 1973) showing that the two macrophage populations differ with respect to fine structure and function is a hint that macrophages may not reflect a homogeneous cell population. Such induced exudates also contain various other cell types. By selecting adherent cells, relatively uniform populations of AM are obtained.

AM exert striking cytocidal effects on tumor cells *in vitro*. On this score all investigators in this area are in full agreement. We sought to explore the essential character of the interaction, i.e. kinetics, nature, and degree of the changes in target cells, direct contact versus elaboration of soluble factors, etc. It became apparent that our inadequate knowledge of macrophage physiology and the limitations of *in vitro* macrophage tissue culture methodology imposed severe limitations on the design of experiments. Most of our own work was based on an *in vitro* model system in which peptone-induced adherent rat peritoneal cells consisting of at least 96% AM were cultured with syngeneic tumor targets. The consequences of the interaction were assessed by morphological alterations, cytotoxicity tests, and by measuring residual tumor cell proliferation. Since macrophages do not replicate under these *in vitro* conditions, quantitative measurement of labeled DNA or RNA precursor incorporation reflects tumor-cell proliferation exclusively. This method is objective, highly sensitive, and provides a reliable measure of the proliferative activity of residual cells. However, it tells nothing about the eventual fate of the remaining cells, i.e., their capacity to resume growth.

Combined use of these varied parameters to assess the consequences of the interaction between AM and syngeneic virus-induced or carcinogen-induced tumor targets provided most of our recent data (Keller, *J. Exp. Med.*, **138**, 625, 1973). Rapid and almost complete inhibition of capacity of targets to incorporate ^{3}HTdR into DNA was the earliest detectable relevant consequence of the interaction. After 4 hours culture with AM, incorporation was reduced to 25% and after 12 hr to less than 5% of controls. This effect was dependent on the ratio of effectors to target cells; whereas tumor cell proliferation was completely blocked by a simple majority (10:1, 5:1, even 1:1 has a considerable effect) of AM, a reverse effector/target cell ratio (1:10) often resulted in target cell proliferation higher than control values. These effects on tumor targets were mediated by adherent cells with the distinctive features of macrophages, i.e., they were phagocytic, radioresistant, and selectively destroyed by silica. The presence of fresh serum was not required for this inhibition of proliferation. Parallel to these incorporation studies, the interaction was also followed by light or phase contrast examination of morphological changes (Keller, *J. Exp. Med.*, **138**, 625, 1973). The alterations observed were analogous to those reported by Remington and colleagues (Hibbs *et al.*, *Nature New Biol.*, **235**, 48, 1972). For example when polyoma-induced or carcinogen-induced tumor cells were grown alone for 12–16 hr, the cells covered most of the dish and were well spread. Identical tumor populations exposed to AM at a ratio of 10:1 were consistently decreased in number and the residual cells were shrunken. After 24 hr interaction, the number of tumor cells was further decreased or all were killed. In some preparations, heaps of agglutinated tumor cells were observed. At no time was cell debris seen.

129

Light and electron-microscopic observations have been made in the course of tumor–AM interaction, in the system involving virus-induced and carcinogen-induced syngeneic rat tumors. After adding tumor-cell suspensions to monolayers of AM, those nearest to a target were seen to migrate onto these cells and were subsequently found in close contact with targets. After 12–24 hr, targets were often shrunken. In a series of experiments performed in collaboration with Bächi, no clear fine structural change in target tumor cells was established, although tight junctions between macrophage and target cells were found occasionally. After 12 hr of interaction, when the number of tumor cells had decreased, neither signs of phagocytosis nor cell debris was seen. Decrease in target cell number did not parallel release in chromium cell label, showing that classical cytotoxicity was not involved in this macrophage effect. This could reflect the operation of either a very effective lytic process or, alternatively, AM are extremely efficient in "mopping up" target cell remnants.

BACH: Is "activation" of macrophages essential for the effects Keller describes, or can he take cells directly from the peritoneal cavity of normal untreated animals?

KELLER: Cells taken directly from peritoneal cavity—"wash-outs" of unstimulated normal rats (or mice)—show variable cytostatic effects. Three points should be kept in mind when these effects are considered. First, during the first 12 hr of culture, peritoneal cell populations are inhomogeneous, consisting of about 70% macrophages, 20–25% lymphocytes and a small percentage of other cell types. Second, in vitro culture, as such, itself leads to some macrophage activation. Thus, the cytostatic effect of normal cells is lower than that of AM during the first 4–6 hr of culture. After 12 hr of culture the cytostatic effect of normal cells is almost as pronounced as that of activated cells. NM cultured for 24 hr or longer yield reestablished proliferation of targets. These findings suggest that while normal peritoneal cells have substantial inherent cytostatic capacity, they are not adequate to support long-lasting cytostasis necessary for target cell killing (Keller, Immunology, in press). Third, many aspects such as intercurrent infection, etc., may lead to either partial or complete activation of macrophages in vivo. Stimulation of exudate formation and emigration of blood monocytes, by peptone, endotoxin, etc., is a means of pushing activation to a maximum level and achieving uniform cytostatic and probably cytocidal capacity. As Alexander and Evans (Nature New Biol., 232, 76, 1971) have demonstrated, macrophages may also become cytocidal by exposure to endotoxin or double-stranded RNA in vitro. We found that supernatants of spleen cells responding to lectins such as PHA or ConA, which contain MIF activity (and presumably other lymphokines as well), also increase macrophage cytostatic capacity. After in vitro contact with these supernatants, normal resting peritoneal cells soon acquire cytostatic capacity comparable to that of exudate AM. Moreover, the loss of macrophage cytostatic capacity which occurs within the first 24–48 hr of *in vitro* culture was much delayed in the presence of such supernatants. These are some of the reasons why the degree of activation and the cytostatic capacity are variable in macrophages taken from untreated animals.

COHN: A major interest in this system lies in the implications of the terms normal and "nonimmune," because the assumption being made here is that there is a "nonimmune" recognition mechanism present in macrophages for all types of transformed cells. Consequently, the first step in trying to understand this system is to be certain that the immune system contributes no specificity elements; this, admittedly, is difficult to establish because the efficiency of killing seems to be spectacular.

CHAIRMAN UHR: I do not understand why Cohn makes that statement. No attempt was made here to demonstrate the specificity of the cytotoxic effect on the target cells.

COHN: Keller claims that macrophages activated nonspecifically kill three independently derived tumors but do not kill normal cells. A mechanism therefore exists for selective killing of tumor cells, the assumption being made that AM recognize all transformed cells via a mechanism independent of the immune system. Is that not the point?

CHAIRMAN UHR: Does Keller know that normal cells are not killed under these circumstances? That was not the thrust of the experiments he has given thus far.

KELLER: A series of experiments now in progress deals with the interaction between AM and "normal" target cells. Hibbs (*Science,* **180**, 868, 1973) and Holtermann and colleagues (*Cellular Immunol.,* **9**, 339, 1973) have reported that the morphologically observable consequences of interaction, such as close contact between effectors and targets and subsequent destruction of the latter, occurs *only* with "neoplastic" and seldom, if at all, with "normal" cell lines. Our preliminary data indicate that incorporation of ^{3}HTdR as a measure of the proliferative capacity of rapidly replicating normal 3T3 mouse fibroblasts and their SV40-transformed counterparts is similarly affected by various ratios of effectors and is consistently totally blocked in the presence of a majority (10:1) of AM. The macrophage cytostatic potential on normal embryonic or adult syngeneic fibroblasts seemed to parallel the proliferation rate of target cells. In early passages, when fibroblasts were growing slowly, no cytostatic macrophage effect was detected. As soon as the proliferation rate of the cell lines increased, i.e., after 7–12 passages, a strong cytostatic effect was obtained against embryonic as well as adult normal fibroblasts.

In contrast to the conclusions drawn from my earlier morphological observations, the data on proliferative capacity indicate that AM have cytostatic potential against *both* normal and transformed cells.

CHAIRMAN UHR: This is clearly a critical issue: What is the differential recognition capacity of the macrophage surface for transformed versus normal cells—independent of overt immune factors.

LANDY: On this point it is appropriate to recapitulate chronologically the essential data emerging from the published work by Remington and his associates. His investigations grew out of studies of host intracellular infection with the protozoan *Toxoplasma gondii* and observations that the chronically infected murine host was immune to reinfection and that this immunity could be passively transferred only by lymphocytes. Such chronically infected mice were strikingly resistant to challenge with any of a spectrum of natural mouse pathogens—both microbial and viral. They were also resistant to an array of autochthonous and transplanted tumors including for example, syngeneic KHT sarcoma, allogeneic Balb/c mammary adenocarcinoma and lymphoma cell lines L5178YE and TLX9. The mechanism of this resistance proved to be generally similar for the microbial and tumor challenges and was closely correlated with the development and prolonged maintenance of a population of AM, markedly effective in destroying tumor targets *in vitro,* whereas macrophages from control mice were quickly overgrown by the tumor cells. No phagocytosis of targets was observed. In contrast, these same macrophages exerted only slight or no cytopathic effects on syngeneic and allogeneic mouse embryo fibroblasts.

What is unique in the Toxoplasma model is the presence of a constant immunogenic stimulus which persists for the life of the murine host in the form of a parasitemia and viable organisms in virtually every organ. This augmented host resistance could be essentially duplicated by administration of killed Toxoplasma in incomplete Freund's adjuvant. These were the basic observations that were followed by extensive *in vitro* studies with macrophages and murine cell strains versus their transformed cell line counterparts. Criteria for transformation of cell strains to cell lines were loss of contact inhibition of cell division, loss of fusiform shape and parallel orientation of fibroblasts, cell overgrowth, saturation density. Macrophages activated *in vitro* (endotoxin) or *in vivo* (infection) did not destroy fibroblast cell strains but were strongly cytotoxic for syngeneic and allogeneic fibroblast cell lines derived from the very same cell strains.

This extensive series of experiments suggested to Remington and Hibbs a mechanism of "nonimmune" recognition by AM, to the effect that surface membrane alterations, whether biochemical or topographical, related to loss of contact inhibition, are important in target cell recognition and destruction by AM. This discriminatory ability of AM to destroy transformed cells and tumor cells did not appear to be based on recognition of foreign target cell antigens, insofar as the H-2 system was concerned. Rather, it seemed to involve recognition of cell properties associated with abnormal growth characteristics. In Remington's view, the results suggest that AM-mediated cytotoxicity represents a nonimmune mechanism of recognition.

KRAHENBUHL and REMINGTON*: Studies from our laboratory have revealed that AM from mice chronically infected with the intracellular protozoa *Toxoplasma gondii* or *Besnoitia jellisoni* or from mice injected with Freund's complete adjuvant (FCA) effect the destruction of a variety of tumor target cells (Hibbs *et al.*, *Nature New Biol.*, **235**, 48, 1972; *Proc. Soc. Exp. Biol. Med.*, **139**, 1049, 1972; *Science*, **177**, 998, 1972). The effect does not appear to be complement dependent nor does it appear to be due to the release of toxic factors from the macrophages into the supernatant medium. This ability of AM to effect destruction of tumor target cells persists after infection with these intracellular parasites, probably for the life of the animal. The data of Alexander and his colleagues serve to emphasize the importance of the presence of specific antigen in the maintenance of a population of AM capable of killing target cells nonspecifically. In the Toxoplasma and Besnoitia models, viable organisms persist indefinitely in the host tissues, thereby insuring continuous exposure to antigen. Thus, extrapolating from the data of Alexander's group and our own *in vitro* macrophage activation experiments (Remington *et al.*, in press; Anderson and Remington, in press), continuous exposure of macrophages and lymphocytes *in vivo* to Toxoplasma or Besnoitia antigens causes a persistent state of activation of the macrophages *in vivo*.

The importance of the persistence *in vivo* of specific antigen (immunogen) in maintaining a population of AM was also affirmed in *Listeria monocytogenes* infections. (Krahenbuhl and Remington, in press). AM inhibit DNA synthesis in tumor L cell targets (measured by quantitating ^{3}HTdR incorporation); macrophages harvested from Listeria-infected mice 2, 5, and 8 days after infection were markedly cytostatic for L cells. However, by days 12–20, these macrophages no longer exhibited significant cytostatic activity. This was correlated with progressive disappearance of viable Listeria, indicating that the nonspecific cytostasis of target cells was only effected by macrophages from Listeria-infected mice during the period when viable organisms were present in the tis-

---

Editors' note: Unfortunately circumstances prevented Remington from actual participation in this conference. Accordingly, the editors invited him to prepare a succinct account of his work, with various colleagues, now spanning some seven years. We believe this account by J. L. Krahenbuhl and J. S. Remington gives a broader perspective to the conference record on the role of the activated macrophage in resistance to tumors.

sues. Only freshly prepared AM were markedly cytostatic (Krahenbuhl and Remington, in press). Thus, in the Toxoplasma or Besnoitia models, AM lose their "activation" relatively early. The reason for the rapid loss of this remarkably effective property is unclear.

Because lymphocytes in very small numbers inevitably contaminate monolayers of peritoneal macrophages, a quantitative evaluation was made of their possible involvement in the effect of AM on target cells. Peritoneal lymphocytes from protozoa-infected mice, added to monolayers of normal macrophages far in excess of the potential number of lymphocytes which might not be removed by washing, produced no cytostatic effect (Remington et al., in press).

Although AM destroy target cells from a variety of mouse tumor cell lines as well as target cells consisting of mouse embryo fibroblasts, which have undergone spontaneous transformation, AM produced only slight or no destruction of embryo fibroblasts which had not yet undergone spontaneous transformation (Hibbs et al., Nature New Biol., 235, 48, 1972; Science, 177, 998, 1972). This discriminatory ability of AM to destroy tumor cells and transformed cells does not appear to be based on recognition of H-2 foreign target cell antigens but apparently involves recognition of cell properties associated with abnormal growth characteristics (e.g., membrane alterations). These results suggest that AM have a definitive role in resistance to tumors and may also function in the homeostatic control of abnormal cell growth in normal hosts. The mechanisms, whereby AM are able to discriminate between cells with abnormal growth properties and normal cells, are unknown. Recently, Hibbs (Science, 180, 868, 1973) reported that AM were not cytotoxic to contact-inhibited nontumorigenic 3T3 fibroblasts but caused marked destruction of tumorigenic 3T12 and SV40-transformed 3T3 fibroblasts, cell lines which have lost contact inhibition. These results suggest that surface membrane alterations (biochemical or topographical, or both) related to loss of contact inhibition are the important factors in target cell recognition and destruction by AM.

The mechanisms whereby macrophages effect destruction of target cells are also not clearly understood. Although the in vitro destruction of target cells by macrophages appears to be accomplished by a nonphagocytic mechanism only after prolonged incubation periods (30–60 hr), within hours after challenge there is a strong adherence to and aggregation of AM around target cells. Although the target cells are not visibly harmed during this early period, measurement of the uptake of ^{3}HUdR by target cells cultured with AM revealed a marked cytostatic effect on the target cells within 4–6 hr after challenge (Keller, J. Exp. Med., 138, 625, 1973; Krahenbuhl and Remington, in press). Target cell DNA synthesis had often practically ceased by 18 hr after challenge, a time when little if any visible destruction of the target cells could be detected.

What are the mechanisms whereby AM are able to discriminate between neoplastic target cells and "normal" cells and the mechanisms whereby these cells effect cytostasis and/or cytotoxicity on susceptible target cells? If these mechanisms are similar to the SMAF controlled reactions demonstrated by Alexander's group in their models, what is the apparently nonimmunologic means by which AM recognize and selectively spare "normal" cells even in the presence of major histocompatibility differences between the macrophages and the target cells? Similarly, the mechanisms operative in the destruction of neoplastic target cells must be more clearly understood.

AM rapidly interfere with the metabolism of the target cells during the early phases of challenge, when their aggregation around the target cells is so apparent. The question arises whether this macrophage-effected cytostasis alone is sufficient to cause the subsequent cytotoxicity, or whether inhibition of DNA synthesis merely reflects other major macrophage-mediated defects on the metabolism of the target cell (a marked inhibition of incorporation of RNA precursors is also demonstrable [Krahenbuhl and Remington, unpublished]).

Finally, it will be important to investigate the relative roles of cytotoxic lymphocytes and AM as an *in vivo* surveillance mechanism in the prevention of the development of neoplasia, in the control of already established tumors, and in the immunotherapy of tumors. *In vitro* studies suggest that the adverse effect of AM on target cells is far more efficient on an effector to target cell ratio basis than specifically cytotoxic lymphocytes. Significant cytostasis occurs with a ratio as low as one activated macrophage per target cell (Krahenbuhl and Remington, unpublished). From what is known about the role of serum-blocking factors, it will also be important to determine whether these factors which inhibit cytotoxic lymphocytes are also operative in macrophage-effected cytotoxicity.

CHAIRMAN UHR: Does anyone have other data relevant to the claim that AM can discriminate between a transformed cell and normal replicating cell?

LANDY: The studies of Holtermann, Klein, and Casale are also relevant to this issue. They reported *(Cell. Immunol., 9,339, 1973)* that peritoneal macrophages of PPD-stimulated rats produced cell destruction of syngeneic and allogeneic tumor cells (PYT polyoma virus-induced kidney sarcoma, MCA-induced sarcoma, LS reticulum cell sarcoma induced *in vitro*) whereas little or no cytotoxicity was exerted on syngeneic or allogeneic second-passage normal kidney cells or fifth-passage FE5 embryonic cells derived from embryos close to term. These authors considered that among their cultures of embryonic cells only the ones that were rapidly replicating were significantly susceptible to the destructive action of AM. The mechanism of this selective destruction of tumor targets was considered to be relevant to the tumor regression they had observed to occur clinically at sites of induced delayed hypersensitivity reactions.

BACH: Just what is an *activated* macrophage? How is it defined?

CHAIRMAN UHR: Will Alexander enlighten us about the criteria for calling a macrophage activated. Are the criteria functional or are there morphological and biochemical characteristics of activated macrophages?

ALEXANDER: The story of the involvement of the macrophage in tumor immunity is an old one. Twenty-five years ago Gorer showed that the rejection of an allograft in the peritoneal cavity was achieved by macrophages. Similarly, Granger and Weiser, and Amos and others demonstrated specific immunological killing by macrophages both *in vivo* and *in vitro*. There was a delay before this was extended to syngeneic tumor systems by Evans, who found that macrophages taken from the peritoneal cavity of mice immunized with syngeneic tumors inhibited the growth of tumor cells in an immunologically specific way. In this process, phagocytosis was a late event, coming after key biochemical changes had occurred in the target cells. I want to emphasize here that the macrophages of normal, uninfected animals are in no way growth inhibitory.

Immune, highly reactive macrophages can be obtained in three ways: First, from suitably immunized animals, where reactivity is directed against the tumor antigen in syngeneic systems, or against histocompatibility barriers in allogeneic combinations. The second way of making such "armed" macrophages is by taking nonimmune macrophages from pathogen-free animals and cultivating them for 24 hr with immune lymphoid cells. This is not achieved with supernatant factors; the immune lymphoid cells must be in contact with the macrophages. These immune lymphoid cells can be obtained from immunized animals or by immune induction *in vitro*. The third way of getting immunologically specific armed macrophages is with a supernatant factor obtained by incubation of immune lymphoid cells with specific antigen. Again, the immune lymphoid cells can be induced either *in vivo* or *in vitro*.

The other class of cytotoxic (i.e., growth inhibitory) macrophages is one that will kill and malignant cells tested, (lymphomas and sarcomas) from a variety of tumors. These cells we designate "activated" macrophages. In our experience, in that of Remington, and in reports from several other laboratories, these AM do not affect the growth of nontransformed, freshly cultured embryonic cells. Such AM can be obtained in a number of ways: by taking "armed" macrophages and exposing them to specific antigen. This is an interesting situation, because one can get activated, killing macrophages by immunizing a mouse with SRBC. Macrophages from mice immunized with SRBC are not armed against the tumor cells and they will, therefore, behave like normal untreated macrophages. If such macrophages from SRBC-immunized mice are incubated for 4 hr with SRBC *in vitro*, one then obtains macrophages which are activated, i.e., they are growth inhibitory for all lymphoma and sarcoma cells. One can also get AM by adding the actual tumor cells to armed macrophages,

136

and then things get quite interesting. Macrophages armed against tumor A will kill *only* tumor A. If, however, such macrophages are incubated for a few hours with tumor A, they are then able to kill *all* tumor cells.

The other mode of activation is pharmacologic, involving exposure to bacterial endotoxin or double-stranded RNA (including poly IC and poly AU), as well as double-stranded RNA of viral origin. In very low concentration, these substances turn normal macrophages into AM, activated being defined by the capacity to kill lymphoma and sarcoma cells.

A final way of getting immune macrophages is by taking them from animals systemically infected with intracellular pathogens. There are many situations exemplifying this approach: Toxoplasma infection, as studied by Remington, BCG—if an American strain is used which is highly infective for mice (with the Glaxo strain which does not persist in mice, one does not get AM, only armed macrophages). As Keller showed, animals infected with certain parasites also yield AM.

To our great distress, we have found that, when a Pasteurella infection spread through our mouse colony, macrophages from these animals were continually activated. The key to all this is the presence in the host of persisting infection. It is tempting to link this with the ''arming'' activation transition, because the persisting infection induces armed macrophages which then meet the antigen *in vivo,* thus yielding AM.

To conclude, I return to what happens in the tumor-bearing animal, which is, after all, the important issue. If one takes a rat and puts a sarcoma in its leg and measures macrophage cytotoxicity in the draining lymph node at 7 days, one finds macrophages which are armed, which kill only that sarcoma and not other syngeneic sarcomas. By 15 days the macrophages which are in the draining lymph node kill all sarcoma and lymphoma cells. The appealing interpretation is, of course, that antigen draining from the tumor into the node makes for the transition from ''armed'' to ''activated'' macrophages. Similarly, in the peritoneal cavity of tumor-bearing animals, one generally finds only armed macrophages, even when the tumor is quite large.

CHAIRMAN UHR: Alexander has described essentially a two-step process for the development of an activated macrophage via specific antigen, i.e., arming and subsequent activation.

ALEXANDER: I would say that the process can be either a two-stage affair (arming followed by activation) or only a single-stage activation (i.e., exposure to endotoxin or double-stranded RNA).

MACKANESS: Concerning the question of defining an activated macrophage, it was recognized some time ago that in the course of some infectious diseases the host develops phagocytic cells which have functional capacities over and above those of the normal animal. Host resistance to infection was shown to depend upon such AM.

It is superfluous to reiterate essentially what Alexander has just detailed, namely that there is a close analogy between host–tumor and host–parasite relationships. There is, in fact, an immunological mechanism for activating macrophages, a specific mechanism in which T cells are the prime movers. The action of antigen on sensitized lymphocytes produces profound local and systemic changes in host macrophages. Once this change has been induced, the resulting macrophages have enhanced functional properties of a nonspecific nature. They are capable of killing a variety of antigenically unrelated organisms.

So what do we mean by an AM? It is presumably a cell which possesses the metabolic attributes which permit it to ingest organisms more efficiently, to kill them and to digest the residue more rapidly. The mechanism of killing is unknown. It is linked metabolically so as to depend on H_2O_2 formation and may involve the generation of free radicals which have a capacity to cause depolymerization of macromolecules. Perhaps they can also destroy the stability of cell membranes. Beyond that, I cannot describe what an activated macrophage is.

CHAIRMAN UHR: Are there differences in morphology or biochemical parameters between a population of activated macrophages and a nonactivated population?

MACKANESS: Conspicuous differences make it possible to recognize immediately whether one is observing a population of normal or AM. The AM spread vigorously on a glass surface. Boyden once gave a picturesque description of a widely spread, activated macrophage which was, he said, "engaged in a gallant if futile attempt to phagocytose a cover slip." A correlative of this urge to spread is an enhanced ability to phagocytose. An AM ingests more particles in a given time than does a normal cell. Morphologically, the AM is likely to contain more lysosomes because it is pinocytically more active, and the natural consequence of increased pinocytosis is the synthesis of more lysosomal enzymes. But an abundance of lysosomes is not a constant feature of the AM. Cells obtained from hyperacutely infected animals, such as Salmonella-infected mice, do not contain large quantities of lysosomes. Yet they are exceedingly bactericidal, highly phagocytic, rapidly spreading cells. Indeed, they are the best killer cells I have encountered. Finally, of course, there are metabolic changes. Oxygen and glucose consumption rates and lactate production are all greatly elevated in the AM; it is an extremely active cell.

CHAIRMAN UHR: Is Mackaness suggesting that the difference between an activated and nonactivated macrophage is the capacity to kill and inhibit and that this capacity may not rest on its lysosomal enzymes but rather on some other yet obscure mechanism?

MACKANESS: There is a strong probability of just that, and consequently there is a risk of artifacts intruding into experiments that purport to show nonspecific killing of tumor cells by AM.
   AM will kill even autologous lymphocytes if cultivated in high density.* I wonder what an appropriate ratio of macrophage to target cells should be in an ideal test system. Remember, we are dealing with an extremely active cell which can quickly compromise the nutritional conditions in the environment and adversely affect the survival of target cells quite inadvertently. The AM also insists on attaching itself to surfaces, thereby tending to displace tumor cells from their anchorage. When a monolayer is used as a target for immunological attack, cells may thus be lost from a population without being killed. It may be, therefore, that cytotoxic effects do not necessarily involve interaction between macrophages and target cells in a way that evokes recognition, whether specific or otherwise.

SMITH: An important element of this definition is surely whether the activated state requires continuous presence of the activating stimulant.

KELLER: Smith has identified a most significant issue. At this stage we do not know for certain whether the continued presence of the stimulant is necessary for typical AM performance. I would point out that the cytostatic effect is of relatively short duration. This could mean either that the continued presence of the stimulant no longer matters or that it may have been metabolized by the macrophage, hence the decline in the activated state. In our experience, *in vitro* activation of macrophages by poly IC or endotoxin, as reported by Alexander, yields no higher a level of cytostatic activity by AM than does treatment of the host with these products. Yet the *in vitro* stimulation should provide a higher concentration of stimulant per cell. So the very little relevant information we do have does not support the notion that the activated state requires the continued presence of the stimulation.

CHAIRMAN UHR: In terms of defining AM, it would be worthwhile to continue to search for a biochemical or morphological landmark for this altered functional state. From experiences in cellular immunology, rapid progress depends on such assays. An example is the elusiveness of T cell immunology compared to what is known about B cells. This is partly because until recently

---

Editors' note: The reader is referred to page 146 where Keller cites further experiments in support of this thesis.

there was no assay for a T cell; we have had assays for B cells and antibody-secreting cells for many years.

WEISS: Gallily and I have observed that macrophages stimulated either *in vivo* or *in vitro* by a tubercle bacillus cell wall derivative ''MER'' show an increase of 20-fold in the concentration of certain lysosomal enzymes, or an increase in the rate of synthesis of these enzymes, although they may not accumulate, as Mackaness has indicated. We have used as a functional criterion for activation in this system total increase in lysosomal enzyme concentration or increase in the rate of synthesis.

How was the measurement made by Keller without inhibition of thymidine or uridine incorporation by target cells, in view of the potential uptake of the labeled precursors by both AM and target populations of cells?

KELLER: Macrophages incorporate neither ^{3}HUdR nor ^{3}HTdR under these conditions and there is considerable evidence that they do not undergo cell division *in vitro*. On the other hand, all target cell lines increased in number during culture; thus, the measured alterations in the incorporation of precursors into cellular RNA and DNA reflect synthesis in target cells only.

CHAIRMAN UHR: Do AM degrade engulfed macromolecules at an accelerated rate?

ALEXANDER: Although AM are defined by the fact that they can inhibit growth of tumor cells and they have increased lysosomal content, these changes are not sufficient characteristics. Macrophages fed protein in high concentration develop an even higher lysosomal content; yet such macrophages will not have the property of killing tumors. I share Mackaness' view that lysosomes have little or nothing to do with growth inhibition of tumor cells. The reason one gets increased lysosomal activity in AM is that these cells have the property, after they have killed cells, to clean up the mess they have created, that is, to phagocytize.

CHAIRMAN UHR: Additional information on the rates of macromolecule degradation in the lysosomes of macrophages would be helpful. Such information could be obtained by feeding labeled material to macrophages and observing the rate at which it is degraded.

ALEXANDER: Such experiments have been done with iodinated albumin, but the findings show no correlation with growth inhibitory properties of macrophages.

140

MANNINO: Differences between "normal" and "activated" macrophages depend upon whether activation was induced by administration of peptone, or was effected *in vitro* by poly IC or by endotoxin. Do "armed" macrophages show the same characteristics as "activated" macrophages?

ALEXANDER: We cannot answer that question. Although it is dramatic, it is a difficult end point to define. The impression is that armed macrophages spread better than the nonimmune macrophages, but this is subjective. Certainly the change in the armed macrophage is of a much lower order than the dramatic changes Mackaness described for the infection-activated cell.

MANNINO: So one can discern different stages among these variously manipulated macrophages.

ALEXANDER: Whether one can detect the armed stage by anything other than the killing mechanism itself remains to be established. Relevant work is under way, but as yet this distinction is not clear.

TERRY: Comparison of AM with the normal macrophage reveals what looks like quantitative shift in activity, rather than a discrete or qualitative difference. Is there any information suggesting qualitative differences are involved in this differentiating process? Do such macrophages demonstrate new properties rather than only demonstrate higher levels of those properties characteristic of nonactivated macrophages?

ALEXANDER: There is a very distinct difference. Peritoneal macrophages from "clean" animals do not interfere with the growth of tumor cells at all; that is the experience of many groups. However, once infection intervenes, then one finds these cells manifesting a background cytotoxicity.

CHAIRMAN UHR: What happens to an activated macrophage if kept in tissue culture without target cells?

ALEXANDER: By the fourth day of tissue culture, activated macrophages lose capacity to kill tumor cells.

KELLER: Alexander is correct, but I do not believe that Uhr's question can be answered so simply. Let me explain why. As mentioned earlier in the discussion, comparison of the kinetics of cytostatic capacity of NM and peptone-induced AM shows that the effect of NM was delayed and of shorter duration than that of AM. Further experiments revealed that the cytostatic potential of

AM depended on the duration of prior culture *in vitro*. Under the culture conditions employed, AM showed full cytostatic activity within the first 12–24 hr of *in vitro* culture followed by a gradual loss. This characteristic pattern of cytostasis was compared with a variety of parameters known to be often associated with macrophage activation. Only the level of protein synthesis closely parallels the macrophage cytostatic potential. Other parameters of macrophage function, such as activity of lysosomal enzymes, glucose oxidation, cellular adherence, pinocytosis and phagocytosis, all manifested a clearly different time course (Keller, Keist, and Ivatt, in press).

Besides handling and optimal culture conditions, a number of other factors could decisively modulate such properties. The role of lymphokines in increasing and maintaining elevated macrophage cytostatic capacity has been mentioned earlier in this discussion; somewhat similar effects are obtained by the increase in macrophage cyclic AMP, as achieved by the combined effects of prostaglandins or catecholamines and theophylline or papaverine.

LANDY: We are being rather simplistic in our approach to an understanding of macrophage performance. The work of Volkman and Gowans established that the monocyte precursors present in the peripheral blood originate in the bone marrow. We know considerably less about how and why these cells normally emigrate to the peritoneum or other serous cavities, nor why or how various agents such as endotoxin, peptone, mineral oil, etc., enhance this emigration and maturation. However, we make a mistake if we regard these cells as a homogeneous population. Realistically, it is far more likely that the normal resident macrophage population, and especially the exudate cells, are functionally heterogeneous. Remember that our primary means for "purifying" these peritoneal or blood macrophages has been via their adherence to glass. Indeed recent work provides evidence for macrophage subsets or subpopulations. This could account for some of the divergent findings mentioned.

COHN: Again, I ask: What is the recognition system here? No paradox arises in how macrophages kill. The question is the origin of the recognition step. In the case of the armed macrophage, the argument is being made that the cell is picking up cytophilic antibodies and is, therefore, specific because its recognition system is antibodies made by the immune system. In the case of AM, if it were true that they distinguish between the normal cells and the tumor cells, then two hypotheses come to mind. Either all tumors share similar recognition sites which are recognized by AM, or activation of a macrophage is a cryptic way of inducing the residual contaminating immune system in the cultures so that the macrophage is actually being armed.

Are any of these systems clean enough to distinguish between "activation" as a very subtle type of arming by antibody, or "activation" as an independent "nonimmune" recognition mechanism? The substances which are being used to activate macrophages are substances which are well known to stimulate the humoral immune system, LPS, poly AU, BCG, PPD and so on. For the moment we need to know how clean these macrophage preparations are in terms of what numbers of lymphocytes are present, and how free the target tumor is of lymphocytes.

KELLER: Cohn's questions point to important issues. We have data pertinent to his major points, but not necessarily final, conclusive answers. With present knowledge, it seems highly probable that the macrophage interaction can have varied consequences for different targets. The present data suggest that the macrophage cytostatic potential affects *all* rapidly replicating cell lines irrespective of whether they are derived from normal or neoplastic tissues or whether they are of syngeneic, allogeneic, or xenogeneic origin. This lack of cell, species, or tumor specificity of macrophage cytostasis suggests, but does not prove, the involvement of a nonimmunological mechanism with homeostatic potential. This macrophage capacity seems to be decisively increased by a large array of nonspecific means known to trigger macrophage activation and by immunologically specific macrophage activation via mediators such as lymphokines. However, our data on this latter aspect are as yet only qualitative.

The second macrophage effect, killing of target cells, is detectable only at a later stage of the interaction. The marked and progressive decrease in tumor cells during the interaction, without overt signs of cytotoxicity, or phagocytosis, or of cell debris, may be indicative of a distinctive and potent cytocidal process. The question arises whether this effect might be mediated by the same factor which produces inhibition of proliferation. So far all investigators unequivocally agree that, in sharp contrast to cytostasis, killing by AM selectively affects transformed cells.

The recognition mechanism involved in the cytocidal process is, as yet, unclear. All data thus far show that AM kill all tumor cells, irrespective of whether or not they are derived from the same cell type or species. Such a concept is incompatible with immunological specificity and suggests the involvement of a more primitive recognition mechanism inherent to macrophages. That antibody is not involved in tumor cell killing is also supported by various observations. First, experiments with various tumor cell lines revealed that their elimination is virtually identical in time course and in degree, irrespective of whether the lines have been branched off from the *in vivo* tumor only recently (5–10 passages) or long ago (50–100 *in vitro* passages). In the latter example, the persistence of host-derived antibody on the surface of tumor cells seems highly improbable. Pretreatment of targets with a variety of proteolytic enzymes did not affect the subsequent interaction with effectors. Moreover, the persistence of host lymphocytes in these tumor cell lines can be dismissed, as lymphocytes do not survive for longer than a few days under these culture conditions. Moreover, regular controls of the cultures have never revealed bacterial and viral contamination. Except for histocompatibility antigens in allogeneic or xenogeneic lines, tumor cell cultures should thus not provide an immunologic stimulus for macrophages.

Whether cultured macrophages are "clean" is more difficult to answer. As mentioned earlier, adherent AM populations contained no more than 4% of lymphocytes and other cells. The observations showing that the cytostatic effect was radioresistant, sensitive to silica, an agent selectively toxic for macrophages, and that the additional presence of a large number of lymph node cells (10^6 to 2×10^6) *diminished* the macrophage cytostatic effect argue against a role for lymphocytes in the present system.

It is more difficult to rule out the presence of antibody passively adherent to macrophage membrane. However, pretreatment of these effectors with a variety of proteolytic enzymes did not alter the outcome of the experiment. The cytostatic capacity of AM taken from mice or rats grown under SPF conditions was similar to that of mice or rats grown under conventional conditions. Accordingly, cytostatic potency would seem to represent an inherent property of macrophages and can be raised by a variety of nonspecific means known to lead to macrophage activation. Thus such observations as are pertinent seem opposed to a decisive role for a system operating through immunologically specific mechanisms.

As mentioned earlier, a certain degree of activation is necessary for acquiring potent and lasting macrophage cytostatic and cytocidal capacities. It is generally agreed that lymphokines such as migration inhibition factor (MIF) or macrophage activation factor (MAF) represent the products of immune recognition by T lymphocytes that can lead to macrophage activation *in situ*. To answer the issue whether the presence of such T-cell-derived mediators is necessary for the acquisition of the macrophage cytostatic effect, the cytostatic capacity of peritoneal macrophages from normal and from athymic, nude Balb/c mice on targets were compared (Keller, in *Mononuclear Phagocytes in Immunity, Infection and Pathology,* Van Furth, ed., Blackwell, Oxford, 1974). AM from nude as well as normal mice diminished proliferation of SV40-transformed Balb/c 3T3 cells to a similar degree. Thus, it appears that macrophages can acquire these capacities in the absence of T cells and such T-cell-derived mediators.

GOOD: For procuring activated macrophages is it always necessary to utilize a system which requires them to phagocytize—like pretreating the peritoneal cavity with oil or peptone? Kramer and Leu found a very striking difference in macrophages obtained by other means, relating to the presence of a receptor for MIF on phagocytizing macrophages. This receptor does not seem to be present on alveolar macrophages or nonphagocytizing cells.

The cells that have phagocytized have the capacity to absorb MIF and can be used almost like an immune absorption column for absorbing MIF from the supernatants of stimulated lymphocytes. Therefore, one wonders whether the surface changes that accompany phagocytosis are necessary. Another question that came to mind was whether the changes referred to as macrophage activation are the ones elicited by injection of endotoxin. In studies during the 1950s and early 1960s evidence was obtained that endotoxin could produce an extraordinary resistance to a wide range of microbial pathogens. The question is whether there is a common mechanism via AM that now seems also involved in tumor immunity. Finally, it would be important to know whether monocytes of peripheral blood, analogously stimulated, can also exert *in vitro* this tumor killing action, or must the cell already be a macrophage to respond.

LANDY: Good is assuming that the array of "inflammatory" agents known to activate peritoneal macrophages *in vivo* are phagocytosed by these cells and that this function is an essential part of the activation process. While that is a possibility, I know of no evidence to support a causal association. The work he mentions on a macrophage receptor for MIF is extremely important and involves reasonable expectations, however, we await its confirmation. I was not aware that only macrophages that had phagocytosed foreign material displayed the MIF receptor; this would seem just the reverse of the needed sequence. How would MIF function as a mediator, converting normal macrophages to effector cells *in vivo,* unless it could first act on these cells; this would require such a receptor. I fully concur with Good's impression that the now 20-year-old observations on the extraordinary effectiveness of endotoxin in enhancing immunity of mice to many microbial pathogens are likely exerted via macrophages. In retrospect, it is hard to believe that all our efforts to elucidate that mechanism were so exclusively focused on humoral factors.

PREHN: It seems to me that there might be a simple explanation for the apparent recognition by macrophages of tumor cells. Is it conceivable that the macrophage, with the possible exception of target lymphoid cells, has a particular capacity to kill only those cells which are not very firmly attached to a substrate? This might be both *in vivo* and *in vitro*. In the *in vitro* situation, tumor cells, in contrast to normal cells, tend to come off the glass as they mitose. It could be at this point they perhaps become peculiarly vulnerable to AM. *In vivo,* I would assume parasites and bacteria are effectively detached while host cells in contrast are attached to a basement membrane and, therefore, would be protected from macrophage attack. This formulation would get us out of the terrible problem of having to have some discrete biochemical signal to distinguish tumor cells from normal cells, an idea that I personally find repugnant.

CEPPELLINI: Either we are dealing with an immune recognition mechanism as Cohn has suggested or, alternatively, it could be that the macrophage antigen receptor sticks on tumor cells, and that the cells that are the recipients of these antigens become sensitive to macrophages. I would also point out that, apart from the possibility that the macrophage in a mysterious way does recognize tumor cells, tissue resorption during embryonic development may involve an analogous phenomenon. In that case, I would expect that these AM would in fact recognize some kinds of embryonic cells or perhaps even PHA lymphoblasts.

KELLER: In response to Ceppellini's provocative prediction about PHA lymphoblast susceptibility to AM, I can say that we explored the susceptibility to AM of rat lymphocytes (from lymph nodes and spleen) replicating under the *in vitro* stimulus of T cell mitogens such as Con A and PHA, as well as LPS—a B cell mitogen. When AM are present in the lymphocyte and mitogen culture at a ratio of 1:1, lymphocyte proliferation is completely blocked. On the other hand, in mitogen controls and where the ratio is reduced to one macrophage to 25 lymphocytes, enhancement of lymphocyte proliferation is seen. It is noteworthy that AM added to already proliferating lymphocyte cultures effect a prompt cessation in ^{3}HTdR incorporation. These observations indicate that mitogen-stimulated cells are especially susceptible targets for AM. Nelson (*Nature*, **246**,306, 1973) has reported that AM elaborate a soluble factor that depresses lymphocyte proliferation in response to LPS, PHA, Con A and GVH.

NOTKINS: On the premise that the immune mechanisms involving macrophages, by which the host eradicates viral infections, may give some insight into his defense against tumors, I shall describe some experiments with herpes simplex virus (HSV).

HSV can spread both *in vivo* and *in vitro* in the presence of high concentrations of neutralizing antibody. There is also evidence from clinical studies and animal studies that the infection is much more severe if the cellular immune response is suppressed. Precisely how cell-mediated immunity acts to stop the spread of the infection has not been clear but if one analyzes the ways in which the virus actually spreads, it appears that cell-mediated immunity can act at several sites. HSV can spread by two different routes, either extracellularly or from cell to contiguous cell as a result of cell fusion. Extracellular virus is readily neutralized by antiviral antibody. However, virus which spreads from cell to cell is protected from antiviral antibody. This is one reason why the infection persists in the presence of a humoral immune response. Moreover, even though the virus induces new antigens on the surface of infected cells and even though the infected cell can be destroyed by antiviral antibody and complement, spread of the virus to adjacent cells takes place before the initially infected cells are destroyed.

146

These observations suggested to us that the host may stop spread of infection not by an effect on the infected cells, but by acting on the adjacent uninfected cells. Previously, we found that peritoneal exudate cells (PEC) from rabbits never exposed to HSV, added to a monolayer of infected rabbit kidney cells (PRK), inhibited viral plaques. The PEC appeared to be mildly toxic to the monolayer of cells and caused a slight rounding of the cells. We concluded that the PEC had broken or prevented cell-to-cell contact so that virus could not spread to the adjacent cells without being exposed extracellularly to neutralizing antibody.

Some unpublished experiments performed in collaboration with Lodmell support and expand these observations. Rabbits were immunized with Freund's complete adjuvant. PEC from these animals were then added to monolayers of PRK cells that had been infected with 10–20 plaque-forming units of HSV, and the virus titer was determined 48 hr later. Table 24 shows that at low concentrations of PEC, viral replication was not inhibited. When the ratio of PEC to PRK cells was increased to 5 or 10, viral replication was inhibited by over 99%. This is similar to what we previously found when PEC's from unimmunized animals were used. It can also be seen that tuberculin (PPD) alone had no inhibitory effect on viral replication. When, however, PPD was added to PEC from animals immunized with Freund's complete adjuvant, viral replication was markedly inhibited with a PEC to PRK cell ratio of as low as 0.1. In contrast to the slightly toxic effect to monolayers observed when high concentrations of PEC were used, no toxic effect was observed with low concentrations of PEC in the presence of PPD. For this reason we suspected that another

TABLE 24

Inhibition of Viral Replication by Peritoneal Exudate Cells (PEC) from
Animals Immunized with Freund's Complete Adjuvant and
Stimulated *In Vitro* with PPD

Ratio of PEC to primary rabbit kidney cells	Concentration of PPD (T.U.)		
	None	50	500
	(PFU, $\log_{10}$)		
Control	6.2	6.3	6.2
0.1	6.3	6.1	5.0
0.25	6.3	5.4	4.2
0.5	6.0	5.2	4.2
1.0	6.2	4.8	3.2
2.0	5.7	3.0	3.2
5.0	4.7	2.9	2.0
10.0	4.2	0.9	0.3

Monolayers were infected with 10–20 plaque-forming units (PFU) of herpes simplex virus and then incubated with different concentrations of PEC and PPD. At the end of 48 hr, the PEC were removed and the monolayers washed and titrated for infectious virus.

mechanism must be involved in inhibition of viral replication. When the cell-free medium of cultures that had been exposed to sensitized PEC plus PPD were placed on fresh monolayers, viral replication was inhibited. Further analysis revealed that the factor in the supernatant fluid was interferon.

Recently we performed a similar experiment using PEC from animals immunized with HSV. When inactivated HSV antigens were added to the sensitized PEC, viral replication was inhibited. Again, an inhibitor was found in the supernatant fluid which we are in the process of characterizing. Presumably, this factor, too, will turn out to be interferon.

These experiments showed that the immune defense to HSV infection can be divided into two phases: one specific and the other nonspecific. The specific phase is concerned with the recognition of virus or viral antigens by antiviral antibody or immune lymphocytes. This results in the activation of biological mediators such as chemotactic actors, lymphotoxin, and interferon which can act nonspecifically on the surrounding uninfected cells and thereby inhibit viral replication.

In conclusion, I shall make several points:

1. In the case of HSV it is not the direct attack by humoral or cellular immunity on the infected cells which appears to stop the infection, but rather the nonspecific attack of inflammatory cells and mediators on the surrounding uninfected cells.

2. There are a number of viral infections in man which seem to require cell-mediated immunity. These include cytomegalovirus, varicella-zoster, vaccinia, and measles. These viruses seem to share certain characteristics in common: the ability to fuse cells and to spread from cell-to-cell in the presence of neutralizing antibody. Thus we suspect that cell-mediated immunity protects the host against these infections in much the same way as against HSV.

3. There is some evidence that immunization of animals with BCG or humans with repeated injections of vaccinia can enhance resistance against HSV. If these observations are valid, the mechanism of action may be through the release of interferon.

4. I suggest the possibility that the cell-mediated response to tumors, especially virus-induced tumors, may act in part through the release of interferon.

CHAIRMAN UHR: The effects Notkins described are effects primarily on cell surfaces of both infected and noninfected cells. How does AM get into the picture? How does Notkins distinguish its effects from the effects of interferon and other mediators?

NOTKINS: The mediators can act on both infected and uninfected cells. Because the virus spreads so rapidly, the major effect of the mediators, in terms of stopping the spread of the infection, must be on the uninfected cells. How lymphotoxin actually damages cells is not clear, but interferon works by inhibiting viral replication within the cell. Chemotactic factors attract inflammatory cells to the site of the infection. In the absence of antigen, in this case PPD, mediators are not released to any appreciable degree. Interferon was characterized by failure to sediment at $100,000 \times G$, resistance to pH 2.0, ability to inhibit virus other than HSV, and species specificity.

The inflammatory cells and mediators can act on both infected and uninfected cells, but, to stop the rapid spread of the infection, I believe these factors must act on uninfected cells.

LANDY: Is it possible that virus-infected cells are normally the proper target for the activated macrophage, without invoking the other factors?

NOTKINS: It would not be a specific effect.

LANDY: I was not alluding to immunologically specific effects in the usual sense but, rather, to the fact that the virus-infected cell displays those membrane changes that are perceived by the activated macrophage, thus, making the virus-infected cell a unique target.

NOTKINS: That is a possibility; that could happen.

COHN: An *in vitro* system is described in which AM kill the uninfected, normal cell. Extrapolate to an animal, is it implied that the macrophage kills those cells which the virus might infect—the normal cells?

NOTKINS: The macrophages may damage both infected and uninfected cells (i.e., increased granularity of the cytoplasm and rounding up of the cell), but cell death does not always occur.

COHN: Rounding up is, presumably by interpretation, a toxic effect preventing the spread of the virus to normal cells. Is it assumed that the activated macrophage is causing a rounding up, i.e., toxic effect, in all normal cells which the herpes virus might infect in the animal?

NOTKINS: We believe that *in vivo* chemotactic factors, induced by the immune response to virus-infected cells, attract leucocytes to the site of the infection where they exert the nonspecific effects that I described for our *in vitro* system.

COHN: I understand the *in vitro* system. I want to understand what the extrapolation is to the *in vivo* situation.

NOTKINS: What happens *in vivo* is a specific response as a result of the viral infection, which in turn brings macrophages into the site of the infection where they act by nonspecific mechanisms.

COHN: It is difficult to understand a normal immune mechanism which inactivates uninfected normal cells in order to prevent spread of the herpes infection.

CHAIRMAN UHR: We have probably reached a dead-end on the problem of specificity. My interpretation is that AM can achieve immunologic recognition by the mechanisms that Alexander has indicated, namely, through cytophilic antibody probably complexed with antigen. In addition, AM have effects on transformed cells and perhaps other cells that suggest another level of recognition. The extent and mechanisms underlying this other type of recognition have not been clearly defined.

ALEXANDER: Whether AM specifically recognize malignant cells as such or rather some surface change which is commonly associated with malignant cells is, of course, the real issue. It is almost certain that it is the latter. For one thing, AM will also lyse certain types of red cells. One guess is that it has something to do with the thickness of the cell wall, because most of the transformed cells have, in fact, got much thinner cell walls than nontransformed cells.

As I see it, the rate of cell division does not determine whether a cell is susceptible to activated macrophages. The 3T3 cell divides as rapidly as the 3T3 transformed cell, but it is only the virus-transformed 3T3 cell which is inhibited by AM.

PREHN: I want to make one point quite clear. My thought, in regard to the role of mitosis, did not concern the rate of mitosis but rather that the transformed cell behaves differently during mitosis than the untransformed cell. The 3T3 cell does not come off the glass during mitosis in the same way as the transformed cell does, and it could be during that coming off process that the transformed cell becomes peculiarly vulnerable to AM, for some unknown reason.

ALEXANDER: Prehn's argument is not acceptable to me because inhibition is evident within a few hours; therefore, it occurs in the S phase. The target cell does not have to go through mitosis to be affected by AM.

COHN: I realize that minds are like parachutes; they have to be open to function. Still I am uncomfortable about the claim for the existence of a nonimmune recognition mechanism present in macrophages and of sufficient specificity to kill pathogens and tumors but not normal cells. No doubt we can envisage mechanisms to recognize factors which might be common to a large array of bacteria, viruses, or tumors which macrophages can destroy, e.g., the type that Prehn has just suggested. Nevertheless, I am rather surprised that all of the agents that activate macrophages are precisely those which enhance very weak humoral immune responses to become very good immune responses. LPS, PPD and poly IC are agents which are known to activate the cooperating system, as well as the B cell immune response. Therefore, we should leave it an open question as to whether the macrophage recognition is via a residual immune system, or whether a new "primitive" system has been discovered to recognize a large array of pathogens which to me, at the moment, seem to be unrelated.

WEISS: For many years claims made have been made by investigators, most recently by Caspari and Field, that there exist on tumor cells some "basic" membrane antigens which distinguish the neoplastic state from analogous normal cells. If one considers neoplastic cells as de-differentiated, more primitive cellular entities, they might indeed express on their surface common archetypes of molecular configurations which could represent early stages in the chain of differentiation events. If so, then what may seem to be a peculiar specificity of AM for tumor cells in general might, in fact, be partly based on a kind of immunological specificity. What seems to be an activated macrophage, in this context, may be behaving as an armed macrophage directed specifically against some such broadly distributed antigen.

CHAIRMAN UHR: Cohn's point would be that this antigen should be widely distributed on a large group of microorganisms ubiquitous in our environment.

WEISS: There is another possibility, however. Certain microbial substances nonspecifically stimulate immunological responsiveness to weak antigens. Thus, exposure to such microbial agents may facilitate an immune response to weak, widely distributed, "protean" tumor antigens, and this response may well be manifested, ultimately, by the appearance of specifically armed macrophages.

LANDY: Mannino, speaking for the Burger group in Basel, could tell us about current investigations there. These studies support their general concept of cryptic sites which are more or less continually exposed on transformed cells, whereas normal cells display such sites only briefly at the time of mitosis, the suggestion just made by Prehn. To me, the attractive notion is that this might well be the very site on transformed cells which is so efficiently recognized by AM.

MANNINO: I shall summarize work done with Professor Burger at the Basel Biozentrum and a concept first formulated by him about six years ago.

In a number of cells a lectin-detectable cell surface change has been shown to accompany neoplastic transformation. A good correlation between the concentration of wheat germ agglutinin, necessary to obtain half-maximal agglutina-

151

tion and saturation density in tissue culture, has been demonstrated (Pollack and Burger, *Proc. Nat. Acad. Sci.*, **62**,425, 1969). The higher the saturation density, the more easily agglutinable it is.

A correlation between saturation density *in vitro* and *in vivo* tumorigenicity was demonstrated by Aaronson and Todaro (*Science*, **162**,1024, 1968). Using tissue culture cells derived from inbred mice, they demonstrated that the final saturation density is roughly proportional to neoplastic potential. The relationship of a cell surface change to the transformed state was also demonstrated, using baby hamster kidney cells transformed by a temperature-sensitive polyoma virus (Eckhart, Dulbecco, and Burger, *Proc. Nat. Acad. Sci.*, **68**,283, 1971). At the permissive temperature (32°C) the cells grew as transformed cells and were highly agglutinable by wheat germ agglutinin. When shifted to the nonpermissive temperature (39°C), the cells returned to normal growth and simultaneously became nonagglutinable. Similar studies in other cell systems, temperature sensitive for transformation, have resulted in the same findings (Burger and Martin, *Nature New Biology*, **237**,9, 1972; Noonan, Renger, Basilico, and Burger, *Proc. Nat. Acad. Sci.*, **70**,347, 1973).

The next question to be asked was: Is this cell surface change solely a measure of transformation or does it play an active role in the maintenance of the transformed state? A functional relationship has been suggested by experiments which showed that a brief treatment of the surface of untransformed cells in a contact-inhibited monolayer with a proteolytic enzyme would bring about both the agglutinable state and a further round of cell division (Burger, *Nature*, **227**, 170, 1970). Thus a treatment which results in the exposure of the agglutinin receptor sites also brings about cell growth and division.

The opposite experiment was also done, i.e., the covering of the lectin sites on transformed cells brought about a return to density-dependent inhibition of growth (Burger and Noonan, *Nature*, **228**, 512, 1970). By incubating Con A with trypsin or chymotrypsin, it was possible to obtain a lectin preparation which was capable of binding to the cell but incapable of agglutination. When this preparation was applied to polyoma virus-transformed 3T3 cells, the cells grew to densities similar to those of untransformed cells. Upon removal of the nonagglutinating Con A, the cells once again grew to high saturation densities.

While investigating the binding of a fluorescent-labeled wheat germ agglutinin preparation to transformed and untransformed cells (Fox, Sheppard, and Burger, *Proc. Nat. Acad. Sci.*, **68**, 244, 1971), it was oberved that untransformed cells in mitosis and the early G_1 phase of the cell cycle bound as much wheat germ agglutinin as did the transformed cells. More recently, it has been shown that although untransformed cells are less agglutinable and bind less lectin than do transformed cells, untransformed cells in mitosis bind five times more Con A than do cells in any other part of the cell cycle (Noonan and Burger, *J. Biol. Chem.*, **248**, 4286, 1973). Untransformed cells in mitosis are also agglutinable with wheat germ agglutinin and Con A.

The fact that untransformed cells in mitosis exhibit the same lectin-detectable cell surface architecture that is exhibited continuously by transformed cells suggested that the cell surface architecture of transformed cells is not solely a property of transformation but a very special part of the normal cell cycle. It has been proposed that the cell surface change accompanying mitosis of an untransformed cell is involved in producing the message which commits a cell to enter the next round of cell division (Fox, Sheppard, and Burger, *Proc. Nat. Acad. Sci.*, **68**, 244, 1971). Because a transformed cell is constantly in the mitotic configuration, it is constantly being induced into a new round of cell division.

If the surface configuration, which is exhibited constantly by transformed cells, is related to the surface change accompanying mitosis of untransformed cells, and the interaction of a nonagglutinating Con A with transformed cells results in lower saturation densities, it follows that the growth of untransformed cells treated with a nonagglutinating Con A should also be inhibited. Figure 19 demonstrates the results of such an experiment. Instead of the enzymatically modified Con A preparation used previously, the present studies were performed using Con A modified by succinylation (Gunther *et al.*, *Proc. Nat. Acad. Sci.*, **70**, 1012, 1973). Our preparations of succinylated Con A (Suc Con A) exhibit essentially the same properties as reported for chymotrypsinized Con A.

The growth of 3T3 cells is terminated prior to the normal saturation density in the presence of Suc Con A. The density at which growth is terminated is dependent upon the concentration of Suc Con A (the higher the concentration of Suc Con A, the lower the final density). The growth termination can be re-

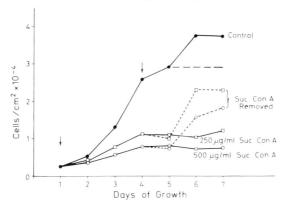

Fig. 19. Suc Con A–induced growth inhibition of 3T3 cells. 3T3 cells were plated into Dulbecco's modified Eagle's medium containing 10% calf serum. On day 1, fresh medium containing 5% serum (O—O), or 5% serum and 250 y/ml Suc Con A (□—□) was added. On day 4, fresh medium and 5% serum with (solid lines) or without (dotted lines) Suc Con A was added. The dashed line indicates the saturation density of cells which would not have received fresh medium on day 4. Each point is the average of 2 plates counted in duplicate.

versed by removing the medium containing the Suc Con A and replacing it with fresh medium. Cells whose growth has been inhibited by Suc Con A accumulate in G_1 in a fashion identical to that of cells in a contact-inhibited monolayer (unpublished observations). An important characteristic of Suc Con A–induced growth termination is that for a given concentration of Suc Con A and a given serum concentration, the cell density at which growth stops is independent of the initial density but highly dependent upon the final density (Table 25).

TABLE 25
Density Dependence of Suc Con A Inhibition of Growth[a]

Initial density cells/cm² × 10⁻⁴		Final density cells/cm² × 10⁻⁴	% of control
	control	2.70	
A	0.13	1.42	52.7
	0.37	1.60	59.3
	control	3.40	
B	0.18	2.27	66.8
	0.35	2.44	71.8
	0.51	2.45	72.1

[a] 3T3 cells were plated into Dulbecco's modified Eagle's medium containing 10% calf serum. One day after plating, the medium was changed to: A—3% calf serum containing 200 μg/ml Suc Con A and replaced every day; B—5% calf serum containing 250 μg/ml Suc Con A and replaced on the fourth day after plating. Final densities were recorded after 7 days of growth. Controls were treated as in A or B minus Suc Con A.

This argues against the effect of Suc Con A being toxic or inhibitory to some metabolic process, e.g., protein synthesis, and suggests the working hypothesis that, in some way, Suc Con A mimics the signal which brings about density-dependent inhibition of growth. Thus, in the case of the termination of growth of 3T3 cells by Suc Con A, two factors are necessary, one is cell–cell interactions and the other is Suc Con A–cell interactions. Another way of saying this is that growth termination is some function of the number of cell–cell contacts and the number of Suc Con A–cell contacts or, growth termination = C[(cell-cell contacts) + (Suc Con A–cell contacts)].

Another prediction, which can be based on the model of Burger *(Fed. Proc., 32, 91, 1973)*, is that Suc Con A should exert its effect at a specific point in the cell cycle, i.e., when the cells are in their mitotic configuration. Figure 20 suggests that this is the case. When 3T3 cells are plated into medium containing 1.5% serum they undergo approximately one round of cell division and accumulate in G_1. If, at this point, the medium is changed to one containing 10% serum, cell growth is stimulated with most cells going through mitosis between 26 and 30 hours after the change to fresh medium. At the concentration

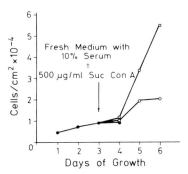

Fig. 20. Interaction of Suc Con A with synchronized 3T3 cells. 3T3 cells were plated into Dulbecco's modified Eagle's medium (DME) containing 1.5% calf serum (●——●). Under these conditions, the cells go through approximately one round of cell division and accumulate in $G_1(G_0)$. On day 3, the medium is changed to 10% calf serum (□—□) or 10% calf serum containing 500 $\mu g/ml$ Suc Con A (○—○). After a lag of approximately 24 hr, the control cells begin growing and grow past their normal saturation density. In the Suc-Con-A–treated cells, growth is terminated after one round of cell division. Each point is the average of 4 plates counted in duplicate.

of Suc Con A (500 $\mu g/ml$) and this cell density (1×10^4 cells/cm²), no cell growth is to be expected if Suc Con A could act at this point in the cell cycle. What is observed, however, is essentially one round of cell division in the presence of Suc Con A before growth is terminated. More recent studies have shown that exposure to Suc Con A for the first 24 hr after the addition of fresh medium and removal just prior to mitosis has no inhibitory effect on cell growth, and addition of Suc Con A to the cells after the first 24 hr with fresh medium i.e., just prior to mitosis, results in the inhibition of cell growth after the completion of mitosis. Thus, exposure to the lectin of 3T3 cells in the mitotic configuration is necessary and sufficient to bring about inhibition of growth once cell division has been completed.

It appears, therefore, that Suc Con A interacts with untransformed 3T3 cells during the time in which the cell surface is in the mitotic configuration, i.e., during mitosis and early G_1, in a manner that mimics the phenomenon that brings about density-dependent inhibition of cell growth.

Accompanying mild protease treatment of normal cells, the transition of interphase into mitotic cells and cellular transformation, is a relatively small (three- to five-fold), but definite, increase in the number of available lectin-binding sites (Noonan and Burger, *J. Biol. Chem.*, **248**, 4286, 1973). These sites appear to exist in a "cryptic" (Rapin and Burger, *Adv. Canc. Res.*, **20**, 1974, in press) form in the membrane, becoming exposed as a result of the change in surface architecture. Thus, these cell surface changes appear to involve a rearrangement of the membrane proteins, exposing some and possibly "burying" others.

To date, there is no evidence implicating the agglutinable surface configuration in the immunologic recognition of neoplastic cells, but such a pronounced difference in the surface architecture can be grounds for speculation. The surfaces of tumorigenic cells expose many antigens not available on the normal cell surface, whose origin and role in host defense against tumor invasion is currently under investigation.

It has been reported that mice immunized against a synthetic antigen containing the presumed receptor site for wheat germ agglutinin could reject five times more transplanted myeloma cells than control, i.e., nonimmunized mice (Shier, *Proc. Nat. Acad. Sci.*, **68,** 2078, 1971).

If the mitotic cell surface change of normal cells is the same surface change accompanying cellular transformation, any theory of immunological defense involving the tumor cell surface for specific recognition must deal with the problem of immunological attack on normal, mitotic cells. In the study by Shier, surprisingly, no deleterious effects on normal cell growth and division were detected.

CHAIRMAN UHR: The changes Mannino described are quantitative and presumably involve the carbohydrate moiety on the cell surface.

MANNINO: We would like to believe that, but we do not have any evidence yet for cell surface involvement.

CHAIRMAN UHR: If one wanted to fit Mannino's findings with those of Keller and of Remington, one could say: Here is further evidence that there are changes in the transformed cell which might allow AM to distinguish it from a nontransformed cell.

COHN: I would like to get a clarification of the experiment showing that the final density is independent of the initial density. Was that experiment done in the presence of an excess of succylinated Con A in the medium so that Mannino is constantly saturating new sites formed, or did he add succylinated Con A, wash it out, and then start the experiment?

MANNINO: Succylinated Con A is present throughout.

COHN: Is not Mannino's finding inevitable then, because he has kept all of the Con A binding sites saturated during the total time of the experiment?

MANNINO: If one wanted to argue that the effect of succylinated Con A is antimetabolic, inhibiting, for example, lipid or protein synthesis not having an effect on cell density, then cells plated at a lower density should be more affected.

MARTIN: In the earlier report by Burger *et al.* on tumor growth control by monovalent Con A, no effect was observed on the growth rate before cell contact. I gather that Mannino is now saying there is such an effect. Does the possibility of cell toxicity, rather than specific nontoxic membrane alteration, need to be considered? Has he, for example, evidence that protein synthesis, membrane transport, and other metabolic phenomena are, in fact, not affected by monovalent Con A?

MANNINO: For one thing this is reversible. We can take off the succylinated Con A and the cells grow fine, but I cannot do that with regular Con A. If one pours it off and puts on new medium, the next day the cells are dead.

The second thing is, if one looks at ^{3}HTdR incorporation, one can find that, as the control cells shut down, the Suc Con A cells shut down also. Upon removal of the Suc Con A, we obtain an increase in ^{3}HTdR incorporation, followed by doubling of the cell number.

CHAIRMAN UHR: Mannino's experiment shows that the affect is reversible, but Martin's question is whether there is any effect on the metabolism of the cell while the Con A is on the cell surface.

MARTIN: Eagle has shown that suboptimal culture conditions could effect the ability of cells to grow beyond contact, without influencing growth up to contact. It seems to me that in Mannino's experiments a mild metabolic depressing effect of Con A could cause the same discriminatory effect, i.e., cells could reach, but not grow beyond, contact.

MANNINO: I think the answer to Martin's query lies in our plating of initial cell densities. It seems to me that if we were dealing only with a toxic effect of Con A, rather than an effect on cell contact phenomena, then the Con A would be more effective against cells at a lower density, but it is not.

MARTIN: In other words, one can have discrimination of a metabolic specificity which will affect cells only at the level they make contact. The point is that some additional metabolic events may be required to grow beyond contact; perhaps that can have an effect on contact rather than on the growth rate.

CHAIRMAN UHR: This is a fascinating subject, but we remain uncertain about the specificity of macrophages, above and beyond there being immunologic factors.

GOOD: I understood from Keller that the nude mouse yielded macrophages that responded to activating agents equivalent to cells from the normal background strain. Why then is Cohn so perturbed about a possible T cell contribution? Doesn't he have confidence in the nude mouse as a T-cell-free source of macrophages?

CHAIRMAN UHR: As I saw that argument, the nude mouse model took care of a possible T cell contribution of mediators such as MIF but left open the involvement of Ig contributed by B cells.

Before we move on to other topics I would like to hear whether there is further information about the mechanism of action of macrophages against tumors: Can macrophages release factors that can carry out the activities of AM i.e., do supernatants of AM have any of the biological effects of the cells?

KELLER: We now have to distinguish between cytostatic and cytocidal macrophage effects. It remains open, however, whether or not these macrophage effects are mediated by the same mechanism. Our earlier observations did not reveal such activities in lysates or supernatants of 4–6 hr cultures of macrophages. However, we have since found that macrophages cultured for a day or two *do* release into the medium a soluble factor which, when appropriately handled, has demonstrable cytostatic capacity. If these preliminary findings are sustained, this would also mean that to obtain cytostatic effects, close contact between effectors and targets need not be essential. However, I would expect that for such a postulated soluble mediator the concentration achieved in the microenvironment of the target cell membrane during close cell-to-cell contact would be much higher than anything we could manage by adding a macrophage supernatant. If this reasoning is valid, the high local concentration obtained on target membrane by intimate effector/target cell contact might result in a cytostatic principle becoming cytocidal.

COHN: I have an experiment to test whether AM are in fact acting via antibody on their surface. One could take bone marrow cells plus colony stimulating factor and get clones of macrophages which are derived in the absence of lymphoid cells. If such a macrophage colony "activated" by LPS or PPD were to kill two cloned tumor cell lines of different origins, but not the corresponding normal cells, then I would be convinced that macrophages are acting via a nonimmunological mechanism and that there is some recognition mechanism common to all neoplastic cells.

LANDY: In principle, Cohn's idea would be a splendid experimental approach, if it were not for technical limitations. It has been sought, without success, to clone mouse macrophages from bone marrow, even with colony stimulating factor. Nor has it been possible to establish normal macrophage cell lines. The only lines thus far reported are those derived from virus-transformed (SV40) macrophages.

NOTKINS: Since immunologically stimulated lymphocytes can produce interferon, it is theoretically possible that some of the tumor-inhibiting effects attributed to cell-mediated immunity might be due to interferon. Interferon could act in several ways. First, there is some evidence that in very high concentrations interferon can directly inhibit the growth of both normal and malignant cells; second, interferon might inhibit the replication of oncogenic viruses; and third, interferon may stimulate or activate sessile or circulating macrophages. Thus, it is important to know what role, if any, interferon plays in the host defense against tumors. I know that Cerottini has performed some experiments along this line, and I wonder if he has any comments.

CEROTTINI: With Lindahl and Gresser, we found that interferon, when injected in large amounts, was able to prevent the proliferation of bone marrow cells and the formation of cytotoxic lymphocytes. These findings indicated that, in contrast to previous claims, interferon does under appropriate conditions inhibit the proliferation of both normal and tumor cells.

ALEXANDER: The interferon situation has been looked at in terms of macrophages that have been activated with endotoxin or with double-stranded RNA. Within eight hours of adding these agents, interferon appears in the medium. However, the levels of interferon attained are quite insufficient to produce any effect on tumor cell division.

CHAIRMAN UHR: Can double-stranded RNA or transfer factor create AM either *in vitro* or *in vivo*? Is there any reason for believing that macrophages are the cells upon which transfer factor has its impact?

ALEXANDER: Double-stranded RNA is possibly the simplest and neatest producer of AM *in vitro*. It is especially convenient because one can be quite sure that, subsequently, the double-stranded RNA is totally removed from the system. In contrast, when one adds endotoxin, it will, of course, stick to the surface of the cells. I know of no work with transfer factor in this context.

MACKANESS: We could exhaust ourselves intellectually on the question of whether there is any recognition involved in the killing of tumor cells by NM or AM. During resorption of the tadpole's tail in the process of metamorphosis, macrophages have been credited with destruction of the vestigial tail. I doubt if this involves a process of recognizing an unwanted self component.

PREHN: How do you know that?

MACKANESS: I do not know with certainty, but resorption stops when it reaches the base of the tail. Secondly, AM do not discriminate between self and non-self when destruction of normal tissues occurs in areas of tuberculous caseation. In tuberculosis, of the kidney, for example, the entire kidney may be destroyed, not through interruption of blood supply, but simply because macrophages become overenthusiastic and damage more than just those tissues that are infected.

The same thing is seen in a tuberculin reaction in guinea pig skin. Normal tissue is violated when specifically sensitized lymphocytes, antigen, and macrophages interact in a skin test site. I cannot see how recognition, other than of the foreign antigen, is involved in this destructive event. I would, therefore, reiterate: When one crowds metabolically active effector cells together with normal cells in tissue culture, the normal cells are likely to suffer, and what we observe in tissue culture may sometimes be an artifact of the conditions of observation.

TERRY: How does Mackaness explain the observations of the apparent destruction of tumor cells and the apparent nondestruction of normal cells by AM?

MACKANESS: In the first place, normal cells can be destroyed by macrophages, especially if conditions do not favor cell survival. So that the issue of cell fragility, raised in the preceding session, becomes important. I do not know what the relative nutritional requirements are for tumor cells and their normal counterparts, but it could well be that tumor cells are more susceptible to damage under adverse environmental conditions.

KELLER: I would like to emphasize once again that our continuing study of various cell lines indicates that there are at least three possible consequences of their interaction with AM.

1. Slowly proliferating cells from normal tissues, irrespective of whether they are of syngeneic or of allogeneic origin, are not attacked by macrophages. At a ratio of ten macrophages per target, neither cytostatic nor cytocidal effects are detectable. It must be conceded, however, that a low degree of cytostasis would not be readily or accurately measured.

2. Rapidly proliferating cells, irrespective of whether syngeneic, allogeneic, or xenogeneic origin or derived from neoplastic or normal tissues, were consistently blocked in their replication in the presence of a small majority of AM.

3. In all tumor cell lines examined by various investigators, the presence of AM leads to a morphologically detectable marked decrease in target cell numbers, indicating that tumor cells are killed. In contrast, the presence of AM was not found to affect the number and morphology of targets derived from normal tissues. Although final conclusions have to wait until results on a variety of other normal and transformed cells are available, the data available now make it probable that macrophages exert both cytostatic and cytocidal effects,

depending on characteristics of the target cells. Whether these effects are in some way related remains to be determined.

   *Experiments performed in our laboratory in recent months have provided additional information highly relevant to the central issue of effects of AM on normal versus transformed cells. In these experiments, the *in vitro* interaction of AM and a variety of syngeneic, allogeneic, or xenogeneic "normal" and "malignant" target cell lines was studied with the parameters of cell proliferation, viability, and morphology.

   Proliferation, the most sensitive and objective parameter assayed, was blocked by AM (in a ratio of 10:1) on all rapidly replicating cell lines examined—ten lines derived from malignant tissues and seven lines derived from normal tissues—irrespective of whether they were of syngeneic, allogeneic, or xenogeneic origin, or showing normal or neoplastic growth characteristics. It was only with very slowly proliferating cells that such an inhibitory effect was not detectable. The data thus relate the macrophage cytostatic effect to the proliferation rate or, more likely, to some cell membrane phenomenon that parallels it. It is noteworthy that marked diminution in target cell proliferation was also achieved with target cells growing in suspension, where close contact between effectors and targets is unlikely; this suggests that a soluble product of AM may participate in macrophage cytostasis. This macrophage effect on cell proliferation is not specific for species, cell type, or tumors, and appears to affect all cell types thus far examined. It is thus differentiated from known inhibitors of cell proliferation such as interferon or the chalones. These potent macrophage effects on cell proliferation are dependent on the ratio of effectors to target cells. Taken as a whole, the findings indicate that macrophages qualify for an important role in host homeostatic regulation of cell proliferation.

   The observation that incorporation of ^{3}HTdR by slowly proliferating human adenocarcinoma cells was more effectively inhibited than that of slowly proliferating syngeneic fibroblasts indicates that, in addition to the criteria already alluded to during the conference, there may well be significant differences in the macrophage reaction against normal and malignant cells, apart from the rate of replication. Despite the lack of the obvious signs of cytotoxicity, of phagocytosis, or of cell debris, morphological observations consistently revealed a striking progressive decrease in the number of tumor cells in the presence of AM. This has also been reported by Hibbs. In every neoplastic cell line examined, there occurred a drastic reduction in the number of targets.

*Editors' note: As is indicated in these proceedings, Keller had experiments in progress at the time of the conference that dealt directly with the central issue of the capacity of AM to discriminate between normal and malignant cells. The editors were further apprised of these ongoing developments during a four month period following the conference. The outcome of this work is that AM have a remarkable and unexpected effect on normal cells; this is relevant to much of the discussion and controversy in Session III. Accordingly, Keller was invited to prepare this brief summary of these experiments. The complete report appears in *Brit. J. Cancer*, in press.

Although the array of lines examined thus far is rather limited (ten tumor and seven normal), the present data seem to attest to tumor targets being selectively killed during *in vitro* interaction with AM. The repeated observations of progressive decrease in the number of tumor cells, without detectable signs of classical kinds of cytotoxicity, phagocytosis, or even cell debris, indicate that the potency of AM in eliminating tumor targets is due to a distinctive, perhaps unique, kind of cytocidal process.

In contrast, parallel studies on cell lines derived from normal tissues showed that the final number of targets was either unaffected or at most diminished by one third in the presence of AM. Some lines, such as syngeneic fibroblasts, were not at all reduced in number, whereas other lines, such as xenogeneic hamster fibroblasts, were significantly diminished.

Finally, the most objective criterion, cloning experiments, showed that neoplastic targets cultured for 72 hr with AM were no longer capable of reestablishing growth, whereas cells derived from normal tissues were consistently able to resume growth.

CHAIRMAN UHR: It seems to me that there is little evidence that recognition by macrophages of differences on the cell surface of neoplastic cells and normal cells is "immune" in character.

Let us now turn to the evidence for involvement of macrophages in tumor-bearing animals. Do such animals have activated macrophages in compartments which are relevant to the problem of tumor immunity? Would Hall comment on this point?

HALL: I wish to present some evidence that cells with the properties of cytotoxic macrophages can be found circulating in the blood of appropriately immunized animals. Much of this work was done by Grant, now in Canberra, who worked with me using the standard Morris model, i.e., a sheep with a cannula in the efferent duct of the popliteal node. The sheep was immunized by a subcutaneous injection of a suspension of murine L 5178Y lymphoma cells which was given into the cannai, just below the hock, so that the efferent lymphatics conveyed the injected lymphoma cells to the regional popliteal node. This is, of course, a somewhat artificial system in that it is a xenogeneic combination and, thus, of restricted biological significance. We are merely using the murine lymphoma cells as a convenient target system, in just the same way as Perlmann uses CRBC. However, the L 5178Y cells grow well in suspension cultures, and the inhibition of their growth can be used as a sensitive test for the cytotoxic activity of lymphocytes or other cells which are added to the cultures.

As with any form of antigenic stimulation we found that after three or four days there was a massive shower of immunoblasts (large lymphocytes) into the lymph, and while these cells were present, the washed lymph cells had a strong

162

cytotoxic activity, judged by growth inhibition (and by ^{51}Cr release), and this was mediated by the complement-dependent lytic antibody which these blasts secreted into the culture system. When the blasts had disappeared from the lymph, and the cell picture had returned to normal, we were somewhat puzzled to find that the small lymphocytes coming from an immunized node had no cytotoxic activity whatsoever, with or without complement, by any method we tried.

We thought that perhaps this was just a reflection of the predominance of antibody-mediated mechanisms in a xenogeneic system. However, we did some further experiments, where we did not cannulate the popliteal node and where the lymphatic pathway between the node and the blood was left intact. When we examined the cytotoxicity of the leukocytes isolated from jugular venous blood, we were surprised to find that there was a strong, non-complement-dependent cytotoxic activity in the blood leukocytes. The question was, of course, what was the nature of these cells; were they lymphocytes or were they something else.

We found very soon that these cytotoxic cells were highly radioresistant *in vitro*, they would resist at least 1000 R, and sometimes 2000 R, and most of them could be removed by incubating the leukocytes in a vessel containing glass beads. This gave us *prima facie* evidence that they could be a macrophage or monocyte type of cell. Of course, there is abundant evidence from the work of Evans that macrophages from the peritoneal cavity of mice can be cytotoxic to tumor cells, but no one had shown that the macrophages or monocytes from peripheral blood can be, as far as I am aware. One cannot easily get macrophages from the peritoneal cavity of sheep. However, one can prepare a very nice monolayer of macrophages by irrigating the milk sinus of an involuted mammary gland of a ewe. We found that such macrophages, collected from an immunized ewe, were indeed highly cytotoxic.

It also gave us the means to raise a specific antimacrophage serum which we then absorbed with normal lymph cells. By using this antimacrophage serum with complement, we showed that it could abolish the cytotoxic activity of the cells in the blood. This was further evidence that we were dealing with a macrophagelike cytotoxic cell in the blood, probably a monocyte, or a promonocyte. So here we have a rather surprising situation. The node that had received the antigenic stimulation was generating cells which were not cytotoxic, and yet these cells in peripheral blood were cytotoxic. Accordingly, we postulated, arguing from the evidence in Evans' system, that the noncytotoxic, efferent lymph cells were conferring cytotoxicity on a subpopulation of the blood leukocytes, probably monocytes.

We were able to demonstrate this by taking these noncytotoxic, efferent lymphocytes and incubating them *in vitro* in the presence of the target lymphoma cells and together with white blood cells from a normal, nonimmune sheep; in this way we produced highly cytotoxic mixtures.

163

In other words, as long as the antigen was present, we could "arm" the mononuclear cells from the nonimmune sheep by incubating them with the noncytotoxic, but sensitized, efferent lymphocytes from an immune sheep. Further, we were able to show that if we took these noncytotoxic lymphocytes from efferent lymph and incubated them in the presence of irradiated lymphoma, a supernatant factor was produced which could activate mononuclear cells from a nonimmune sheep in just the same way that Alexander described activation of the macrophages from the peritoneal exudates of mice. We conclude, therefore, that this is fairly good evidence for the existence of a radioresistant, glass-adherent cell in the blood of these animals that can be armed by contact with specifically sensitized lymphocytes, which have encountered their target antigen. In the immune sheep, there is also present complement-dependent lytic antibody and cell-dependent antibody, but these are separate considerations. For the present, I only want to make the point that when one is considering tumor immunity, one must look for cytotoxic cells either in the milieu of the tumor itself, or in the circulating body fluids, the cells of which have some chance, under physiological conditions, of making contact with the tumor. In the particular system just described, the cytotoxic, circulating monocyte seems to be an important factor. It is necessary, however, to stress that although the lethal event is mediated by the monocyte or macrophage, the recognition and specificity are determined by the lymphocyte. It is the lymphocyte that premeditates the kill, the monocyte or macrophage is the nimble and indiscriminate assassin.

CHAIRMAN UHR: Does the armed macrophage phagocytize its surface antibody and become disarmed?

HALL: We do not know whether or not it is antibody that confers this activity on the monocyte. Obviously, in this system it is very hard to exclude the presence of antibody molecules, but as far as we can see this does not involve the phagocytosis of an antibody molecule. All evidence points toward its being a factor released by the lymphocytes which have contacted the antigen. In the experimental system, this is carried out in medium containing heat-inactivated fetal calf serum which does not contain complement. The killing activity of these adherent cells is not dependent on complement.

CHAIRMAN UHR: *In vivo*, complement is present. It would be expected that surface antibody, in the form of antigen-antibody complexes in the presence of complement, would be rapidly phagocytized, necessitating continual re-arming.

HALL: Yes, I have checked this point, and I think it is because we are dealing with an artificial system, i.e., a xenogeneic tumor; the actual mechanism, by which the sheep gets rid of this irrelevant rubbish we inject, is by means of complement and antibody.

COHN: I was led to believe that in order to function, the macrophage required interaction with an antigen–antibody complex or aggregated antibody. Can deaggregated antibody, mixed with macrophages and then washed, carry out, in an efficient way, a specific function? For example, to get cell killing or phagocytosis, one would have to coat the target cell, and it is this antigen–antibody complex that the macrophage acts upon. This seems *a priori* obvious, since "normal" immunoglobulin must be in 1000 to 10,000 fold excess over the specific antibody being studied in a tumor situation. Consequently, the macrophage Fc receptors for any given antibody would be blocked by unrelated immunoglobulin. This argument applies to all cytophilic antibody systems.

CHAIRMAN UHR: In response to Cohn, I would say that *in vitro*, cytophilic immunoglobulin, without antigen, can also bind to macrophages.

HALL: Whatever it was that was released from our lymphocytes, after they contacted the antigen, was adsorbed onto the macrophage.

COHN: In the absence of the target?

HALL: The lymphocyte only produces this arming material in the presence of antigen and, as far as we can discern, antigen does not participate thereafter.

COHN: I am asking about the arming—are macrophages armed in the absence of added antigen?

HALL: Yes.

CEROTTINI: Could we have more information about the nature of the arming factor described by Alexander? From the published data, it appears that armed macrophages can be treated with trypsin without apparent loss of activity.

ALEXANDER: As our chairman has said, Ig binds to macrophages. If one takes ordinary antibodies, in allogeneic systems, adds them to macrophage monolayers, and washes these monolayers, the macrophages are *not* armed.

CHAIRMAN UHR: I did not make the statement that Alexander attributes to me. I do not believe that the kind of negative evidence presented in any way excludes the concept that the sole antigen-specific factor on macrophages is conventional immunoglobulin but not necessarily any class of immunoglobulin.

165

ALEXANDER: Uhr's point is one which I would accept. The material which is released by T lymphocytes into the tissue culture supernatant, which binds and confers on washed macrophages the property of being armed, is certainly different from normal cytophilic antibody.

Cohn raised the issue of trypsinization. Fischer and Matthe-Lohmann say they can trypsinize armed macrophages and the cells recover cytoxicity. We were puzzled why macrophages armed *in vitro* should retain their armed status for days, when one knows that the rate of turnover of the macrophage membrane is extremely rapid. Therefore, we had to postulate that there was some exocytosis of arming factor which had been internalized. When Matthe-Lohmann found that 2–3 hr after trypsinization the cells had recovered their armed state, that seemed to resolve the problem as to why these cells persisted. If this material was merely adsorbed on the surface, we were at a loss to explain why it stayed on, but if the material was inside and was being regularly exocytosed, that, of course, would provide a more acceptable interpretation.

CEPPELLINI: In the case of K lymphocytes of Perlmann, I understand that antibodies cannot be fixed on the lymphocytes if antigen is not present. In the case of macrophages, in contrast, it is probable that they are armed by immunoglobulin, without antigen being present. Is that correct?

CHAIRMAN UHR: Yes, that is so.

PERNIS: My comment is in response to Alexander. His point, if I got it correctly, was that one can disarm armed macrophages by trypsin treatment, and that they will subsequently recover their specific activity. Now, it is very difficult for me to understand that something which had been endocytosed and presumably went into a lysosome or a phagosome could be put once again on the membrane and retain its specificity and biological activity. In dealing with lymphocytes, when we see something reappearing on the membrane after its disappearance by capping or by trypsin treatment, we take this to be evidence of new synthesis, of the appearance on the membrane of something that is being synthesized by the cell.

Accordingly, I wonder whether once again we are not in a situation similar to the one Cohn suggested. The macrophages are not a pure population; the immunocytes or lymphocytes present could be providing a very minute amount of a specific molecule. This amount may be, in fact, exceedingly small, but the driving force beyond all this is specificity, and in all systems this proves to be immunocytes.

CHAIRMAN UHR: I want to back up Pernis' comments. Even an occasional plasma cell would be sufficient to account for specific sensitization.

ALEXANDER: My comment on Pernis' and Uhr's point is as follows: The trypsin experiment is not ours; however, all our experiments are in agreement with the conclusion Uhr stated, that the factor which conveys specificity comes from the lymphocytes. The actual chemical nature of the molecule involved remains to be resolved.

CONE: In terms of the chemical nature of the factor arming the macrophage, I believe Feldmann's experiments suggest that T-cell surface immunoglobulin molecules can arm a macrophage. Moreover, Feldmann, Marchalonis, Nossal, and I have found that the monomeric IgM-like immunoglobulin isolated from T cells is indeed cytophilic for a nonlymphoid cell population in the peritoneal exudate. Interestingly, in marked contrast, it has been our experience that B cell surface immunoglobulin is not cytophilic.

COHN: The cooperating activity (associative antibody) is what was measured in Feldmann's case. But we are discussing macrophage killing activity.

CONE: That is indeed the case in Feldmann's work. But in my own experience, we have not yet ruled out the possibility of this antibody being involved in cooperating or killing.

CHAIRMAN UHR: In my view, this issue remains controversial, and these experimental results will have to be confirmed and extended before the interpretations that have been made can be accepted.

HOWARD: There is relevant information about the fate of molecules reaching a macrophage surface from studies on the fate of antigens. There are two kinds of findings. First, Unanue and his colleagues' finding was that antigens can be bound to macrophage surfaces and sit there for a long period in an unaltered form (*J. Exp. Med.*, **127**, 915, 1968; *Nature*, **222**, 1193, 1969). The fact that a molecule gets on to a macrophage surface does not necessarily imply immediate endocytosis. The second point is Kölsch and Mitchison's finding (*J. Exp. Med.*, **128**, 1059, 1968), that antigen which is taken in by macrophages is segregated into two compartments, one compartment rapidly degraded and the other compartment apparently preserved. These two pieces of information may be relevant to the fate of any molecule reaching a macrophage surface.

CHAIRMAN UHR: We have already heard from Hall that one can find armed macrophages in the circulation of the tumor-bearing animal. We should next ask: Can we find macrophages at the site of the tumor? Would Alexander summarize his findings in this regard?

167

ALEXANDER: The findings are those of Evans *(Transplantation,* **14,** 468, 1972), who used as criteria for defining a macrophage not morphology but rather physiological properties such as ability to adhere to glass in the presence of trypsin, phagocytosis, and sensitivity to antimacrophage sera. By these and still other criteria, all of which agree rather well, Evans was able to show in a series of different rodent sarcomas and lymphomas that the number of macrophages present in these tumors varied widely. Some tumors had as few as 5% macrophages whereas, in others, more than half the cells present were macrophages. The reason why this was not previously apparent is that morphologists only recognize the macrophages after they have phagocytized foreign material. Evans' experience now exceeds some 18 tumors, where he has seen that the proportion of macrophages in them range from 60% down to 5%. The question arose of how the macrophages get into the tumor, and Evans was able to show, quite clearly, that they were of host derivation.

The next question was why these macrophages go into the tumor. Is it that the blood vessels in the tumor are so altered that they permit the transudation of macrophages to a different extent? Would the blood vessels of the 50% macrophage tumor be different from that of the tumor with only 5% of the cells? Or could it be that these cells come into the tumor as part of an immune response? The latter issue was resolved by Sue Eccles, who took rats and immunosuppressed them without, however, damaging their bone marrow. She used two methods: One was prolonged thoracic duct drainage, the second was whole body irradiation, thymectomy and bone marrow restoration. These two ways of immune suppression leave the bone marrow function reasonably intact. It is interesting that, when she grew the tumors in these immunosuppressed animals, the macrophage content was low. This deals with the proposition that the macrophages might go into the tumor to a different extent because of some alteration in the anatomical structure of the tumor. Rather, they go in as part of the immune response. Indeed, we can think of the tumor as reflecting a delayed hypersensitivity reaction, in which macrophages play a familiar role. The corollary is that the tumors of low macrophage content should perhaps evoke a smaller immune response. That this may be so is indicated by the fact that, by and large, the tumors which have the low macrophage content metastasized spontaneously from their subcutaneous implant readily, whereas those tumors with the high macrophage content remained localized.

CHAIRMAN UHR: The tumor plays a role in determining the extent of macrophage infiltration, given an appropriate immune response?

ALEXANDER: Yes. All evidence points in that direction.

CHAIRMAN UHR: Is there any evidence, on the other side of the coin, that there are differences between strains of mice in the capacity to mount this type of macrophage response? Is there any evidence for genetic differences in the control of these macrophage populations?

ALEXANDER: The data are not yet in. These various tumors are scattered throughout a whole range of strains of mice and rats.

CHAIRMAN UHR: Is there any evidence for physiologic changes in the capacity of a mouse to produce this population? For example, is there involution with aging of the capacity to generate this type of population?

ALEXANDER: I do not know. The point which is important is that monocytes move into an area of an immune reaction, remove the immune reaction, and there is no infiltration into the tumor. It is noteworthy that those animals, which had been immunosuppressed by either of two ways, possessed normal monocyte production. The number of macrophages in the peritoneal cavity was the same as in normal rats, both before and after stimulation.

SMITH: Do you have any idea why the macrophages within the tumor do not kill the tumor cells? You claim the tumor can be over half full of them. Have they been deactivated? Does something secreted by the tumor turn off the activation process? Does this signify that those macrophages are in any way impotent?

ALEXANDER: As somebody said, your glass can be either half full or half empty. Clearly, a tumor that grows has escaped host control. Whether the tumor would have grown even faster had macrophages not been present is a difficult question; indeed, it may be the crux of this entire problem.

CHAIRMAN UHR: The data presented by Hall and Alexander are amply suggestive that macrophages may well be critical components of tumor immunity. Clearly, more data are needed, particularly from *in vivo* experiments.

CHIECO-BIANCHI: In microscopic sections of some human tumors it is possible to note a high percentage of macrophages. This is particularly true for neoplasms characterized by a high rate of cell multiplication and loss, as in the case of Burkitt's lymphoma.

The question that arises is this: Are these macrophages there simply to remove the products of cell death? In experiments with immunosuppressed animals, it may be that the reduced number of macrophages is due to the fact that the tumor can grow easily without immune reaction and consequently less cell destruction occurs.

In this regard, I would like to ask whether individuals bearing tumors with marked macrophage infiltration have been examined for specific activity of blood monocytes against target tumor cells.

LANDY: As implied by the work of Alexander, Evans, and Eccles, in the tumor-bearing host, a critical issue may be the capacity to mobilize effectively macrophages at the tumor site. In this regard, I asked Rebuck some months ago whether his skin window technique had ever been utilized for studying such cell mobilization capability in experimental animals carrying tumors, or in cancer patients. He recalled a publication by Dizon and Southam (*Cancer,* **16,** 1288, 1963), in which it was reported that cancer patients had a significantly impaired ability to mobilize macrophages. Now, it may be that this technique is not at all suitable to the need, and I do not cite this as proof of the macrophage thesis. I only want to emphasize the issue as one being worthy of attention and experimentally feasible.

An adjunct approach, and one perhaps a bit closer to the mark in immunobiologic terms, is the following: During the past few years, several investigators, notably Turk, Pick; Schwartz, Catanzaro, and Leon *(Am. J. Path.,* **63,** 443, 1971), have reported that in experimental animals the local injection of mitogen-induced lymphokines elicits a cellular infiltrate histologically similar to the classical DTH reaction, i.e., a characteristic preponderance of large mononuclear cells. Assuming that these cells are the effectors of tumor regression, it would be interesting and informative to ascertain whether in tumor-bearing animals and in cancer patients authentic lymphokine preparations would elicit such a local infiltrate and whether the kinetics and temporal aspects of the response are defective or abnormal.

E. KLEIN: We have made several attempts to find macrophages in the blood of Burkitt patients which would react with the tumor cells or with derived cell lines; as yet we have no evidence for such cells being present. As regards the "starry sky" appearance, it is not necessarily a sign of an immune response. When we transplanted a Burkitt-derived cell line into neonatal rats, widely disseminated growth occurred in one animal. The histology of the resultant tumor was characteristic of the human tumor, with the presence of macrophages. There was no other sign of immune response in this animal. Therefore, these macrophages can either be considered as the single sign of an immune attack by the host, or regarded merely as scavenger cells.

LANDY: Part of our problem in assessing the basic biologic role of macrophages in host resistance to tumors is that, given a functioning bone marrow, there appears to be no way, selectively, to deplete the host of macrophages. This is a crucial issue, as depletion or ablation experiments would offer the least ambiguous means for assessing the macrophage contribution to tumor resistance. I had thought, some time ago, of still another way of exploring this point, i.e., by implanting in rodents a depot of a gram or so Trydimite (hydrofluoric acid-etched quartz) which is selectively cytotoxic for macrophages; moreover, these quartz particulates cannot be eliminated by the host. However, in discussing this approach with Pernis, who has had much experience with the effects of silica, he was of the opinion that the prospects of achieving macrophage depletion were minimal, as the host has an inordinately high capacity to regenerate these cells. This maneuver might, nonetheless, be worth exploring.

ALEXANDER: In actual fact, the host bearing tumors with a high macrophage content *is* depleted in monocytes.

CHAIRMAN UHR: The major insights, which have emerged thus far from this aspect of our session, are as follows:

It was established that activated macrophages can limit the proliferative capacity of tumor cells *in vitro*. The reaction seems to require intimate contact between macrophage and tumor cell. There is no hard evidence that macromolecules released by macrophages play a role in this effect, but this possibility has not been entirely excluded. It is also clear that macrophages can be "armed" by antigen-specific factors released from antigen-stimulated lymphocytes. In tumor situations, the type of lymphocyte involved and the factor released have not been definitively characterized. Such armed macrophages are also activated when specific antigen is introduced. Once they are activated, however, they no longer display immunologic specificity in their effect on target cells. Rather, they are inhibitory to many kinds of tumor cells. Activated macrophages appear to be able to affect transformed cells *in vitro*, under conditions in which normal replicating cells are unaffected. It is not clear, however, whether this is due to the recognition of differences between the surfaces of transformed and normal cells. Rather, the difference may reside in different functional and/or structural properties of transformed cells which render them more susceptible to the untoward effects of activated macrophages. In fact, it was noted that there are circumstances in ontogeny (resorption of tadpole tail) and in pathological situations (tuberculin lesion with necrosis) where macrophages appear to play a major role in the destruction of normal cells.

There is *in vivo* evidence consistent with the possibility, but not yet proven, that macrophages play a role in tumor immunity. Two major problems in investigations regarding macrophages and their function in tumor immunity have been brought out. First, there are no current experimental means for abolishing the function of macrophages *in vivo* for a significant time span and, yet, retaining normal lymphocytic function. Second, in the so-called highly purified populations of macrophages, there may still be a minute lymphocyte component which could be sufficient to sensitize the macrophages.

Let us now shift the subject of attention to the host or cellular factors which affect or control metastatic spread of tumor *in vivo*. The problem of metastasis in general, particularly the problem of dormant metastases, is of critical importance in clinical cancer. An example of this problem might be a patient we have observed who had a melanoma removed ten years earlier; after a short course of corticosteroid therapy for unrelated reasons, he suddenly developed a solitary brain metastasis. One can speculate that, at the time the primary lesion was growing rapidly, malignant cells invaded adjacent blood vessels, and dissemination of large numbers of melanoma cells occurred via the systemic circulation. Most of these cells were probably killed in the circulation or in the tissues after seeding. Foci in some tissues must have persisted for a decade, however. Either the seeded cells were in G_0 or they were dividing and being killed at the same rate during this interval. The latter possibility is not fanciful, because dermatologists occasionally observe malignant melanomas in which the lesion had not recently grown. Histologically, such lesions show numerous mitoses and considerable infiltration of surrounding lymphoid cells. Presumably, rapid rates of replication are balanced by rapid killing. In the example under discussion, corticosteroids may have upset the balance in these small foci between growth and host defense mechanisms.

The point to be made from this anecdote is that such dormant lesions may represent examples of the temporary success of host mechanisms and an opportunity, par excellence, to influence favorably the outcome. It should also be stressed that the "ground rules" of host defense against such foci could be quite different from those concerned with growing, primary solid tumors: Namely, the host is immunologically experienced with the tumor, i.e., the immune response is anamnestic. The foci may be quite small, perhaps even single cells. A primary tumor would have to grow to a considerable size, perhaps the cell number would be measured in thousands or millions, in order to have similar immunologic impact on the host. The tumor cells are in a different environment from that in which they arose. Sufficient time has elapsed for mutation and selection of tumor cell variants. The critical components of immunity could differ in this situation from those operative in a large primary tumor. Nonimmunologic mechanisms might play a very critical role in this highly dynamic equilibrium. These are among many fundamental questions to be asked concerning the biology of these dormant metastases.

VAAGE: Immunologic factors are among many that predispose to and influence metastatic dissemination and tumor growth.* The first experiment indicating this to us was a rather simple one. C3H mice with syngeneic MCA-induced

*Editors' note: The related subject of concomitant immunity is discussed, in another context, in Session IV.

172

sarcomas or spontaneous mammary carcinomas were divided into three groups: irradiated, normal and presensitized. Tumor cell suspensions were injected via subcutaneous, intraperitoneal, and intravascular routes. Injected *in vivo*, growth is almost exclusively in the lungs; injected into the left ventricle, growth is distributed everywhere. At autopsy, tumor growth patterns in the normal presensitized host differed significantly from one site to another. For example, the liver is apparently immunoresistant to tumor growth, since reduction from normal to sensitized host is very great. Lung distribution was also effectively reduced in sensitized mice. In general, the visceral organs from immune animals with the exception of the kidney resisted tumor growth. Such resistance was not apparent in subcutaneous sites, intramuscular sites, in the myocardium, mediastinum, and in other areas. These observations indicate that in considering the immunology of metastases, we must realize that there are pecularities that distinguish it from classical transplantation immunology. We cannot approach cancer clinically by simply extrapolating from classical cutaneous and subcutaneous transplantation studies.

Second, the protective effects of antibodies against solid tumors also differ according to the route of injection. When tumor cell suspensions are inoculated subcutaneously, it is difficult or impossible to demonstrate the protective effects of antibodies. However, if a primary immune response is first precluded by sublethal radiation, and the animal is then challenged intravascularly, together with antiserum given in large amounts over a period of five or six days, bracketing the time of challenge, antiserum alone protects against establishment of the injected tumor cells. This may have some practical significance in terms of the biology of metastatic dissemination, which is the most serious aspect of neoplastic disease. The protective role of immune serum factors may have been underestimated, and it may develop that the relative importance of cellular immune factors has been overemphasized.

A third point follows from the observation that the concomitant immune response to a tumor implant increases as the tumor grows, but, as the tumor mass becomes large, a kind of immune depression seems to take hold and resistance declines progressively as the animal becomes moribund. If the tumor is resected in the stage of immune depression, resistance recovers rapidly within 24 hr. If, however, one attempts "immunotherapy" by injecting killed tumor cells, the depressed state of specific resistance is sustained, judged by growth of challenge tumor.

This may have relevance to both past and current attempts at clinical use of specific immunotherapy. Tumor cell injection procedures started at the time of biopsy or surgical removal may have the unwanted effect of causing continued depression rather than the intended immunostimulation. After a period has elapsed, as short as seven days after surgical removal, injected tumor tissue no longer causes continued depression of resistance. In fact, after a longer interval injected killed tumor tissue actually boosts the declining specific immune response.

How do these experiments relate to metastases? The reactivation of dormant foci of tumor cells may be caused by a shift in a balance of host resistance and tumor growth potential, which could be reached at a certain point of a declining antitumor immune status. If by storing tumor material one could give booster vaccinations at appropriate intervals, one might maintain immune resistance, and, hypothetically at least, might prevent the reappearance of dormant cells.

STJERNSWÄRD: Only in the time interval before a manifest tumor is established and in the time interval before metastases occur, can immunity have a realistic tumor limiting effect. Immunologic reactivity toward an established tumor may rather represent an epiphenomenon.

Before a tumor is clinically recognizable, it is 0.5 to 1.0 cm^3, which represents about 10^9 cells. The time interval for a primary tumor usually takes 150–300 days, but necrosis, tumor cell shedding, tumor stroma considered, it probably takes a much longer time. Analysis of clinical doubling times for tumor volume indicates that, from a single cell to 10^9 cells with a doubling time of 23 days, it takes 2 years; with a doubling time of 3 months, 8 years are required before a clinically detectable tumor appears.

We may overemphasize, by wishful thinking, the effect of immune responses which fail to eliminate tumor cells during this long time interval. We center our analysis on the tumor-bearing state and the time immediately after tumor removal, ignoring the often long interval before manifest metastases. The interval between tumor removal and manifest metastases is a realistic situation where we can adapt all the knowledge we have and seek the task of eliminating tumor (metastases) through manipulation of immunity.

In the most common tumor in women, breast carcinoma, about 50% of women considered to have a localized, operable tumor are dead in five years of distant metastases. We thus have a crucial interval in which tumor cells are present, during which time the immune response has not eliminated a relatively few tumor cells, at least an amount not clinically detectable. Are tumor cells dormant, multiplying slowly or circulating around? In leukemia and Burkitt's tumor we know seeding from immunologically and chemotherapeutically privileged sites occurs.

Important mechanisms may be indicated by rare occurences. For example, X-ray therapy occasionally appears to facilitate local spread of tumor growth within irradiated skin, even in irradiated skin areas far removed from the primary and many years after removal. May I describe briefly one of 9 similar patients, seen in a large oncological clinic during a 5 year period. Radical mastectomy for a moderately differentiated ductal cancer was followed by postoperative irradiation, ^{60}Co irradiation in the amount of 4400 R over a period of 30 days. Six months later multiple tumor nodules appeared in the irradiated field, including an area in the opposite healthy breast, which also had received some irradiation. The nodules coalesced to a homogeneous growth of tumor covering but limited to the irradiated skin area, both on the side of the primary and the skin of the contralateral breast. Constant occurrence of circulating tumor cells in such patients is suggested by observation that such recurrence is known in irradiated areas far from the primary. Sixteen years after removal of a primary, localized, poorly differentiated mammary carcinoma, tumor appeared in a suprapubic skin area, far away from the primary. The extent of tumor in this skin corresponded to the area that had been irradiated 2 years previously for stage 2A cancer of the cervix.

Trauma to tissues has been also correlated with unusual distribution of metastases from various tumors. This includes metastases in distant surgical scars, occurrence of metastases in distant skin grafts, and unusual distribution of metastases from a larynx carcinoma to skin exposed to plaster of paris. Nidation of tumor cells may thus be facilitated in traumatized tissue.

Another mechanism or additive factor facilitating the outgrowth of tumor cells may be that host ability to destroy tumor cells in such tissues is decreased. Diminished ability to mount a delayed hypersensitivity reaction was found in irradiated skin. This may, however, only represent a secondary phenomenon reflecting decreased vascular supply and skin fibrosis.

The patients described indicate one among many factors that determines ultimate localization of metastatic tumor cells. They also suggest that tumor cells are around for many years in small amounts, indicating the failure or limited effect of postulated host-tumor-limiting immunity. Where are the tumor cells? Are they constantly in circulation and not being eliminated or are they locally dormant or slowly replicating?

CHAIRMAN UHR: There are numerous side effects of X-irradiation; for example, damage to blood vessels can decrease blood supply. Does X-irradiation affect the number of tissue macrophages in the irradiated areas?

STJERNSWÄRD: The answer to the first question is yes. As to the second question, we know that irradiation can result in fibrotic changes in irradiated skin. Metastases from melanoma may be found only in the scarified tissue where the skin graft was taken in order to cover the excision area of primary melanoma removal. There must be many nonimmunological factors that are of relevance for metastases, besides immune mechanisms.

STUTMAN: The story of steroids and metastases also presents an important point. Tumors of animals that are normally nonmetastasizing produce showers

175

of lung metastases after steroid treatment. Such results are very difficult to reproduce with other immunosuppressive procedures. Perhaps steroids are producing permeability changes, etc.

Our experience with either life-long immunosuppression with ALS (*J. Nat. Cancer Inst. Monograph* **35,** 107, 1972), or tumor induction in nude mice (*Science,* **183,** 534, 1974), is that such animals develop tumors, but these tumors rarely metastasize. The experience with xenogeneic tumor transplantation from humans to nude mice, also show that the tumors may grow to enormous size locally but rarely metastasize.

ALEXANDER: Do they elicit antibodies in nude mice?

E. KLEIN: Yes, they do.

CHAIRMAN UHR: Do the tumor cells enter the circulation?

STUTMAN: I do not know. However I conclude that the metastasis problem is much more than a simple immunological one.

E. KLEIN: I suppose Stjernswärd does not want to ascribe this regional effect to local immunocrippling. When we started to work with Burkitt's lymphoma, I was told that after regression tumors reappeared, they would very seldom develop at the same site. It is possible that local immunity develops and when relapse occurs, the first site remains tumor free.

CHAIRMAN UHR: There certainly are many examples of local immune responses. These can occur in sites of previous immunologically induced inflammation.

STJERNSWÄRD: A more likely explanation than local immunity for the observation that Burkitt's lymphoma does not often recur at the primary site is the much greater chance of cells nidating somewhere else.

KLEIN: Burkitt's lymphoma is a very interesting model of dormancy. We believe that it is due to the slipping through of a single clone across the otherwise efficient barrier of immune surveillance.

There is a peculiar predilection of lymphoma sites as far as the primary lesion is concerned, depending on the age of the patient. Between ages 4 and 6, most tumors locate in the jaw. Between 10 and 12, testicular and ovarian tumors appear, and in teenagers there are often long bone tumors. Perhaps high proliferative activity in a given area facilitates outgrowth of neoplastic clones. The mechanism of this can be only subject to speculation; for example, local immunosuppression and local growth proliferating stimuli acting in a promotion capacity. One of the two documented cases of spontaneous regression occurred in a 22-year-old woman who developed huge tumors in both her breasts during lactation. These turned out to be typical Burkitt's lymphoma on biopsy. She refused therapy, and both tumors regressed. It suggests that local tissue proliferation played a role in promoting the outgrowth of essentially dormant clones.

MARTIN: Relevant to the chairman's comments are experiments by Ketcham and his colleagues at the National Cancer Institute. They confirmed the observation that excision of subcutaneously growing MCA tumors can lead to resistance to a second subcutaneous implant of the same tumor. If the so-called immune mice were challenged with an intravenous inoculum of tumor, an increased growth ratio of lung metastases was observed. These experiments indicate an important distinction between tumor growth control in subcutaneous tissues from that in parenchymous organs.

VAAGE: To counter this train of evidence it is appropriate to give some data supporting immunological involvement in control of metastatic spread. The experiments involve mice sensitized to an intermediate level of immunity with an immunogenic tumor, then challenged intravenously to get growth in the lungs and also challenged interperitoneally. Shortly after challenge, the animals are divided into three groups, then irradiated. In one group the thoracic area but not the abdominal area is radiated. In the second the abdominal but not the thoracic area is radiated, and the third is a nonirradiated control. Tumor growth in the lungs was least in the first group, greatest in group two and intermediate in group three. Growth in the peritoneal cavity was greatest in group one, lowest in group two and intermediate in group three. In other words, while radiation of an area implanted with tumor cells has a therapeutic effect, radiation of an extensive area like the thorax or the abdomen will damage systemic immune resistance and influence the ability of an animal to resist tumor growth in other, unradiated parts of the body.

CHAIRMAN UHR: Perhaps the increased availability of nucleotides increases tumor growth, analogous to the effect of X-irradiation in enhancing antibody formation.

HOWARD: The local effects that have been described, in which tumor unexpectedly reappears in the irradiated field, is most interesting. A possible explanation is that irradiation is acting in this context as an immunosuppressive, and the tumor reappears in the irradiation field because some local antitumor immunity has been suppressed, and the tumor breaks through. If this is right, the implications are twofold; first, that the tumor was already in the irradiation site, and second, that some kind of immune mechanism preexisted in that site. If it is a specific immune mechanism, then a lymphocyte or macrophage is involved, and if it is radiosensitive, it is probably a lymphocyte. If that is the case, it implies something about the ecology of a lymphocyte subpopulation for which we do not have any information at present, i.e., whether specific lymphocyte localization in the skin may be permanent or persistent. Do we know anything about the way in which potentially immune lymphocytes enter normal skin?

CHAIRMAN UHR: A half century ago, Von Pirquet (*J. Pharmacol. Exptl. Therap.*, **1**, 151, 1909) described the retest reaction. Tuberculin injected into a previous site of a tuberculin reaction elicits an inflammatory reaction that appears within several hours and is accompanied by an enormous infiltration of eosinophiles. Later, lymphoid cells infiltrate. The retest reaction is immunologically specific. Apparently, lymphocytes with specificity to tuberculin remaining from the previous reaction have made this piece of skin different from a virgin area of skin with regard to tuberculin reactivity.

HOWARD: Do we know that release is due to lymphocytes; could it be due to a tissue-fixed antibody?

CHAIRMAN UHR: The lesion has components both of cellular immunity and antibody. The simplest explanation is that both T and B cells are involved in the production of the lesion.

TERRY: For several years, Prehn has been tweaking us with the idea that small increments of immune responsiveness may actually facilitate tumor growth. In the present circumstances, there is tissue damage, and it is reasonable to assume that a low-level immune response occurs in these sites. If the Prehn hypothesis is correct, this immune response might be facilitating tumor growth.

STJERNSWÄRD: What can be done to attack or analyze the problem of metastasis. The immune status at time of the primary tumor, which we have been discussing intermittently, is in my opinion of less interest and practical importance than the interval from discovery or removal to manifest metastasis. There must be constructive ideas for attacking this problem. Selection of tumor cells with propensity for metastasis may occur but we have no data on changes of tumor-associated antigens or of HL-A on metastatic cells as compared to primary tumor cells.

KLEIN: The analysis of metastasis is certainly possible, and, to some extent, it has been carried out experimentally. It is a very complex phenomenon;

some of the elements are certainly not immunological. There are questions of adhesiveness, of penetration into the vascular space, and of localization by tumor cell arrest in the vascular system. Some years ago, Coman showed that the very specific localization of a metastasizing rabbit tumor was entirely explainable in terms of tumor cell arrest in the capillaries, because stained dead cells ended up in the same organ as the living cells that later grow into metastases.

Following vascular arrest, there is the problem of invasion into the tissue and the question of dormancy. Dormancy can have an immunological and a nonimmunological basis. There are beautiful examples of nonimmunological dormancy, e.g., the classical experiment of Gardner—an estrogen-dependent testicular tumor. When grafted into nonestrogenized males, the tumor can lie latent one or two years, but starts promptly growing, at the site of inoculation, when the host is estrogenized. Regarding immunologic mechanisms of dormancy, one should ask the question whether there is local cytostatic immunity to dormant tumor cells, rather than cytocidal, and examine the defect in mechanisms there that mediate cytotoxicity.

STJERNSWÄRD: If dormant tumor cells are multiplying very slowly during a long time interval, why are they not eliminated? Are they in an immunologically privileged site? Are they not antigenic, or are they not expressing their antigen during this phase?

KLEIN: There is suggestive evidence that EBV-carrying clones remain at a constant relative level in normal individuals through their life span. This is suggested, among other things, by their highly constant EBV antibody titers, from year to year. In contrast, EBV titers increase strongly on immunosuppression. Recently, Aiuti and colleagues have reported the converse situation; high EBV titers in congenitally immunodeficient (T cell deficient) children, which decreased to normal levels when thymus grafts were given and a normal T cell picture was reestablished.

PREHN: Experiments done several years ago by Billingham and his colleagues with allogeneic melanophores and their transplantation in guinea pig skin seem pertinent. They found that if transplantations were done very carefully into the superficial layers of the skin, foreign melanophores would survive indefinitely. Furthermore, animals could be immunized; this reduced the melanophore population but did not necessarily get rid of it—it persisted for years this way.

It is quite apparent that there are sites, and the superficial layers of the skin represent one such site, where the immune mechanism is deficient. These are the so-called privileged sites, and there are many others. The mouse breast, for instance, is another such site. There is very good evidence that tumors in their early stages do not immunize in this site; that the afferent limb of the immune response is defective. They can, however, be destroyed by effective immunization. Thus, the efferent limb is intact. Tumor cells may thus be secreted in such privileged sites and persist for years, kept in homeostatic balance by nonimmunologic mechanisms.

MARTIN: I refer to spontaneous mouse lung tumors described earlier. In partially resistant strains of mice, such as C3H, one finds benign lung tumors in about 30% of one year old mice. These small tumors seemingly do not express the antigen expressed on the malignant lung tumor cells. Can dormancy of tumors represent a few nonantigenic or benign cells which coexist with a few malignant cells? The reason that the cells stay dormant is because they are benign.

CHAIRMAN UHR: Would you not expect the metastasizing cells to be the ones that had been rapidly growing and which had invaded the blood vessels?

MARTIN: Tumors may contain cells with different degrees of malignancy, growth rate, and antigen expression. Tumor dormancy may reflect a predominance of benign tumor cells. Any malignant cells developing may derepress additional tumor antigens and be eliminated immunologically. The tumor would not be completely destroyed, however, because of the reservoir of benign cells.

PREHN: What is Martin's evidence that these benign tumors are nonantigenic or nonimmunologic?

MARTIN: The high incidence of benign lung tumors in C3Hf mice in the face of the resistance, by these mice, to challenge with a malignant lung tumor suggests that there may be antigenic differences between benign and malignant cells.

PREHN: If these benign tumors are nonantigenic, this is really very interesting. In several other systems that we have looked at, the earliest benign tumors that we can get hold of share the antigens with the malignant tumors that eventually come from them—for instance, in the mammary tumor system in the mouse, where one has hyperplastic nodules, and in the skin with papillomas that can be induced with chemical agents. So, if you indeed have a system in which the benign tumor expresses less antigenicity or less immunogenicity, or what have you, than the ultimate malignant tumor, this is highly interesting and perhaps an exception to a more general rule.

DELLA PORTA: What is Martin's definition of a benign tumor?

MARTIN: The criteria we use are size (<2 mm), scanty mitosis, no evidence of compression of surrounding lung tissue or of infiltration. More important, however, is the long term behavior of these tumors. They change little in size or incidence in adult C3Hf mice over an observation period as long as 1–2 years.

VAAGE: To add to Prehn's comment on dormancy, we should consider the concept of tumor establishment vis-a-vis immunosensitivity. After tumor cell injection, there is a period of about four days when the implant is immunosensitive; at that point, a clear change occurs into a state of immunoresistance. This can be observed experimentally in two ways. First, if one follows resection of a large tumor, which depresses immune resistance by continued injections of killed tumor tissue, the depressed state is sustained. If sustained for four or five days after challenge, accelerated tumor growth occurs. If tumor tissue injections are stopped about the third day after challenge, the recovery is quick and most tumors are rejected. Thus, about the fourth day immunosensitivity changes.

This can be demonstrated in another way. If an existing immunoresistant state is depressed by irradiating the whole body or a significant portion of the body of the mouse, immunoresistance is at least partially restored by passive transfer of antiserum. If antiserum is given shortly after the challenge, the number of tumor cells that grow in the lungs is decreased. After the fourth or fifth day no protective effect occurs. The fourth day after challenge coincides with the usual time of vascularization of most grafts. Consequently, the establishment of the tumors may be associated with a loss of immunosensitivity. Such establishment may in turn have something to do with dormancy and a change in the dormant state.

WEISS: The microenvironment around a latent or small tumor focus may be special in two ways. On histological grounds, Witz of Tel Aviv and Black of New York suggest that tumor cells may be able to produce factors which seem to be specifically toxic to lymphoid and macrophagic cells. Certain tumor cells elaborate enzymes which rapidly digest immunoglobulin (Keisari and Witz, *Immunochemistry*, in press; Black, in *Immunological Parameters of Host-Tumor Relationships*; D. W. Weiss, ed., p. 80, Acad. Press, N.Y. 1973). Perhaps then, in the immediate vicinity of a small tumor island, such a "toxic microenvironment" prevents final attack and total disruption of the focus of neoplastic cells; any cells from the tumor island that break away from this immediate environment would then be destroyed.

The second possibility, for which we have some evidence in our laboratory, is that, in the immediate vicinity of certain tumor foci, there may be gradients of either shed or secreted antigenic factors through which any immune element would have to traverse and could become inactivated (i.e., neutralized) in the process. By such mechanisms small tumor foci may be capable of maintaining themselves for years in a seemingly static equilibrium with the host, until something changes in the interaction between host and isolated focus and facilitates either breakthrough by the cancer cells or a final solution by the organism.

BALDWIN: With respect to the issue of dormancy, there are many good examples in the literature on chemical carcinogenesis, and Prehn has already brought out the problem of skin tumors. Many years ago, we did some studies where we treated mouse skin with subthreshold doses of skin carcinogens. No tumors occurred in the treated mice until they received a promoting agent such as croton oil. The latter treatment could be delayed for as long as 12 months, but even then multiple skin papillomas arose within 2–3 weeks. Since croton oil is not a potent immunosuppressant, we have here a model with transformed cells after exposure to a carcinogen, which presumably lie dormant and then following some trigger mechanism (in Stjernswärd's case this would be irradiation) rapidly evolve into preneoplastic lesions.

WEISS: Slemmer, working in Prehn's laboratory, showed in a mouse mammary tumor system that transformed cells, which some call preneoplastic, may be dependent on intimate association with wholly normal cells for their maintenance (Slemmer, *J. Nat. Cancer Inst. Monograph*, **34**, 57, 1972). The suggestion was made by Slemmer, at one time, that there may be a mechanical protection of these isolated, low-grade neoplastic cells, as they are completely surrounded by the normal ones on which they are dependent for their continued survival and maintenance and are, thus, removed spatially from immune attack.

Does Prehn think that there may in fact often be such physical or mechanical protective barriers for the persistence of preneoplastic or premalignant clones, which could break out and initiate progressive cancer only when a host containment mechanism fails or a change occurs to higher malignant potential and invasiveness in one of the sequestered clones?

PREHN: The experimental evidence that Weiss cites from Slemmer's work is that hyperplastic-nodule-transformed tissue, in most instances, is dependent upon the presence of a normal component for its survival. That is correct. But the inference that this is in any way due to a shielding from the immune response is, I think, incorrect, primarily because Slemmer has been able to show elegantly in his own work that the immune response is really not active at all in these very early lesions in the breast.

WEISS: My suggestion was not that premalignant cells need, in the first place, normal tissue association in order to be protected against immune attack but that, once such an association was established, it would form a shielding against later immune attack—which is quite different.

PREHN: Slemmer himself has suggested the hypothesis Weiss raised, but it may be wrong in this case because the same tissues taken outside the breast and still presumably shielded in the same way now immunize perfectly well. So I think that, in this particular system, it may be the site rather than the tissue that is at fault.

GOOD: Regarding the croton oil experiments, the active ingredient of croton oil, phorbol myristate acetate, has been investigated by Estenson at the University of Minnesota. He found that this substance is an active mitogen in certain lymphoid cell systems. It increases the amount of cyclic GMP in stimulated cells by a factor of 20- to 40-fold, within a matter of a few minutes, in the cell systems where it acts as a mitogen. In addition, and apparently based on a similar mechanism, it causes liberation of specific granules from leukocytes. Thus, the possibility is that phorbol myristate acetate could contribute to the balance as cocarcinogen by driving proliferation, altering circulation, or nonspecifically changing cell surfaces.

CHAIRMAN UHR: Are the granules from macrophages?

GOOD: The granules are from neutrophils, but possibly other cells may be involved as well.

CHAIRMAN UHR: How about the possibility that the histamine released turns off cytotoxic lymphocytes à la Kenny, Plaut, Klaus, and Lichtenstein?

GOOD: That is a possibility.

PREHN: The immune response is probably not involved in any way in the skin carcinogenicity system for the following reason. In experiments done in my laboratory several years ago by Lappe and by Andrews, the promoting agent used was not a chemical but rather simple skin transplantation, which produced a stimulus to hyperplasia in the skin and evoked the papillomas that were latent in that carcinogen-treated skin.

One can do this sort of experiment in immunologically suppressed animals, and the sequence of events is identical. The papillomas come up, and then they regress in the usual fashion without any immune response. Curiously, they will sometimes go through waves of regression, also in the immunologically suppressed animal. So, we are really straining hard if we wish to invoke an immunologic explanation for the latency of papilloma formation in two-stage oncogenesis. Immunologic suppression was by irradiation and thymectomy and, in fact, the papillomas were induced on skin allografts to make sure the hosts were immunologically suppressed. The whole experiment was done on the skin allografts.

CHAIRMAN UHR: In this discussion it has become clear that dormant metastasis is an experimentally approachable problem. I am convinced that there is significant information to be obtained from what probably are very small foci in an immune animal, in contrast to relatively large solid tumors.

STUTMAN: There are few good animal models of spontaneous metastases. The majority of the mouse tumors we work with grow as localized tumors for a long time and can be easily cured surgically. Also the majority of the published metastasis work consists of injecting intravenously suspensions of nonmetastasizing tumor cells. That approach can be extremely misleading if other factors, such as membrane changes or other surface determinants, are involved.

BALDWIN: We are injecting tumor cells intravenously as part of an immunotherapy program specifically aimed at treating metastases. There are some good model tumors that metastasize spontaneously. In the rat, we study a spontaneously arising squamous cell carcinoma which, on implantation, always kills the host with pulmonary metastases. If one eliminates pulmonary metastases the animals will then die of massive visceral or skin metastases.

WEISS: With Treves at the Weizmann Institute, using a spontaneous C57BL pulmonary carcinoma which metastasizes spontaneously, if one stimulates by (seemingly) nonspecific means the base line of cellular immunological capacity of such animals, the incidence of metastases and the number of metastases found is consistently reduced.

CHAIRMAN UHR: Are circulating tumor cells a routine aspect of the growth of primary tumors, human or experimental? The example we heard suggests that immune surveillance does not eliminate tumor cells from the circulation. It clearly is not an immunologically privileged rate. Is this an unusual situation or a routine one?

SMITH: There are a variety of data concerning this point in the literature; in aggregate they establish that circulating tumor cells are the rule, rather than the exception (reviewed in *New Eng. J. Med.*, **287**, 439, 1972).

184

CHAIRMAN UHR: Is there evidence that bears on the question whether tumor cells in the blood are under attack by any mechanisms? Can they grow out *in vivo* after transplantation?

ALEXANDER: In reply to Uhr's second question, yes, one can, at times, transplant animal tumors by injecting blood from tumor-bearing animals.

CHAIRMAN UHR: It seems to me that our discussion of the problem of metastatic cancer and dormant metastases, in particular, has brought out the following points: There may be possible differences in the host–tumor relationship between dormant metastatic foci and solid primary tumors of larger size. Tumor cells from primary lesions probably enter the circulation very frequently and, in some instances, circulate chronically. We know little about the biology of these events. It is of fundamental importance to establish the relationship of the dormant metastases to the primary tumor, with regard to such factors as the immunogenicity and density of tumor antigens, cell division, etc. We need to know what is happening at the interface between these foci and neighboring cells in the particular organ of their residence. The opportunities for modulating the immune response and increasing host resistance at this interface might be exploited with decisive effects on the clinical outcome. It is also possible that nonimmunological factors play a critical role in this host response.

The problem appears approachable, at least in terms of the immunological aspects. There are already several spontaneous and experimental tumors which appear to be likely candidates for suitable experimental models. The cell sorter of Herzenberg might be useful in a study of disseminated tumor cells.

GOOD: The point was made by Landy that there are no models in which we can study an animal who lacks macrophages but possesses normal lymphocytes. Twomey studied clinical situations where, after prolonged cytotoxic therapy, a dearth of macrophages existed while granulocytes and lymphocytes seem to be present in normal numbers and to have normal function. It seems it would be possible to create such models if we would only work at the problem.

LANDY: Good is referring to studies on a "drug-induced" macrophage deficit, but I was alluding to "inborn errors" involving this cell type.

GOOD: Rodey, in my laboratory, did such studies and showed that the same kinds of abnormalities were present for these cells that had been established with respect to granulocyte function. Thus, phagocytosis and killing of catalase-positive bacteria in monocytes of patients with fatal granulomatous disease are as defective as the granulocyte function. The abnormalities of phagocytic func-

185

tion, which have been demonstrated, for example, in the Chediak-Higashi anomaly, also extend to macrophages.

LANDY: In reply to Good, I would say that the work he cites on defects in macrophage function deals primarily with phagocytic activity. However, I thought that discussion earlier in this session had made it clear that macrophage destruction of tumor targets is quite independent of phagocytic mechanisms, so, the work he alludes to may be wide of the mark. The crux of the matter is that our present criteria are too few and far too primitive to disclose more subtle but, nonetheless, important alterations in these cells. Again, the analogy with Good's own studies on the cell defects in fatal granulomatous disease may be apt in that some of those defects proved to be not so obvious.

CHAIRMAN UHR: An issue of considerable importance is the effects of tumor bearing on the lymphoreticular system. What is the status of T and B cells and their functions in tumor-bearing animals?

SMITH: Konda, Forbes, Nakao, and I (*Cancer Research*, **33,** 1878, 1973; **33,** 2100, 1973; *Proc. Eighth Leucocyte Culture Conference*, Lindahl-Keissling and Osoba, eds., p. 673, Acad. Press, N.Y., 1974) have been interested for some time in the problem of the apparent immunodeficiency in tumor-bearing man

TABLE 26

Effects of Tumor Bearing on the Mouse Lymphoreticular System

Cell mass	Effects
PBL	Decrease concentration T cells (θ bearing, PHA, Con A stimulation)
	Increased B cells
	PMN leucocytosis, lymphopenia
Lymph nodes	Increased total T cells (2-3x) (θ, PHA, Con A, MLC, GVH)
	Increased total B cells (2-3x) (IG, CRL, adoptive anti-SRBC)
	Increased indeterminent lymphoblasts (50-100x)
	Increased sessile macrophages
Spleen	Greater increases than LNC
	Increased CFU (10^2-10^3x)
Thymus	Decreased cortical cells (95%)
	No change in Th-2
Bone marrow	Slight decrease in T cells
	Increase in B cells
	Decreased CFU (2-3x)

and animals. We developed a model to examine the elements of this situation in terms of T cells and B cells, their interactions, and related parameters of lymphoreticular function.

After the model was developed, it was tested in 8 mouse strains carrying over 50 different primary and syngeneic transplanted tumors. Our findings can be summarized briefly (Table 26). First, as recorded in man, the PHA dose response in mouse peripheral blood lymphocytes is reduced significantly (Fig. 21). This apparent deficiency in peripheral blood lymphocytes appear very early in tumor-bearing animals, within 7–10 days. Thus, the model appeared to be appropriate for examining the whole body "lymphon" for an explanation of apparent deficiency in terms of the state of T and B cells.

We examined all cells harvested from the various lymph node masses by a rigorous and quite reproducible technique, and from the spleen as well as peripheral blood. We enumerated T and B cells in terms of θ- and Ig-antigen bearing and in terms of various established functions of these subpopulations and their subclasses and evaluated their interactions. These studies were made with tumors of varying immunogenicity at varying intervals.

The data obtained are summarized in Table 26 and were not wholly expected. The data on T cell numbers (anti-θ sensitive) and T cell functions gave the expected reduction when expressed per 10^6 responding cells. However, a great increase occurs in cell content or the lymph node mass and the spleen during the course of tumor bearing. It seems possible that the observed reduction might represent dilution of T cells in a larger mass of non-T cells. When the data were corrected to the size of the cell mass involved, quite a different picture emerges with respect to both spleen and lymph nodes. Tumor bearing

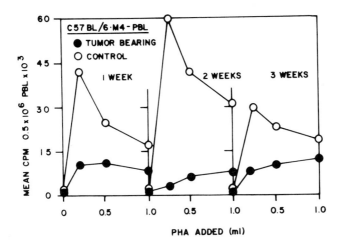

Fig. 21. Diminution by tumor bearing of PBL responsiveness to PHA.

appeared now highly stimulatory of both T cell and B cell subpopulations. During tumor growth, the lymphon, therefore, is not stable; it changes in numbers and distribution of subpopulations throughout the lymphoreticular system, and not uniformly. The number of spleen cells increase up to 8-fold over the course of bearing some tumors we studied. Regional lymph node cell numbers increase in number up to 20-fold. Nonregional and mesenteric node cell numbers increase also but not so much as regional lymph nodes or spleen.

Calculation of data on stimulation by PHA, LPS, PWM, and alloantigens in MLC, or soluble tumor-specific antigens, in these various subpopulations of lymphoid cells, indicates clearly that stimulation greater than controls was a constant finding. Most extraordinary were the LPS and alloantigen responses in the tumor-bearing hosts. In MLC, the recognition subsets stimulated by targets representing multiple alleles are increased, as tested in congenic tumor-bearing systems. This suggests that, whatever the origin of the stimulatory effect of tumor bearing, it has a broad effect on recognition responses, not a narrowly focused one. Corroborating augmented alloantigen-reacting T-cell subsets are data showing that cells, which give rise to GVH in F_1 newborns, are very greatly increased per cell mass as well. An important, but incompletely understood aspect of this phenomenon, is that augmentation of alloantigen-responsive subsets is greater than would be predicted by an increase in the number of θ-positive cells. Conversely, the increase in PHA responses in the same cell mass is generally proportionate to that of the θ-bearing cells. As we have reported elsewhere, the total immune response to several antigens is augmented in both *in vivo* and adoptive *in vivo* tests, provided it is accounted for in relation to the total lymphon. Except as viewed through the transients of the peripheral blood-cell subpopulation, therefore, immunologic deficiency is not demonstrable; by every measurement, hyperreactivity, not only in respect to the tumor but with respect to every other measure of T or B cell function, is the key feature of tumor bearing in this system.

Worthy of emphasis is the finding that LPS responses occur practically *de novo* in lymph node cell subpopulations of the tumor-bearing host and of an intensity greatly exceeding the proportionate increase in the number of Ig-bearing cells. This suggests that LPS responses are not only augmented but that the proliferative process has brought about an extraordinary susceptibility to B-cell triggering by LPS. We believe that we have a possible explanation for this unexpected observation. Since the response is out of proportion to the Ig-bearing cells in lymph nodes, we cannot account for it in the usual simple terms of direct triggering. Both lymph node and thymus cell subpopulations, normally unresponsive, are triggered to respond to LPS by interactions between alloantigens, Con A, or tumor antigen and the immunocompetent T cell subpopulations therein. Even submitogenic amounts or subthreshold interactions trigger large LPS responses. We postulate that the special subclass of T cells, responsive to alloantigens, Con A, or tumor antigens (also low θ, high H-2, low density), are greatly increased in the nodes of the tumor-bearing host, and their ongoing stimulation by tumor antigens is responsible for LPS triggering. This does not explain LPS triggering *per se*, of course, it merely provides the triggering mechanism.

CHAIRMAN UHR: What is the status of these animals with regard to rejection of skin grafts and sensitization to DNCB?

SMITH: That is not something we have examined critically.

TERRY: I will report two sets of experiments. We do not quite agree with the interpretation outlined by Smith. I hope that during the discussion we can determine some reasons for the differences. The first series of experiments is from Glaser and Herberman at the NCI. Three rat tumor systems were used: (C58NT)D in W/Fu rats, the Murphy–Sturm tumor in Lewis rats, and the Dunning tumor in Fisher rats. The data were calculated in every case on the basis of CPM/10^6 cells. Spleen cells of either normal or tumor-bearing rats were stimulated *in vitro* with PHA, Con A or PWM. In all instances, spleen cells from tumor-bearing animals were less stimulable than normal spleen cells.

It seems unlikely that recalculation of the data would give another answer. Mixtures, made from varying proportions of the spleen cells from tumor-bearing and normal rats, show inhibition of stimulability in mixtures of 10% tumor-bearing spleen with 90% normal spleen. This result seems more compatible with the conclusion that spleen cells from the tumor-bearing animal are suppressing the stimulability of the normal spleen cells.

The second experiment dealt with the response of spleen cells to PHA from normal B6 mice compared with the response of those from B6 mice at various times after inoculation of MSV. Normal mice showed a constant level of ^{3}HTdR incorporation over the 20 days of the experiment. Virus-inoculated animals start at the same level, but between day 8 and 12, the tumor becomes palpable and PHA responsiveness decreases to a minimum at about 14 days when the tumor has reached maximum size. The tumor then regresses spontaneously, and the level of PHA responsiveness returns to normal at about day 20.

In other experiments, the spleen cells were harvested at the time of maximum suppression of PHA response (day 14) and passed over a rayon column (rayon removes adherent cells). The cells passing through the column were compared with precolumn cells, and the results showed that the nonadherent cells were just as stimulable as normal spleen cells. The interpretation of these data is that within the adherent cell population there are cells capable of suppressing the responsiveness to PHA of nonadherent cells. The suppressor cells appear to be phagocytic, since they can also be removed by an iron filing ingestion-magnet technique. Finally, suppression appears to be specific for T cells, since there is no suppression of responsiveness of spleen cells to LPS, a presumed B-cell stimulant.

The last relevant work is from Wunderlich's laboratory. The system compares the capacity of tumor-bearing or normal spleen cells to generate effector cells following *in vitro* immunization. Spleen cells are harvested from C57BL/6 animals that are either normal controls or bearing MCA tumors. Spleen cells are immunized *in vitro* with spleen cells from normal C3H mice using the Mishell–Dutton culture system. After five days of culture, the C57 spleen cells are examined for their capacity to kill ^{51}Cr-labeled C3H spleen cells in a 4 hr assay. (In some experiments a C3H polyoma-induced cell line— 4198—was used as the labeled target.) In all experiments, spleen cells from tumor-bearing animals caused less lysis than those from normal animals. Moreover, nylon columns were used to separate spleen cells into adherent and nonadherent cell populations. Mixtures of the various populations (e.g., adherent cells from normal spleen mixed with nonadherent cells from ''tumor'' spleens) were then immunized *in vitro*. In all cases, the adherent cells from tumor-bearing animals suppressed the capacity of nonadherent cells to generate ''killer'' cells while the nonadherent cells from the spleens of tumor-bearing animals gave normal levels of lysis when they were mixed with adherent cells from normal spleens.

The conclusion we reach from these data are that adherent cells in the spleens of tumor-bearing animals have the ability to actively suppress the development of effector cells against immunogens other than the tumor.

BACH: We have data in man which confirms Terry's studies. We examined a large number of tumor-bearing patients with varying types of tumors with and without metastasis, and three control groups matched for several variables. Initially, MLC data from these patients suggested that tumor-bearing patients have a much reduced response in MLC. Analysis of variance of these data, however, considering variables that include cancer, age, sex, and the percentage polymorphonuclear leukocytes in the culture, gave a highly significant correlation only with the percentage of neutrophils in the peripheral blood—not cancer status. No decrease in reactivity in MLC was found when the decrease caused by neutrophil contamination was taken out of the data. This is apparently in accord with what Terry just told us about experiments in mice.

HOWARD: This remark is directed to Smith. It does not seem to me fair to assume that because the excess lymphoid mass of the tumor-bearing animals seems to be competent in *in vitro* and cell-transfer assays on a one-per-cell basis, that *ipso facto* these cells are capable of engaging in immune responses *in vivo* in the tumor-bearing animals. It is fairly well established that the normal induction of immune responses by lymphocytes requires that they be participating in the lymphocyte circulation stream. From what I understand him to say, the intravascular lymphocyte concentration was not increased in the hyperlymphoid tumor-bearing mice. The correct estimate of the potential immunological activity of an animal's lymphocyte population is surely by whole-animal *in vivo* assays. For example, in tumor-bearing mice, what is the magnitude of the splenic SRBC response after intravenous immunization.

SMITH: It seems most accurate to assess stimulatory responses in terms of the cell mass. We measure not only *in vitro* functions, but *in vivo* functions such as GVH reactions, and the data do correlate. Moreover, in both direct *in vivo* assays of SRBC responses and in an adoptive model, we observed increased numbers of anti-SRBC plaque forming cells.

In response to Terry, we do not claim that all tumor systems are stimulatory, but in the system we examined involving 12 mouse lines and about 50 tumors, this generalization is soundly based. Not only is the phenomenon highly reproducible in both primary and transplanted syngeneic tumors, but similar effects are induced by BCG vaccination, by injection of large numbers of SRBC, irradiated allogeneic lymphoid cells or irradiated tumor cells. The explanation for the widely observed and carefully documented evidences of deficiency in expression of delayed hypersensitivity, we have concluded, is not T cell or B cell deficiency, but some factor or factors related to the effector systems, perhaps concerning macrophage function. As PHA or alloantigen stimulation of the peripheral blood leukocytes does not reflect the T cell status of the tumor-bearing mice, I doubt that it does so in cancer patients.

CEPPELLINI: We compared skin homograft rejection time in normal individuals and tumor patients. In normals the rejection time was the expected 9 to 11 days. In tumor patients, this time was 18 to 20 days. Another consideration which is less well known, the lymphocytes of tumor patients are not only poor responders in MLC but also poor stimulators and that must be taken into account.

CHAIRMAN UHR: There are many reports which indicate that cancer patients may have reduced *in vivo* immune responsiveness. The interesting point is to try to explain the relationship of such data to the *in vitro* data of Smith.

STJERNSWÄRD: I do not think the data of Smith and Terry are contradictory at all as they involve two different tumor systems, one chemical induced and the other virus induced and virus releasing. This in itself may explain differences. A lot of examples of virus-induced immunosuppression are known. In Smith's system, the data do not surprise me, because if you have an antigenic tumor, as documented, it may, of course, stimulate host immunity or act as a general adjuvant. It would surprise me if it did not. Stimulation of a host for a long time with any antigen, even tumor associated, can have such effects. However, again, immune status at the tumor-bearing stage, even if not an epiphenomenon, cannot be of the same importance as that *before* a manifest tumor appears.

CHAIRMAN UHR: The *in vitro* assays are not properly assessing the immune reactivity of these patients. What is the reason?

GOOD: The regional lymph nodes draining tumors may show quite different responses from patient to patient. Furthermore, the total lymphoid system may show nonuniform changes. I do not think everything can be explained on the basis of macrophage or poly excess as compared to the numbers of responding lymphoid cells. The important point is that prognosis and outcome of malignancies can be related to the immunological deficit in man.

BACH: Of course we must assess the total immunological capacity of the animal or the human bearing a tumor. These *in vitro* tests are simply meant to dissect the system into component parts and ask which ones react normally or abnormally and under which conditions. The MLC response is normal if we eliminate polys. What Terry has told us is, possibly, the same story. We are saying that one component of the immune system is normal, tested under these conditions. If the lymphocyte is normal, the macrophage may be the deficient section of the immune apparatus. We are not trying to prove that any one *in vitro* test is prognostic of the *in vivo* situation.

ALEXANDER: My colleague Evans found that the macrophage content of various transplanted tumor lines studied ranged from 4 to 56% of the total viable cell population and were found to be related to the biological behavior of the tumors *in vivo* (*Transplantation*, **14**, 468, 1972). Low macrophage-content tumors were generally of low immunogenicity with a high incidence of spontaneous metastases, whereas high macrophage content tumors were more immunogenic and less likely to metastasize. Further work by Eccles and me (*Brit. J. Cancer*, **30**, 42, 1974) showed that the percentage of macrophages in tumors could be influenced by manipulation of the host's immune response. When rats were immunosuppressed by severe depletion of T lymphocytes via prolonged thoracic duct drainage or by adult thymectomy followed by irradiation, the numbers of macrophages appearing in tumors grown in these animals were much reduced. Yet animals immunosuppressed in this way had normal bone marrow and their macrophage and monocyte response to i.p. inflammatory agents was normal. The incidence of metastases after tumor excision in these rats was much increased, showing that effective immunosuppression had occurred. Also, when the host's immune response was stimulated by various means, the macrophage content of tumors could be raised and the incidence of metastases decreased. Thus, macrophage infiltration into tumors appeared to be a T-cell-dependent immune phenomenon, and a high percentage of macrophages in a tumor (whether naturally or artificially stimulated) represented good host immune responsiveness, which also was expressed in a low incidence of metastases.

It was found that sequestration of macrophages in tumors could explain various degrees of immunological "anergy" often seen in cancer patients or tumor-bearing animals. The delayed hypersensitivity skin response to antigens (Table 27) and i.p. inflammatory response to irritants (Fig. 22) were depressed in tumor-bearing rats, but the suppressive effects were greatest in the presence of high macrophage content tumors. Lymphocyte responsiveness to unrelated antigens was normal in the tumor-bearing rats. The observed deficiencies in DTH of tumor bearers to antigens like SRBC (Fig. 23) and BCG (Fig. 24) could be restored by passive transfer of normal peritoneal macrophages with antigens used to elicit DTH. We suggest that growing tumors interfere with the expression of DTH and related phenomena by competing for available blood monocytes to a varying degree, depending on the intensity of macrophage infiltration which they invoke. The capacity to mount DTH to antigens like BCG and to give a macrophage-rich inflammatory exudate returned within six days of excising a tumor.

CHAIRMAN UHR: Stutman will present his data on the effect of tumor bearing on the migratory patterns of lymphocytes, as it is pertinent to understanding lymphocyte function in the tumor-bearing state.

STUTMAN: Our experiments were to analyze the migratory patterns of ^{51}Cr-labeled thoracic duct lymphocytes derived from tumor-bearing mice after intravenous injection into normal animals. Instead of the 10–20% of normal thoracic duct lymphocyte radioactivity found in the liver 4 hr after injection, 50–55% of injected cells from tumor-bearing animals was found in the liver. We called this phenomenon "liver sequestration" (Stutman, Transplant. Proc., 5, 969, 1973). We thought we had a possible explanation for the immune deficit of the tumor-bearing host, in that the host was sending his immune lymphocytes to the wrong place. However, the problem is not this simple. If recirculating lymphocytes from tumor-bearing mice are incubated in vitro for 6 hr, they thereafter recirculate normally. The tissue culture fluid from such cultures converts normal lymphocytes to liver migrators. This abnormal migration is also dependent on the presence of tumor and/or tumor mass. Abnormal migration returns to normal within 12–29 hr after tumor resection.

The same effect can be accomplished in vitro with any antigen–antibody

TABLE 27

Delayed Cutaneous Hypersensitivity Responses to BCG in Rats Bearing HSBPA or MC3 Sarcomata, and the Effect of Tumor Excision[a]

Tumor inoculated	% increase in foot thickness 24 hr. after PPD					
	Days after tumor inoculation			Days after tumor excision		
	7	14	21	1	3	7
None (controls)	33.0 ±5.9	28.8±4.2	30.7 ±5.0	25.9±6.2	32.5±3.1	31.8±4.8
MC3 (low macrophage content)	30.05±3.1	19.0±4.1	12.40±1.4	N.T.[b]	N.T.	29.8±4.8 18.4±2.6[c]
HSBPA (high macrophage content)	23.2±1.8	10.1±2.2	1.5±0.8	16.5±8.4	17.9±5.3	28.6±3.2

[a] Eccles and Alexander, *Brit. J. Cancer*, **30**, 42, 1974.
[b] NT = not tested.
[c] Animals with recurrent tumor or metastases.

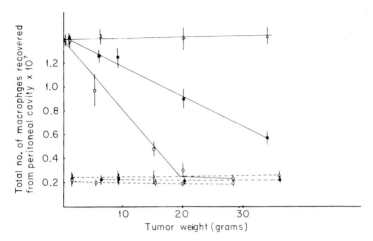

Fig. 22. Kinetics of intraperitoneal oyster glycogen response in HSBPA and MC-3 tumor-bearing rats.

Δ — Δ : normal control rats.
●: MC-3 tumor-bearing rats.
○: HSBPA tumor-bearing rats.
– – – – unstimulated peritoneal cavities
——— oyster glycogen (4 mg) stimulated peritoneal cavities
(Eccles and Alexander, *Brit. J. Cancer*, **30,** 42, 1974)

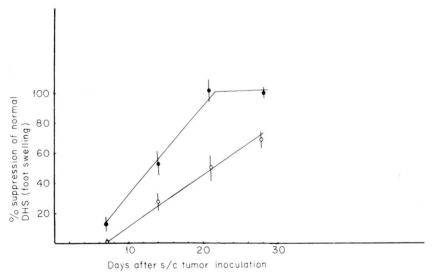

Fig. 23. Kinetics of suppression of delayed hypersensitivity response to SRBC in HSBPA and MC-3 tumor-bearing rats.

○: MC-3 tumor-bearing rats.
●: HSBPA tumor-bearing rats.
(Eccles and Alexander, *Brit. J. Cancer*, **30,** 42, 1974)

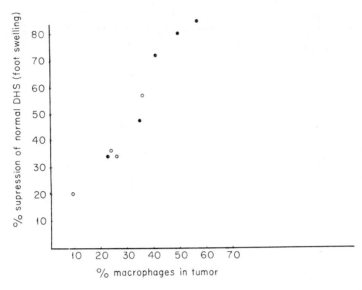

Fig. 24. Degree of suppression of delayed hypersensitivity reaction to BCG in rats bearing tumors of different macrophage contents.
●: Primary benzpyrene-induced tumors.
○:Transplanted methylcholanthrene-induced tumors.
⊗: Transplanted benzpyrene-induced tumors.
(Eccles and Alexander, *Brit. J. Cancer,* **30,** 42, 1974)

complex. Using BSA and anti-BSA antibody, complex-treated cells gave the "wrong" migratory patterns. All the liver migrators could be removed by passage on nylon wool columns. Removal of B cells plus adherent cells accounted for 70% of the liver migrators. Using a double transfer, through newborn syngeneic hosts, we found that 6–10 hr after liver sequestration the lymphocytes regained their normal migratory patterns. Liver sequestration might represent a beneficial instead of a detrimental effect for the tumor-bearing host.

CHAIRMAN UHR: The pattern Stutman described is reminiscent of the pioneering work of Gessner on enzyme-treated lymphocytes going to the liver before returning to the recirculating pattern. It seems to me that the difference between the findings of Smith and the *in vivo* immune responsiveness of cancer patients, could be explained by the Alexander experiments, i.e., a deficiency at the macrophage level. The macrophage is, thus, at the root of two problems: Macrophage infiltration of tumors diverts macrophages from participating in immune phenomena to exogenous antigens. In addition, in some of the *in vitro* assays, macrophages can alter the results. Is this an agreeable summation?

TERRY: You must prove to me that the experiment, in which a mixture is made of 10% spleen cells from a tumor-bearing animal and 90% normal spleen cells and gives marked reduction in PHA stimulation relative to the control, does not involve some sort of active suppression. We do not understand the nature of the suppression but in two different systems, it appears to be mediated by the adherent cell population. The data show only a decrease in function. Since a small admixture of spleen cells from the tumor-bearing animal decreases function, I do not believe that this is due to infiltration of the spleen with leukocytes in sufficient quantities to dilute out some necessary cell population. If you wish to argue that the spleen might contain a subpopulation of adherent cells which are themselves cytotoxic, or which release toxic substances into the medium,thus interfering with either lymphocyte stimulation or generation of killer cells, then I will accept that possibility.

If these systems really do show active suppression, which is the way we are tentatively interpreting the results, one might speculate that the spleen of the tumor-bearing animal is similar to the spleen of a hyperimmunized animal (data supporting this part of the speculation have previously been published by Smith) and that one of the consequences of hyperimmunization is the generation of suppressor cells. These cells would have the function of limiting T cell stimulability and might serve as a feedback control and be representative of the normal biology of the lymphoid system.

CHAIRMAN UHR: Is it possible that suppressor T cells, which could represent a minor population, are adherent cells?

TERRY: It is certainly possible that any minor population of adherent cells could account for these observations.

BACH: In the data from studies I described, there is no evidence for suppression. I interpret your remarks to mean that that is how you are currently looking at your data and that you do not have any evidence for it. You have a time-sequence study of course, in which you show that, at a given time, reactivity does go down. We would not have seen that in our work even looking at a large amount of data.

NOTKINS: I think that at this point we should mention the fact that certain oncogenic and nononcogenic viruses can also suppress immune function. Many of these viruses produce a more or less generalized suppression of the immune response. When one is dealing with a murine system, one just does not know what viruses are present. Attention is now being directed to the specificity of the viral attack. For example, do viruses affect: (1) different classes of lympho-

197

cytes (i.e., T versus B cells), (2) specific subpopulations of T or B cells (e.g., suppressor T cells), or (3) clones of lymphocytes making an immune response to a specific antigen. The amount of information in this field is still quite limited, but there are several provocative observations that should be mentioned:

First, EBV replicates in B cells but not T cells. Moreover, there is some evidence that the atypical lymphocytes observed in this disease are T cells and may represent a blastogenic response to viral antigens. Work from several laboratories has shown that other viruses (e.g., vesicular stomatitis virus) will replicate only in activated lymphocytes (presumably T cells) but not in normal lymphocytes.

Second, lactic dehydrogenase virus can suppress the cell-mediated immune response in mice while enhancing or leaving the humoral response intact. On the basis of morphologic evidence, the infection seems to deplete the thymic-dependent areas of the lymph nodes and spleen during the acute stage of the infection.

Third, Woodruff and Woodruff have shown that there are receptors on lymphocytes for myxo- and paramyxo-viruses and that these viruses can alter the surface of lymphocytes and the recirculation pattern of these lymphocytes. It will be interesting to determine whether purified subpopulations of lymphocytes have different receptors for viruses. Thus, one might visualize the situation where a particular virus might destroy suppressor T cells and leave other T cells more or less intact. Destruction of suppressor T cells by viruses could, for example, be one of the factors responsible for autoimmune phenomena associated with certain diseases, including tumors.

Finally, McFarland, using a hapten-carrier system in mice, found that measles virus suppressed the T cell but not B cell immune response. Thus, there is the possibility that certain viruses might act in somewhat the same fashion as cyclophosphamide; that is, they might destroy lymphocytes that are actually making an immune response to a specific antigen. Theoretically, at least, this might be one of the factors responsible for the persistence of certain types of viruses or tumors. For example, when a cell becomes transformed, the lymphocytes of the host will respond to the foreign antigens associated with the transformed cell. If these lymphocytes are in a blastogenic state, they may be more susceptible to viral attack. The clones of cells making antibody to specific tumor antigens might be destroyed while leaving nonactivated lymphocytes intact. This might allow the tumor to survive. In my opinion this area deserves further attention.

ALEXANDER: Some patients with large carcinomas do not give a good Mantoux reaction. I must stress that in Britain everybody gets immunized with BCG, so the level of Mantoux positivity is high. The lymphocytes from these patients perform normally in the MLC and are stimulated by BCG. However, when one comes to lymphoma patients, there is occasionally also a failure of lymphocytes to transform with PPD. Therefore, we must not oversimplify or jump to conclusions.

CHAIRMAN UHR: Is there evidence for a serum factor that is immunodepressant in tumor bearing?

GOOD: Plasma from cancer patients will interfere with normal isolated lymphocyte responses to PHA and in the MLC. One of the generalizations that should come out of this set of arguments is that there is no simple single explanation for the complex forms of immunodeficiencies in humans with cancer. One can define circumstances in which morphological depression of the regional nodes is seen. Circumstances exist, as Alexander has convincingly showed us, where macrophages in the circulation are grossly depleted. We also know circumstances in which depletion in the circulation of T lymphocytes unquestionably exists. For example, Hanson had a case where we could find essentially no lymphocytes in the circulating blood. This patient had a pleural effusion associated with cancer in the chest cavity, and the effusion fluid was loaded with responsive T lymphocytes. In this instance, the pattern of recirculation may have accounted for the apparent deficiency of T lymphocytes. Lastly, there are the noncellular substances in the circulation of cancer patients which suppress the responses of the lymphocytes nonspecifically. We are, therefore, dealing with a great multiplicity of influences that do not permit easy generalization.

SESSION IV

FACTORS THAT INTERFERE WITH OR PREVENT EFFECTIVE DESTRUCTION OF TUMORS VIA IMMUNE MECHANISMS

Tumor cell escape mechanisms from host control—Blocking factors in DTH—Blocking factors in various models of tumor immunity—Character of blocking factors in tumor-bearer sera—Blocking by tumor antigen and by Ag–Ab complexes—Antibody-mediated antigen release from tumors—Blocking in tumor–virus systems—Blocking in alloantigen systems—Molecular models for blocking phenomena—Concomitant immunity—Blocking in the MLC—Theoretical framework for immune responses to transformed cells.

CHAIRMAN KLEIN: If strong limitations are imposed on a population of living organisms—e.g., by treating bacteria with drugs, flies with DDT, or by closing down the border of a country—methods of escape will develop through which some organisms will pass. The methods of escape are not uniform. It is the effect, the escape itself, that is common—not the mechanism. Crossing a closed border can mean infinite variations on a common theme, ranging from cutting through barbed wire to being driven out in a government car.

We can draw up a list of known mechanisms of escape from surveillance for tumor cells that have been demonstrated experimentally in one system or another, and, I am sure, the list is very incomplete:

1. Immunodeficiency of the host.
2. "Sneaking through."
3. Immunoresistance.
4. Lack of recognition (synonymous with lack of antigenicity or absence of surveillance).
5. Malfunctioning of the immune mechanism.

The largest part of present experimental work in tumor immunology is devoted to the last item. This is reflected in the topics of discussion we shall be developing later.

With due respect to current interest in this area, I would suggest that much of the phenomenology of tumor bearing may be a *consequence* of successful tumor growth, rather than a *cause* of it. Perhaps it would be important to consider the question of how early events in surveillance breakdown could be studied. The importance of the dormancy problem came out clearly during the preceding discussion. The study of oncogenic latency is also very important, a variation on the same theme. Among questions we should consider are: What is the relative contribution of antigen, antibody, and antigen–antibody complexes in relation to each system studied? This will be important also, with regard to the related question whether T cells, non-T cells, with or without antibody, or macrophages are responsible for cell-mediated killing. Other equally important questions concern if, and to what extent, these *in vitro* systems are relevant to corresponding *in vivo* phenomena.

I would first say a few words about each of the escape areas, proceeding from the beginning of the list. We all know the effects of neonatal thymectomy, ALS treatment, X-irradiation and treatment with immunosuppressive drugs in facilitating tumor growth in one system or another. Perhaps less attention is given to genetic unresponsiveness to certain tumor antigens. This is deplorable, because the question of tumor-antigen recognition is *the* key question of all tumor immunology. I cannot emphasize strongly enough the importance of this topic. Let me provide some examples.

Marek's disease in chickens is due to a highly oncogenic, lymphotropic herpes virus. Other than feline leukemia virus, this is the only known viral agent that causes tumors under natural conditions by horizontal contagion. Genetically resistant lines of chickens have been selected where viral infection leads to self-limiting disease or no disease at all. Neonatally thymectomized resistant chickens lose their resistance to the malignant disease. On the other hand, susceptible chickens can be vaccinated with a closely related, but apathogenic, turkey herpes virus. Prevention of tumors by vaccination is not a matter of antiviral immunity but of the ability of the immune system to reject potentially neoplastic cells. Resistant chickens can do this without vaccination.

Resistance is often due to a single dominant gene. Since the action of this gene is abolished by neonatal thymectomy, it is fair to assume that genetically determined resistance acts through the T-cell system. This does not say whether it acts via the differentiation of specific, killer T cells, or through T-cell-dependent antibody formation, but it certainly says that genetic resistance acts through the immune system. It is possible, and likely, that the gene in question is akin to the immune response (Ir) genes. It is becoming increasingly clear that Ir genes influence virtually every type of immune response. They can act at the T cell or at the B cell level, or at the level of cooperation of T and B cells. In some situations, they can make all or none of the difference between responsiveness and unresponsiveness, whereas in other cases they determine the promptness and magnitude of the response. All this must be very relevant to tumor immunology.

Other examples can be considered. The high leukemia incidence of AKR mice is due to vertically transmitted Gross virus. This virus is often referred to as the natural leukemia virus, because it is found in wild mice. It is not often added, however, that the virus is not known to cause leukemia in wild mice.

AKR mice have been established by continuous inbreeding and selection for leukemia. We know that this strain carries a special susceptibility gene or, more precisely, a susceptibility allele at a locus that normally determines resistance to Gross virus-induced leukemia. This locus is called Rgv-1 and the resistance and susceptibility alleles carry the superscript r and s, respectively.

The Gross virus does not induce leukemia in mice unless the host carries the s allele in double dose. Perhaps even more importantly, the Rgv-1 gene is localized in the K region of the H-2 complex, the same region where a major Ir locus is found. It is, therefore, possible that Rgv-1 is an Ir gene, involved in the recognition of (or development of efficient rejection mechanisms against) the Gross leukemia virus-determined surface antigen. The specificity of this gene is also reinforced by the fact that it plays no role in the reactivity of mice against leukemias induced by the Moloney agent. Moloney and Gross are closely related agents or, perhaps, even variants of the same agent, but the Moloney surface antigen does not cross react with the Gross virus surface antigen.

If Rgv-1 is an Ir gene and its s allele is a deficient (unresponsive) variant of it, Jacob Furth may have selected a deficient mutant at this locus when he established the AKR strain. The strain C3H that is sensitive to the Gross virus (but only if inoculated soon after birth) carries the same H-2^k complex and the same Rgv-1^s alleles as AKR.

In the Moloney system, we have preliminary evidence that one or several Ir-like genes also play an important role in recognition and/or rejection. These genes are not H-2 linked, however. In relation to the induction of mouse mammary tumors by the Bittner agent (MTV), Muhlbock and Dux discovered an H-2-linked resistance gene, derived from the strain selected for low mammary tumor incidence in C57BL. In contrast to Rgv-1, this gene is localized to the D region of the H-2 complex. This has been discovered by comparing the mammary tumor incidence of congenic resistant sublines of mice with a C57BL background, where the major histocompatability locus, H-2 or non-H-2 loci, has been substituted by intercross and repeated backcrossing. All congenic resistant lines that had the original H-2^b of C57BL, but were substituted at other loci, were resistant to mammary tumor induction by MTV, whereas the H-2 substituted lines were susceptible. It is not yet known whether the H-2–linked resistance gene against the MTV induction of mammary carcinomas is an Ir gene, but this is one of the important alternatives that is being considered.

Polyoma virus causes tumors only if inoculated into newborn mice, within 24–48 hr after birth, and if the mice have not received maternally transmitted antibody. Under these circumstances, it can induce a wide variety of tumors. Polyoma is also a widespread natural contaminant of wild mice. However, Huebner has shown that virus-infected wild mice, when put into cages in the laboratory, do not develop tumors. He, therefore, concluded that this was neither a natural oncogenic agent for mice nor for any other species.

Polyoma-induced tumors have relatively strong TSTA. It is possible to build up considerable resistance against polyoma tumors, either with the virus or with irradiated, polyoma-induced tumor cells. The resistance of adult mice to the oncogenic effect of polyoma virus is due to prompt recognition of the polyoma-associated surface antigen. Because wild mice are usually infected with the virus, mothers transmit antibodies to their young and they are protected during the critical first 24 hr of their life. Upon later infection, they can respond promptly to the TSTA. Again, we have a situation where a highly oncogenic virus and its host species evolve a symbiotic relationship and exist together in balance. What is important here is not so much the mere presence of a potentially oncogenic virus, but the way it can act when this balance is disturbed. Obviously, the main question is what happens when the immune system is depressed.

Law and, more recently, Allison and their collaborators have shown that adult mice become susceptible to the oncogenic effect of even small doses of polyoma virus spread by room infection, if they receive total body X-irradiation or are treated with ALS. Obviously, it would be of the greatest interest to know whether polyoma-infected wild mice can develop polyoma tumors upon exposure to various kinds of immunosuppressive treatment. Man is the only wild species that experiences immunosuppression for prolonged periods of time (kidney graft recipients and children with various congenital immunodeficiency diseases); under these circumstances he develops a significantly increased incidence of tumors.

The next escape mechanism, "sneaking through," is essentially a trivial "numbers game," rather than a special mechanism, but it may be important nonetheless. The issue is whether an efficient rejection reaction can occur in response to an incipient tumor focus before it has reached an irreversible size. "Sneaking through" has significance as a situation lending itself to preventive measures. Virtually complete prevention of tumors can be achieved in hamsters inoculated with polyoma or SV40 virus neonatally by a second inoculation of the same virus, or this can also occur when irradiated tumor cells, induced by the same virus, are inoculated toward the end of the oncogenic latency period. Successful reduction of tumor incidence in susceptible chickens infected with Marek's virus, by a related nonpathogenic turkey herpesvirus already mentioned, probably belongs in the same category.

Drug resistance is known to evolve by many different ceullular mechanisms. I am convinced that the same is true for immunoresistance. In fact, by somatic cell hybridization, we have obtained evidence for two different mechanisms. One is "dominant" and another is "recessive" in the hybrid cell. Stable variations in immunosensitivity are demonstrated by the development of immunoresistant sublines. These lines also show physiological variations in immunosensitivity, depending on the growth cycle. Conceivably they also have a role in the escape of tumor cells from what otherwise might be efficient rejection.

"Lack of recognition" is closely related to the question of whether nonantigenic tumors actually exist. Baldwin has told us that he encounters a number of tumors, spontaneous and chemically induced as well, that are not recognizably antigenic in their host. Doubt was expressed in *in vivo* rejection tests were sufficiently sensitive, and it was suggested that *in vitro* lymphocytotoxicity tests always measure responses that are relevant *in vivo:* I regard the *in vivo* tests as the more significant.*

Editors' comment: It should be reiterated that the usual transplantation-type assays (immunogenicity rejection) for presence of tumor antigens have been judged relatively insensitive. The *in vitro* tests can add a further dimension by virtue of their sensitivity and the capability they provide for juggling variables and, thus, further analyzing the phenomena involved. Alexander's argument, elsewhere in this session, is that the burden of proof for tumor nonimmunogenicity should not rest upon the single criterion of a transplantation-type assay, despite its *in vivo* character. His emphasis is that the presence of immunoblasts and specific cytotoxic cells in the draining lymph nodes of the tumor-immunized host, in the absence of other more obvious manifestations of rejection, provides an objective criterion that "nonimmunogenic" tumors can, in fact, engender resistance in the recipient.

Another point that can be made about *in vitro* tests is related to the question of timing, in relation to tumor development. The host may become sensitized to tumor-associated antigens, but only at a time when it is too late. This is more analogous to tissue-specific antigen sensitization in autoimmune disease, a probable consequence of antigen release and subsequent sensitization from damaged tissues, rather than a mechanism preexisting but breaking down, thereby allowing the tumor to emerge.

Herpesvirus saimiri (HVS) is the most oncogenic tumor virus known, but only in species other than its natural host, the squirrel monkey. Here it is regularly present. Virus can be isolated from and antibodies demonstrated in 100% of adult animals when captured in the jungle or kept in the zoo. Like polyoma-infected wild mice, squirrel monkeys never develop tumors. When inoculated into two New World monkeys, the marmoset or owl monkey, the virus induces progressively growing lymphoproliferative malignancy in 100% of the recipients, irrespective of age. The potency of this virus is so great in these two experimental host species that attempts to vaccinate have broken down so far. Heat-killed vaccines contain enough live virus particles to induce lymphoma and kill the monkey.

We have studied the immune response in the squirrel monkey and the 2 susceptible hosts in terms of induction of early and late viral antigens. All 3 species responded with high antibody levels. Primary infection in the squirrel monkey induced high antibody titers in 10–12 days, but in the marmoset and the owl monkey this happened only after 30–50 days. The timing is too late, however, because lymphomas are already growing progressively by this time. This illustrates the importance of timing in recognition. It brings us back again to the question of Ir genes that may influence the timing of the response. The timing factor can make the difference between tumor or no tumor and between detectable or nondetectable antigenicity of the tumor.

The surveillance mechanisms have limitations. While antigens associated with tumors induced by viruses ubiquitous in their natural host species are promptly and efficiently recognized, as I have pointed out, this does not mean that a surveillance mechanism exists which can recognize *every* conceivable membrane modification cells undergo in the course of neoplastic change. It is, therefore, not surprising that we encounter tumors not detectably antigenic by rejection tests. In trying to deal with this problem by immunological means, we

---

A further argument can be made on *in vivo* grounds that failure to demonstrate resistance in the transplantation model cannot be taken, alone, as evidence of nonimmunogenicity of a tumor. Certain tumors, judged nonimmunogenic by transplantation tests, have been shown to be rejected when reimplanted into the tumor-bearing host in the demonstration of concomitant immunity (see pp. 258–260 for a detailed discussion). Taken together, the data suggest that our devotion to the transplantation model for demonstrating tumor immunogenicity may have more of a traditional than an objective foundation.

must take a close look at the beautiful experiments concerned with the genetics of immune responses against chemically defined antigens. Here Benacerraf and his colleagues have shown that unresponsive animals respond when the relevant antigen is coupled to an appropriate, immunogenic carrier.

At least one virus-induced tumor—murine sarcoma virus (MSV)—lacks detectable virus-determined surface antigens, despite containing the viral genome, demonstrable by co-cultivation. As a rule, MSV and MLV occur together. In the absence of MLV, MSV is noninfectious. MSV- or MLV-induced sarcomas are highly antigenic and regress spontaneously in the autochthonous host. A few years ago, we tried to identify antibodies specifically directed against surface antigens induced by the sarcoma virus by absorbing appropriate antisera with MLV-induced lymphoma cells. To our surprise, absorption was complete, suggesting that the sarcoma had no surface antigen not also present on the lymphoma cells, carrying a nontransforming MLV virus. MSV genome alone is apparently unable to bring about an antigenic surface change with a distinctive specificity. This was shown by our failure to identify any tumor-associated antigen in the MSV-carrying, but MLV-free, S+L-line. Strong membrane antigenicity was readily induced, however, by superinfecting the S+L-cell with MLV.

This does not imply that MSV brings about and maintains neoplastic behavior of its target cell without any membrane change. Lack of contact inhibition is presumably due to a membrane change, and there may be others. However, the host immune mechanism apparently does not recognize this particular membrane change as an antigen. This might well be related to the fact that the host does not encounter, under natural conditions, MSV virus or MSV-induced transformants, in the absence of MLV. Whereas when recognition occurs of MLV-induced surface antigens, present both on sarcomatous and on leukemic target cells, apparently no selective pressure is present for the recognition of MSV-related antigens.

The human Epstein–Barr virus/Burkitt system is also relevant to our present topic in a number of ways. In all probability, the relation of man to EBV is comparable, *mutatis mutandis*, to the relationship of the natural resistant host species, the squirrel monkey, to HVS.

Primary EBV infection of sero-negative individuals can either lead to seroconversion without disease, like the HVS infection of squirrel monkeys, or, if it affects teenagers or young adults, it may induce infectious mononucleosis (IM). Antibody formation during mononucleosis has been followed carefully. Response to virally determined late (VCA), early (EA) and membrane (MA) antigens is very rapid, reaches high titers within a few weeks, and is then maintained at moderate titers throughout life. In contrast, antibodies to the EBV-determined nuclear antigen come very much later, often after several months, and are then maintained. This may signal the effects of ongoing immune surveillance, eliminating virus-carrying potential transformants.

The distribution of EBV antibody in different human populations is significant. In low socioeconomic groups throughout the world, the early infection of young children predominates. This infection does not cause mononucleosis, as a rule, although it may induce a fever syndrome of ill-defined type. However, after early conversion, infected individuals are protected from IM. From their peripheral blood cells, permanent lymphoblastoid cell lines can be established, which carry the viral genome, in multiple copies, and, when inoculated into immunologically crippled animals, can grow as heterotransplanted malignant lymphomas. Similar lines cannot be established from the peripheral blood of sero-negative individuals. Mononucleosis is a "college disease" because it is restricted to the hygienically protected high socioeconomic classes where primary infection often occurs in adolescence. The possibility that the virus is transmitted by "cellular kissing" is well established, and it agrees with the fact that biologically active (transforming) virus preparations can be isolated from the throat washings of mononucleosis patients and also from sero-converted normal individuals, long after the disease. Good hygiene is a late development that could hardly have played any role during human evolution. This suggests that analogy with the prompt response of the squirrel monkey to the HVS disease is even closer. One important difference between HVS infection and EBV infection is that HVS appears to infect and convert T lymphocytes, whereas EBV appears to be exclusively restricted to B lymphocytes. All established EBV genome-carrying lines, having B cell characteristics and only B, but not T lymphocytes, have virus receptors on their surface.

To study the biological effects of the virus, the surest source of EBV-free lymphocytes is cord blood, since the virus is not transmitted vertically. Cord blood cells are never found to grow into established lines unless EBV is added, although this has been tried extensively. Certain preparations of EBV can transform B lymphocytes in cord cell populations, at very high efficiency, into established lines. These lines have the characteristics of multiple genome loads, nuclear (EBNA) antigen and malignant potential on heterotransplantation. This shows that the virus has, at least in this artificial system, oncogenic potential.

Is the virus involved in human malignant diseases? A strict distinction must be made between an association between high antiviral antibody titers and disease, on the one hand, and evidence for the proliferation of EBV genome-carrying tumor cells, on the other. The former condition accompanies the latter, as a rule, but the reverse is not true. With the exception of the African Burkitt lymphoma (BL), occurring in the high endemic regions, and nasopharyngeal carcinoma (NPC), irrespective of geographic localization, no tumors have been found to carry the viral genome.

In Hodgkin's disease (HD), particularly the lymphocyte-depleted form in chronic lymphatic leukemia and in undifferentiated lymphocytic lymphoma, anti-EBV titers are often elevated. None of these tumors were found to contain the viral genome by nucleic-acid hybridization, nor do they carry EBNA. In contrast, 97% of African BL cells carry EBV genome. The clonal nature of the tumor has been shown by Fialkow, via G6PD marker analysis. This applies even to cases with multiple tumors. The number of genomes carried per cell is similar to the established nonproducer lines (38 on an average in the materials so far studied). The presence of the EBNA antigen is regularly correlated with the presence of the viral genome. No antigen-positive, genome-free lines, or antigen-negative, genome-positive lines, have been found either in biopsy or in tissue culture materials. What is the mechanism of high EBV antibody titers in patients whose tumors do not carry the viral genome?

The best probable explanation is suggested by two patients with congenital thymic deficiency, recently described by Aiuti *et al.* in Rome. These two children lacked demonstrable T lymphocytes but had very high anti-EBV titers, including both VCA and EA antibodies. Presence of EA antibodies in normal individuals is very rare. It is usually associated with the acute phase of infectious mononucleosis, with BL or with NPC. Upon thymus transplantation, the T-cell count in both patients rapidly normalized. At the same time, the anti-EA titer disappeared and the VCA titers went down to the normal range. This suggests that proliferation of the virus, or what seems more likely, of virus-carrying cells, is restricted by a T-cell-dependent mechanism in normal individuals. It may be noted, however, that the two thymus-deficient children did not develop lymphoma. Their surveillance mechanism was not completely deficient, however, as is also reflected by their high antibody titers against the EBV antigens. Antibodies alone or antibodies acting with non-T cells may play an important role in surveillance.

Johansson in Stockholm has recently obtained evidence in Hodgkin's disease showing that patients with a depressed immune reactivity, as determined by a battery of lymphocyte stimulation and skin tests, have elevated VCA and EA titers. The interpretation is that the relatively moderate and irregular increase of EBV titers in HD patients is a consequence of the relative immunosuppression, caused by the disease.

In African BL the situation is quite different. Nucleic acid hybridization studies, conducted on biopsy materials, and corresponding EBNA antigen tests collated from three different laboratories, (zur Hausen, Germany; Nonoyama and Pagano, United States; and our laboratory, Sweden), show that 81 of 83 cases studied had genome-positive tumors. On the other hand, the genome was not found in four American BL by Pagano, nor could we detect the EBNA antigen in three European Burkitts. In the African material, two genome-negative cases were found out of 83 patients. They might well represent a disease that corresponds to the genome-negative, non-African cases. If so, the genome-positive tumor would be superimposed on the worldwide background provided by the ubiquitous genome-negative cases in the high endemic regions of Africa.

Recently, we have succeeded in establishing a cell line from one of the genome-negative African tumors. The line, called B-JAB, does not carry EBV-DNA or EBNA. It is a B cell line, with surface immunoglobulins and other B cell markers. It also contains receptors for EBV, like other B cells. For this reason, it can be superinfected with EBV *in vitro*. Superinfection leads to the regular induction of EBNA. Moreover, the patient from whom the line was derived was sero-positive for EBV antibodies, at a relatively high level. This illustrates one important point: The virus does not readily "jump" upon an established tumor *in vivo*, even if the tumor cells are susceptible to superinfection. This is probably due to the high neutralizing antibody titers that develop soon after primary infection. Presumably, neutralizing antibody is an effective barrier against the spread of the virus between the cells, including the jump from normal to established lymphoma cells.

Similar evidence is now available for two Swedish lymphoma cases, studied by Nilsson and Sundström in Uppsala. They established EBV genome-free lines *in vitro*. The lines come from sero-positive patients, but they are not equally sensitive to superinfection *in vitro*, as the B-JAB line. It may be also mentioned, in this connection, that Minowada has established two cell lines with T cell characteristics from *all* patients. These lines are also genome free, but this is, perhaps, less surprising because T cells do not carry virus receptors.

If it can be reasoned that EBV does not readily infect lymphomas and leukemias that appear at a time when the patient already has neutralizing antibodies, it implies that in the genome-positive African Burkitt tumors, the genome is present from the very inception of the tumor clone. This essentially leaves us with two hypotheses. First, the African Burkitt patient is exposed to the same primary EBV infection as normal individuals but, unlike the latter, is not capable of restricting the outgrowth of all clones. Perhaps, due to a temporary deficiency of the surveillance mechanism, one clone breaks through and grows into a tumor. After having reached irreversible size, it would no longer be amenable to immune restriction. Burkitt himself has postulated that chronic holoendemic malaria might be responsible for this or similar series of events. A combination of T cell suppression and stimulation of B lymphocyte proliferation, such as in chronic malaria, may achieve this, although adequate studies to demonstrate this have not yet been performed. As an alternative, one could imagine a situation where the transition of the immunologically restricted EBV-carrying cell to a full malignant cell requires an additional change. This change would be induced by another virus or be akin to the mutation-like cellular changes collected under the phenomena designated as "tumor progression."

According to this reasoning, the non-African BL and the rare EBV genome-negative African would have another, probably unrelated, etiology. Because the distinction between Burkitt and non-BL is very tenuous, and often quite subjective, it would not be surprising if two different viral agents would

211

cause lymphomas with a fundamentally similar histological and cytological picture. The morphologically indistinguishable Gross and Moloney lymphomas in mice may serve as an example to show that this situation can indeed occur.

Nasopharyngeal carcinoma has provided us with even less knowledge than BL. It is clear, that NPC is the only known tumor, besides African BL, that is *regularly* associated with high anti-EBV titers. The tumor also contains EBV genome in biopsy material. Association appears to be independent of geography. No ambiguity exists in histological diagnosis: The poorly differentiated or anaplastic type of NPC is a very distinct entity.

Until recently, the extensive lymphocytic infiltration that characterizes these tumors was thought responsible for their content of EBV genome. Zur Hausen found, however, that there is an inverse correlation between genome positivity and lymphocyte infiltration of different NPC biopsy specimens. Moreover, *in situ* hybridization, which he carried out with cRNA, suggested that EBV-DNA was present in the large carcinoma cells and not in the small lymphocytes. Working with Giovanella and Lindahl, we have recently obtained evidence that NPC biopsies, when inoculated into nude mice and carried as serially passaged human carcinoma lines, maintain the EBV genome. Moreover, the EBNA antigen is clearly present in the large, carcinoma cell complexes.

Therefore, another cell type carries the genome. It has been a matter of some discussion whether NPC represents the proliferation of a highly anaplastic, epithelial carcinoma cell or is a reticulum cell. At the least, we have one other cell, in addition to the B lymphocytes, that carries the viral genome. It will be particularly important to establish whether the association between this genome and the host cell is comparable to the relationship between the EBV-carrying lymphoblastoid cell and the virus, also whether the NPC-associated viral genome has the same characteristics as the virus associated with BL.

The specific immune status of the BL patient, in relation to his own tumor, is particularly relevant to the question of tumor cell dormancy and latency. By several criteria, the Burkitt patient has a relatively strong immune response against his tumor. This is, in all likelihood, the reason why about 25% of cases have long lasting and apparently total regression after chemotherapy, often despite mild or insufficient chemotherapy. What immune effector mechanisms are responsible for inhibiting the regrowth of BL cells in such a patient?

Surprisingly little evidence exists for T cell killing in BL. On the other hand, the patients have high antibody titers, including anti-MA directed against the EBV-determined MA complex regularly present on the surface of the tumor cells. It is conceivable that antibodies, alone or with non-T cells, exert a cytostatic and, to some extent, perhaps also cytolytic function. Gunven has carried out extensive studies on MA-antibody levels of treated patients, during different stages of the disease. Patients with total tumor regression who became long-term survivors have, as a rule, steady anti-MA levels maintained over many years, quite like normal EBV sero-positive individuals, although at higher levels. On the other hand, patients whose tumors recur may show a precipitous fall of the anti-MA titer, 4–6 months prior to the reappearance of the disease. It is one of the fastest growing human tumors known, and it is unlikely that it would grow undetected at a high rate 4–6 months prior to diagnosed recurrence. It is possible, therefore, that the fall of anti-MA antibody titer is not merely a consequence of antibody absorption by a recurrent but undiagnosed tumor. Gunven has shown, moreover, in several prerecurrence sera, that MA decrease already had occurred and that antigen–antibody complexes with MA specificity are present at recurrence. If the complexes were dissociated at low pH and if high and low molecular fractions were separated by filtration through Amicon filters (No. 100), the anti-MA titer in the immunoglobulin-containing supernatant clearly increases, suggesting that it was bound to a low-molecular antigen fraction in the serum. However, after the tumor had recurred clinically and continued to grow progressively, a secondary rise occurs in anti-MA titer. This suggests that a massive release of antibody-binding, but nonimmunogenic, MA fragment is characteristic in prerecurrence patients. The reservoir from which this antigen is released is completely unknown, but one hypothesis is that release, together with the subsequent fall of the membrane antibody titer, may be instrumental in promoting recurrence.

This brings up the final question I would raise: What types of antigen–antibody complexes are maintained in the circulation through long periods of time, and how does the presence and maintenance of such complexes relate to tumor recurrence?

SMITH: With respect to Klein's last point, he will recall that working together in 1966 (Smith, Klein, Clifford), we found that MA on human LCL derived from BL is shed or modulated from the membrane surface in the presence of anti-MA antibody at 37°C. As long as the antibody was present in the cell environment, the membrane antigen did not reappear. After removal of the antibody, a 24–36 hr lag phase preceded MA reappearance. Is it not possible that during the prerecurrence phase of BL, when anti-MA dropped to low levels and antigen–antibody complexes appear, an *in vivo* equivalent of this *in vitro* shedding process is occurring?

CHAIRMAN KLEIN: It *is* a model for antigen release, but it does not clarify the puzzling presence of antigen–antibody complexes, with virtually no free antibody, 4–6 months before the tumor reappears. Subsequently, when the tumor has reappeared, excess antibody is rapidly induced. Incidentally, sera from a minority of all EBV positives are negative for MA antibody but positive for EA and VCA. These discordant sera were found *only* in BL and NPC patients with large tumor loads. It is likely that they have a great antigen excess, since there is no other reason the MA-antibody level should be selectively paralyzed, in comparison with the antibodies directed against EA and VCA

UHR: I would like to comment on the apparent low molecular weight of the membrane antigen in the circulation. One possible explanation is that the antigen has been degraded by the tumor cell just prior to release. The reason I suggest this is that the BL line, which Klein kindly sent to us, shows degradation of the immunoglobulin on its surface during cell lysis.

CEPPELLINI: Does the difference between African Burkitt and non-African Burkitt involve environmental or genetic factors?

CHAIRMAN KLEIN: The African and non-African BL are probably different diseases. They have nothing in common except histological resemblances. Every pathologist will tell you, if pressed hard, that the distinction between Burkitt and non-Burkitt lymphomas is not based on any strict criteria. NPC is a different proposition altogether, because the typical, poorly differentiated or anaplastic NPC can be diagnosed easily, irrespective of geography.

CEPPELLINI: Klein's reply is not a complete answer to my question. Even if it is a different disease, why do we have the African BL in Africa?

CHAIRMAN KLEIN: This depends upon the elements of one's working hypothesis. On the first alternative (the slipping through of an EBV genome-carrying clone in the Burkitt patients otherwise restricted by immune surveillance), one can consider genetic or environmental reasons for breakdown of the rejection mechanism. Evidence for an environmental factor is rather strong from the time-space clustering so marked in all the epidemiological studies on BL. This is what led Burkitt to postulate that an insect-mediated factor is involved. In his up-to-date view, this would be a malaria carrying mosquito, but a cofactor would not be just malaria but chronic holoendemic malaria, which is quite a different thing. In fact, holo-or hyperendemic malaria is strongly stimulatory for a large part of the lymphoreticular system, and it is also immunosuppressive. If one imagines an adequate combination of, say, T cell suppression and a stimulation of neoplastic B cell proliferation, this could make sense. It is a reasonable proposition, but not conclusive, because the insect VC factor could obviously carry many other things.

CEPPELLINI: A third possibility from our studies is significant correlation between the distribution of malaria in different regions and some HL-A types. Because malaria defense has possibly selected some Ir genes and, as a consequence, linked Ir genes, it may be responsible for the genes of BL.

CHAIRMAN KLEIN: I agree that all this has to be analyzed.

DELLA PORTA: Has Klein had the opportunity to study IM in Africa with respect to the host cell genome?

CHAIRMAN KLEIN: If one looks at the distribution of EBV titers in a normal African population, one can easily see why IM does *not* occur in Africa. The vast majority of the population acquires the infection at a very early age. IM is a disease of young adults, living in a protected socioeconomic environment, who have not been previously exposed to the virus. Early infection does not lead to recognizable IM.

MARTIN: Can Klein detect the nuclear antigen in nonmalignant cells of a BL patient?

CHAIRMAN KLEIN: I cannot answer Martin's question, because to look for an antigen-positive cell among many antigen negatives is really looking for a needle in a haystack. It is very difficult to do all the necessary controls to show that one is dealing with the EBV-specific nuclear reaction, unless one deals with a relatively homogeneous population.

MARTIN: But is it a fact that the vast majority of cells do not have the antigen?

CHAIRMAN KLEIN: We have found an antigen *in vivo* only in the homogeneous BL biopsy preparations. We have not found it in other lymphomas, Burkitt-like or non-Burkitt-like, occuring outside the high endemic areas of Africa, irrespective of anti-EBV serum titers. A lymphoma patient can have very high anti-EBV titers but still an EBV genome-negative tumor.

MACKANESS: There will be much sophisticated talk about blocking mechanisms later. It may be appropriate to start at a very mundane level with a subject which Uhr and Smith had much to do with many years ago. The subject concerns the conditions of immunization that lead to induction of cell-mediated or delayed type hypersensitivity (DTH). It has been known, since the early studies of Uhr, Salvin, Pappenheimer, and Smith in the fifties and early sixties, that dose and route of antigen injection profoundly influence the type of immune response that ensues. The level of T cell activity, measured as DTH, in mice immunized with varying doses of sheep red blood cells (SRBC) is shown in Fig. 25. When the dose was varied from 10^3–10^9, DTH increased to a maximum at a critical intravenous dose of 10^5 SRBC. As the dose was increased into the range which gives maximum antibody formation (10^8–10^9), all evidence of T cell

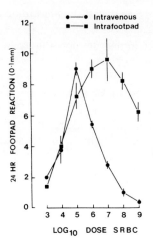

Fig. 25. Level of DTH generated in response to varying doses of SRBC. Antigen was administered i.v. or into a hind footpad; reactions were measured on days 4 and 5, respectively. Means of 5 ± SE. (*J. Exp. Med.*, **139,** 528, 1974).

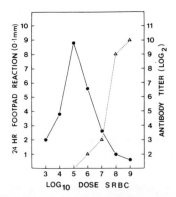

Fig. 26. Mean levels of DTH measured on day 4 (●—●), and of hemagglutinin titers (△----△) in pooled serum, also obtained on day 4. Mice were immunized intravenously with the indicated doses of SRBC. Means of 5 (*J. Exp. Med.*, **139,** 543, 1974).

activity was lost. Animals sensitized by footpad injection were obviously much less sensitive to whatever it is that blocks the induction of DTH at high antigen doses.

Figure 26 shows an inverse relationship between T cell activity, as measured by DTH, and the prevailing levels of mercaptoethanol-sensitive hemagglutinating antibody in circulation on day 4—the day when footpad sensitivity

216

was measured. Obviously, doses of antigen, which caused progressive blocking of T cells, caused increasing antibody formation.

If one allows the serum, taken on day 4 of the immune response to intravenous immunization with 10^9 SRBC, to react with SRBC, a process that removes most of the antibody from the serum, two interesting products are obtained: opsonized SRBC and serum with a reduced antibody titer. The former are completely ingested by macrophages within 1 hr of injection into the peritoneal cavity; nevertheless, they are apparently unaltered antigenically, for the antibody-treated SRBC were exactly like nonopsonized SRBC, they both produced maximum DTH at a dose of 10^5 (Fig. 27). The serum, on the other hand, after most of its antibody had been removed, suppressed the induction of DTH almost completely, regardless of the dose of SRBC. This implies that when antigen and immune serum interact, they produce a product which interferes with the induction of T cells.

Figure 28(a) shows that unabsorbed immune serum (US4) also partially suppresses the induction of DTH but is less active than absorbed serum (AS4). Moreover, the absorbed serum almost completely abolished an existing state of DTH when given to previously sensitized mice (Fig. 28b). It appears, therefore, that a product of the interaction of antigen and antibody has the capacity to prevent the primary induction of T cells and to block the mediators of DTH once they have been formed.

ALEXANDER: Can Mackaness get the same depression of delayed hypersensitivity with an unrelated serum that he got with the absorbed anti-SRBC?

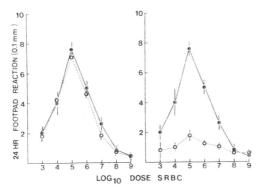

Fig. 27. Blocking of footpad reactivity to SRBC with absorbed immune serum. Left: the identical dose-response relationship for opsonized and unopsonized SRBC given i.v. Right: after absorption with an equal volume of SRBC, immune serum lost most of its agglutinating activity (from 1:1024 to 1:16), but nonetheless powerfully blocked induction of DTH when given i.v. (0.2 ml) just prior to antigen O----O. Absorbed normal serum control ●—●. *J. Exp. Med.*, **139**, 543, 1974).

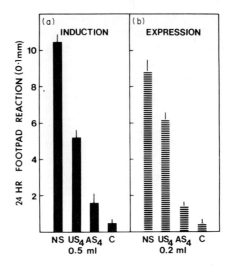

Fig. 28. Effect of absorbed and unabsorbed immune serum on the induction and expression of DTH. (a) Unabsorbed 4-day serum (US4) from mice immunized intravenously with 10^9 SRBC caused partial blocking of DTH when given immediately before a sensitizing footpad injection of 10^8 SRBC. After absorption with an equal volume of SRBC the same serum (AS4) blocked induction of DTH almost completely. DTH was measured 5 days after immunization. NS refers to recipients of normal serum absorbed with SRBC. C refers to unsensitized controls. Means of 5 ± SE. (b) The same absorbed and unabsorbed serum had a similar suppressive effect on previously established DTH in mice which had been sensitized 5 days earlier with 10^8 SRBC in one footpad. Serum (0.2 ml) was given intravenously 1 hr before the eliciting injection of SRBC (also 10^8). Means of 5 ± SE (*J. Exp. Med.* **139**, 543, 1974).

MACKANESS: The interference with established DTH is totally specific, provided that one uses antigens which do not cross react at the T cell level. It is interesting to note that red blood cells tend to cross react at the T cell level to an unsuspected degree. Sheep and burro, and sheep and goat, give cross reacting DTH reactions, but chicken and sheep do not. The blocking factors produced with chicken cells and serum of animals immunized with chicken red blood cells do not block hypersensitivity to sheep red cells.

CHAIRMAN KLEIN: At this point, Sjögren, Baldwin, and Alexander will describe some tumor-associated systems. Later we shall again return to MLC and H-2 models.

SJÖGREN: I shall summarize, in a condensed form, work performed on blocking in various tumor systems. This work was done with use of the colony-inhibition assay and then with the microplate lymphocyte-cytotoxicity assay. Two principal types of blocking have been studied by means of these assays.

The first detects blocking at the target cell level. Tumor target cells are plated and allowed to fix to the bottom surface of microwells. To study blocking at the target cell level, we add the serum to these tumor cells, and then we incubate for a period of time varying from a half-hour to one hour, after which excess serum is washed away. Then the effector lymphoid cells are added, and the extent to which the lymphocyte effect is abrogated is recorded as a measure of blocking.

The other method assays blocking at the effector cell level. This is performed by mixing the serum, or material under study, with effector cells, incubating, and then either adding this mixture to the target cells or adding lymphocytes *after* excess serum has been washed off. If the serum-lymphocyte mixture is added, the assay detects blocking both at the effector cell level and at the target cell level. When effector cells are first washed free of serum, before they are added to the target cells, the assay only detects effector cell blocking.

Table 28 summarizes the results obtained in a number of different animal systems and also with human tumors. The presence or absence of lymphocyte effector activity, blocking activity, homologous C'-dependent activity, and unblocking activity is indicated. In animal systems, the chance exists to predict the appearance of a tumor, and we can assay at various times before primary tumors are evident. Lymphocyte effector activity appears before the tumor can be detected by palpation or by giving discernible signs. Blocking activity can occasionally be detected a few weeks before a tumor is palpable, but in other cases blocking activity is not detected even a few days before the first nodule is felt. On the other hand, lymphocyte effector activity and blocking activity are present at the first appearance of visible tumors. This occurs in 100% of cases in some animal systems, in other systems, in less than 100%. In human

TABLE 28

Summary of Tumor Immune Status at Various Stages
of Tumor Growth

Status of tumor-bearing host	Lymphocyte effector activity	Blocking activity	Homologous C'-dependent activity	Unblocking activity
Before appearance of detectable tumor mass	+	±	?	?
In the course of progressive tumor growth	+	+	−	−
At final stages with widespread tumor growth	±	+	−	−
After complete tumor excision	+	−	+	+
At tumor recurrence upon incomplete tumor excision	+	+	?	−

systems, the figure is about 80% although this frequency varies in different reports.

In final stages of tumor growth, detectable lymphocyte effector activity is usually lower than in earlier stages. Blocking activity, on the other hand, does not seem to disappear or decrease, at least not as studied at the target cell level. After complete tumor excision in all experimental tumor systems studied and in most human patients, lymphocyte effector activity stays constant, even increases in some, but not all tumors. Blocking activity, in contrast, disappears rapidly after excision of tumor, tested either at the effector cell level or the target cell level. Even in instances in which the tumor is destined to recur, blocking disappears upon excision and then reappears. This means that, even when a limited number of cells remain after excision, blocking still disappears.

The nature of blocking factors in serum is defined by several pertinent items. First, blocking has the same specificity as lymphocyte cytotoxicity. This means that when virally induced tumors, which have common antigen(s) are studied, "cross blocking" is demonstrable from one tumor to the other. If the tumors have individually distinct antigens, no "cross blocking" is found. To study the nature of blocking factors, we absorbed sera with cultured tumor cells. We could show that the relevant tumor cells, but not unrelated tumor cells, absorbed all blocking activity from the sera. Most absorption studies were made testing blocking on the target cell level. In other experiments, blocking was tested on the effector cell level, and here cultured tumor cells were shown also to absorb blocking activity.

We next attempted to elute blocking activity from those tumor cells used for absorbing this activity. Blocking activity was indeed recovered in the supernatant after incubation of the cells in glycine buffer at pH 3.1. The characteristics of this activity were the same as those of the original blocking sera. Eluates, maintained at low pH, were then subject to Amicon filtration on filters with a cutoff level of either 100,000 daltons or 10,000 daltons. This gave filtrates or fractions of high (above 100,000) and low (10,000–100,000) MW.

In two different, but not cross-reacting, mouse-tumor systems, we tested such fractions for blocking at the target cell level. Neither of the fractions had any blocking activity. However, if we mixed the high and the low molecular weight fractions, blocking was demonstrable at the target cell level. When tested on the effector cell level, however, the high MW fraction had no blocking activity, while both the low MW fraction and the mixture were active. By using two non-cross-reacting tumors, we could also show that the specificity of blocking resided not only in the high MW fraction but also in the low MW fraction.

The conclusion from these studies was that the low MW fraction contained a tumor antigen (accounting for the specificity), and the high MW fraction contained an antitumor antibody. When these fractions were mixed, antigen–

antibody complexes were formed which blocked at the target cell as well as the effector cell level. Free antibody did not by itself block in the same concentration. This conclusion is strongly supported by recent experiments of Baldwin, which he will describe. Klein has asked whether we felt blocking was important *in vivo*. As I see it, there is, in the tumor-bearing individual, a balance between free tumor antigen(s), antigen–antibody complexes of various kinds, and free antibody. In different clinical situations, this balance may be shifted in different directions, depending on the level of antigen release and the rate of antibody formation. My experience so far is that, when an individual has a large tumor, most of the blocking activity seems to be in the form of complexes rather than as free antigen.

The question of the significance of blocking *in vivo* is an important question, but also a most difficult one to clarify. No definite proof of its *in vivo* function exists, but we know of three indications that this is the case. One is that antitumor antibodies or complexes can be shown to be absorbed onto tumor cells *in vivo*. This is a rather important finding, because it indicates that the tumor antigens expressed *in vivo* are accessible to antibodies. This has been shown by various techniques, including elution experiments with fresh tumor tissue taken directly from *in vivo*. Under circumstances which excluded passively trapped antibodies, antitumor antibody complexes could be eluted and shown to have blocking activity.

Further, passive transfer of blocking factors contained in tumor-bearer sera and tumor eluates at the same levels, giving readily detectable blocking activity in the sera of the recipients, result in specific facilitation of tumor-isograft growth. Animals with facilitated tumor growth developed lymphocyte cytotoxicity against the tumors in the same way as animals receiving control serum. This finding argues against afferent enhancement as the mechanism of the facilitated tumor growth.

A third piece of evidence, pointing to the importance of the blocking phenomenon for tumor growth *in vivo*, comes from studies on so-called "unblocking" activity of certain antitumor antisera. The sera are defined by their ability to counteract the blocking activity of tumor-bearing sera when admixed with them *in vitro*. When such sera are inoculated in rather large quantities into animals bearing the tumor in question, the serum blocking activity of the recipients may disappear completely. When this occurs, it is accompanied by tumor growth inhibition. This tends to indicate the importance of blocking factors in progressive tumor growth *in vivo*. These results do not give conclusive proof, since other effects of the "unblocking" sera might also be instrumental in tumor inhibition. As an example of such an alternative mechanism, one can mention that these sera are known to contain antibodies which are cytotoxic in the presence of complement.

We do not find antibody free of antigen that blocks. On the other hand, we can produce antisera by hyperimmunization that can, indeed, block. Baldwin has a similar experience. My interpretation of this is that tumor-bearer serum has not sufficient antibody concentration to block by itself but can block when the antibodies are forming complexes with soluble tumor antigen. A hyperimmune serum would contain enough antibodies to block at the target cell level without participation of antigen–antibody complexes.

CHAIRMAN KLEIN: In what system did you get these data?

SJÖGREN: The blocking activity of hyperimmune sera has been demonstrated in polyoma rat and mouse systems and also in adenovirus type-12 tumors in mice.

CHAIRMAN KLEIN: Was T cell killing rather dominant in that situation?

SJÖGREN: The microplate cytotoxicity assay was used and, according to present views, that would mean that both T and B cell killing were possible. Our experiments did not clarify which was the effector cell. While it is evident that antibodies may block by themselves, in the tumor-bearing individual they usually do not, probably because of insufficient concentration.

MACKANESS: In the system I have described, antibody does not block, and antigen does not block. It takes *both* antigen and antibody to prevent or suppress DTH.

In varying doses (10^6–10^9) of SRBC are given intravenously to normal or splenectonized mice, the normal animal, which produces antibody, shows progressive blocking with increasing antigen dose. The splenectomized animal, which produces almost no antibody, develops DTH in response to very high doses of antigen. The fact that DTH exists in the presence of vast quantities of antigen (10^9 SRBC given intravenously) shows that DTH is not suppressed by antigen alone.

Secondly, and I will bring out this point in greater detail later, BCG-infected mice develop very high levels of specific antibody but show no evidence of T cell blocking, except at the very highest levels of antigenic stimulation. For this and other reasons, I am equally sure that DTH is not suppressed by antibody alone.

HOWARD: It occurs to me that the antigen–antibody complex which appears to block even on the target cell, may be operating through the mechanism related by Eva Klein earlier. Antibody directed towards an antigenic constituent of the cell surface could sponsor antibody-mediated lymphocyte cytotoxicity, while the same determinant separated from the surface by a single layer of protein

222

could not serve as an adequate lytic target. Clearly an antigen–antibody complex could "inactivate" a cell surface in just this way without any significant change in the visibility of the antigen.

My problem, in the case of Sjögren's data, is that we have a target cell which expresses an antigen, then you put antibody and a second antigen on top of that, after which it is still antigenic. So what would be the explanation for the blocking activity? It might be a spacing effect, such as Eva Klein suggested.

SJÖGREN: This is a possibility, but what causes the blocking may be the antigen that comes off from the complex or, without coming off, reacts with lymphocytes directly. But we have no evidence, as yet, to support this view.

VAAGE: During the investigation of immune depression by excess tumor antigen, experimental animals showed specific immune depression in the presence of a large tumor. After the tumor was removed, the depression was maintained by injections of tumor antigen. The question was: Could the depression be maintained by injections of even large (1.5 ml) quantities of serum from a tumor-bearing, depressed animal? The answer was no!

In a second test, similar animals, recently cured of a large specifically depressing tumor, were injected with serum from non-tumor-bearing animals. The latter animals had been irradiated to preclude a primary immune response and then had been repeatedly injected subcutaneously and intraperitoneally with large quantities of killed tumor cells to flood their system with tumor antigen. The serum from these animals, presumably containing soluble tumor antigen, was injected into depressed mice recently relieved of their tumors. Under these conditions depression was sustained.

CHIECO-BIANCHI: It may well be significant that the serum blocking effect is detectable only by the microplate assay, whereas the other tests, particularly the ^{51}Cr-release assay, do not pick it up at all.

SHELLAM: I will be giving some evidence later on that. In the T cell cytotoxicity system, blocking occurs in a short-term assay; this is due to the effect of the serum antigen alone.

UHR: These data raise major problems for people interested in the biological role of the presumed antigen–antibody complexes in the circulation. We really need a good deal more information about the kind of complexes, not only their size, but also the class of immunoglobulin involved.

CHAIRMAN KLEIN: It seems to me that it is rather remarkable the way the field has been moving. We had been led to believe, mainly by workers who demonstrated enhancement in the H-2 system, that antibody was responsible for enhancement. It was, therefore, natural to think that antibody was also responsible for blocking lymphocytotoxicity *in vitro*. In fact, antibody could be shown to inhibit T cell cytotoxicity in the direct, short-term killing systems. When experiments were started, on tumor-associated antigen systems in animals and also in patients, using *in vitro* lymphocytotoxicity, the first thought was that serum blocking was due to antibody as well. However, it was hard to understand why the blocking effect would disappear when the tumor was removed. As you will recall, it was thought that perhaps a different kind of antibody appears as immunization proceeds and that it blocks no longer, perhaps due to a change in affinity. It was hard to see, however, how this could happen relative to tumor removal in so many different species and so many different tumors. The more recent evidence, as we have heard here, points in a different direction. It now seems that antigen rather than antibody alone or in the form of antigen–antibody complexes, is responsible for the blocking in the tumor-associated antigen systems. This would be much easier to understand, because antigen is what a tumor can produce, and a change in blocking status with removal of the tumor burden would be entirely rational. Moreover, antigen–antibody complexes could block T and B cells as well, and this would be a nice model. Antigen as such would be able to inhibit both T and B cells, even though there remains some question about whether antigen alone can do this, as far as T cells are concerned.

Can antibody alone really block *any* tumor-associated antigen system? With the antibody-dependent cytotoxicity, as described by Perlmann and by MacLennan, it seems that antibody, at least certain classes of it, would be beneficial, rather than harmful. Is it, therefore, possible that the H-2 system has introduced a rather important bias into this field? This would be due to the close linkage between H-2 and the very strong T-cell stimulator locus that is designated by various names. If T cell stimulation and differentiation into killer cells dominates lymphocyte-defined, H-2–linked differences, this will perhaps lead to the overwhelming impression that only T cells can kill (as was believed a few years ago) and, in relation to this, that antibody blocks. I am specifically asking questions concerning the relative role of antibody in blocking versus promotion of antibody-dependent lymphocytotoxicity, the relative roles these effects play in tumor-associated antigen systems, and, of course, whether all this is related to the relative roles played by T and non-T cells in the killing of tumor cells carrying tumor-associated or tissue-specific antigens. I would very much like our conferees to state their position on this.

PERLMANN: Klein should put a parenthesis (or question mark for antigen inhibition) around T cells rather than B cells. There is good evidence that cell-mediated *in vitro* killing of tumor cells by non-T effector cells can be inhibited by soluble antigen, most likely by neutralization of the antibodies involved and by formation of inhibitory antigen–antibody complexes. To my knowledge, there is less unequivocal evidence for inhibition of T killer cells by soluble antigen *in vitro*.

UHR: There are many techniques that could be brought to bear on the nature of the complexes in the circulation of tumor-bearing animals. It would be very interesting to attempt to fractionate these complexes by sedimentation. High speed centrifugation in gradients would allow fractionation of complexes of different sizes. The relationship of size of complex to particular biological functions could then be determined. The binding of radioactive complement by complexes of different sizes could be studied, and the role of complement, if any, in causing the different biological functions of complexes could be determined.

At a simpler level, more evidence is needed that the various blocking phenomena described are all due to antigen–antibody complexes and not to free antigen. By means of ammonium sulphate precipitation, antigen in the form of antigen–antibody complexes can be precipitated and, thus, separated from "free" antigen. Heterologous antibody to immunoglobulin can also be used to precipitate antigen bound to antibody. In fact, there is a large immunochemical armamentarium that could be brought to bear on this problem. I believe that such an approach is essential to an understanding of the biological effects of tumor antigens in the circulation.

CHAIRMAN KLEIN: I agree, but I would add that this approach would be really efficient only if the antigen–antibody system is well defined. It will not be really feasible with the relatively clumsy lymphocytotoxicity assay. I cannot escape the conclusion that the development of serological systems, with identified antigens and antibodies, are needed to work this out.

UHR: I agree that it would be optimal to have purified characterized antigens, but I do think we can obtain significant information from the systems available.

MARTIN: Before attributing too much suppressive activity to complexes and blocking factors, it should be noted that the presence of any immune cells *to be blocked* indicates the overall ineffectiveness of blocking factors.

CHAIRMAN KLEIN: This may be related to the fact that lymphocytes are washed and incubated in the course of these tests. It is conceivable that they may free themselves from attached antigen, perhaps by capping or cappinglike mechanisms, and recover rather quickly, whereas they might still be relatively inefficient *in vivo*.

225

MARTIN: Assuming continual production of tumor antigen, then in order to maintain complexes, continual antibody production must be occurring in parallel. These cells, at least, are not being switched off by complexes.

BALDWIN: Studies, which I shall now present, relate to aminoazo-induced tumors in syngeneic rats where individually distinct rejection antigens are demonstrable, making them ideal for studying modification of immunity in tumor-bearing hosts. Serum factors in tumor-bearing hosts which modify cell-mediated immunity may be measured in two ways:

Blocking may occur by binding of serum factors to neo-antigens expressed upon tumor cells, thus preventing cellular recognition by sensitized effector cells. This we view as being mediated in the tumor-bearing host by tumor-specific immune complexes, although antibody alone can elicit this effect.

Inhibition of effector cell reactivity may also occur. We view this to be produced by circulating tumor-specific antigen or immune complexes.

The evidence for the involvement of tumor-specific immune complexes in blocking by heat-inactivated serum from tumor-bearing rats is as follows:

1. Tumor-bearer sera, showing blocking activity, do not usually contain significant levels of tumor-specific antibody, demonstrable by complement-dependent cytotoxicity or membrane immunofluorescence.

2. Surgical excision of a developing tumor rapidly (within 72 hr) results in the almost complete loss of serum blocking activity. At this stage, however, these postexcision sera contain demonstrable levels of tumor-specific antibody, since they show complement-dependent cytotoxicity for cells of the appropriate tumor.

3. In comparison with the lack of blocking activity in postexcision sera, sera taken from rats having rejected several challenges with viable tumor cells (i.e., hyperimmunized hosts), block tumor cells from attack by sensitized lymph node cells. These sera contain tumor-specific antibody demonstrable by membrane immunofluorescence staining of viable tumor cells or by complement-dependent cytotoxicity. This suggests that the failure to observe blocking by antibody in postexcision sera reflects concentration differences, although the alternative possibility that these sera contain different classes of antibody has not been excluded.

4. Probably the most conclusive evidence that the blocking factor in tumor-bearer serum is immune complex is provided by "unblocking" tests (Fig. 29). Thus, the blocking activity of tumor-bearer serum can be specifically abrogated by the addition of either postexcision (PE) or tumor-immune (TI) sera, the latter being most effective. In this case, it is highly significant that mixing two sera, namely tumor-bearer and TI, both of which block alone, neutralizes this reactivity. These observations are interpreted to indicate that addition of TI serum, containing specific antibody, neutralizes an antigen-containing factor in the tumor-bearer serum.

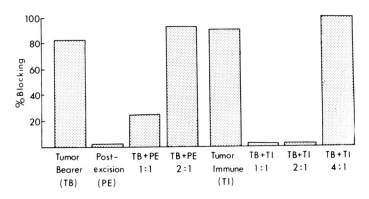

Fig. 29. Reversal of blocking activity of tumor-bearer serum by post-excision serum or tumor-immune serum. Cytoxicity was determined by the reduction of survival *in vitro* of tumor cells exposed to lymph node cells (LNC) from tumor-immune rats compared with controls exposed to LNC of normal rats. Blocking activity was then determined from reduction of the cytotoxicity following preexposure of tumor cells to serum or serum mixtures, these being removed before addition of LNC. Tumor-bearer serum was obtained from rats bearing established hepatoma grafts. Postexcision sera were taken 10–14 days after surgical resection of hepatoma transplants, while tumor-immune sera were from rats immunized with γ-irradiated (15,000 R), hepatoma tissue and immune to challenge with viable hepatoma cells (5×10^5). All of the sera were inactivated at 56°C for 30 min (*Cancer*, in press, 1974).

This conclusion, that immune complexes are involved in blocking *in vitro* cytotoxicity of sensitized lymph node cells for the appropriate tumor, is also supported by our published studies, showing that addition of purified hepatoma D_{23}·antigen to post-excision serum (which contains antibody but at a level where blocking is not observed) results in the appearance of this activity.

Serum from tumor-bearing rats can also interfere with cell-mediated immunity by specific inhibition of sensitized effector cells. This is illustrated in Fig. 30 which shows that, as with blocking, preexposure of sensitized lymph node cells (from a tumor-immune donor), to tumor-bearer serum inhibits their reactivity. Again, these factors are rapidly eliminated from the host after total resection of the tumor, but, unlike blocking sera, tumor-immune sera are inactive. This indicates that the effects are not mediated by antibody, and the view is held that this is due either to free circulating antigen or immune complexes. In support of this, it can be seen (Fig. 30) that the inhibitory factor in tumor-bearer serum is neutralized by the addition of appropriate amounts of either post-excision or tumor-immune sera, the latter being most effective. The specific factor in tumor-bearer serum still has to be characterized, but there is convincing evidence that fractions containing soluble tumor-specific antigen are effective. This was emphasized in model studies showing that addition of purified hepatoma D_{23} antigen to sensitized lymph node cells specifically inhibited their reactivity. Comparable studies with human tumors (melanoma, carcinoma

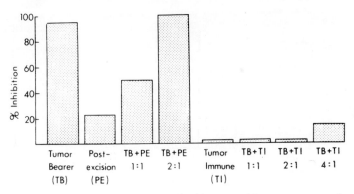

Fig. 30. Inhibitor in tumor-bearer serum is neutralized by postexcision serum or tumor-immune serum. The cytotoxicity of hepatoma-immune lymph node cells was inhibited by preincubation with serum from tumor-bearing rats (see Fig. 29 for details of serum donors). Postexcision sera did not inhibit LNC reactivity. On the contrary, these sera, when added to tumor-bearer serum, reduced the latter's inhibitory capacity (neutralization of inhibition). Tumor-immune serum did not itself inhibit LNC cytotoxicity, and these sera were more effective in neutralizing the inhibitory reactivity of tumor-bearer serum. (*Cancer*, in press, 1974).

of the colon and breast) have established that the reactivity of peripheral blood lymphocytes can be neutralized by adding papain-solubilized tumor membrane.

These findings indicate that a variety of serum factors, including antigen, antibody, and immune complexes, may act to modify cell-mediated immunity. For this reason, it becomes necessary to specify which reactants are present in tumor-bearer serum. This is illustrated by the data in Fig. 31 showing that, during the growth of hepatoma D_{23} at a subcutaneous site, circulating tumor-specific antigen is early demonstrated in the serum. At the time when a significant immunity begins to develop (days 10–14), there is rapid loss of tumor antigen, and, at this time, immune complexes become detectable. Finally, in the late stages of tumor growth, excess free antibody is present in addition to immune complexes.

The total contribution of these factors in the serum of tumor-bearing hosts has yet to be resolved; because blocking reactions can be observed with sera from tumor-*immune* rats, it is, however, felt that free antigen or immune complexes operating against effector cells are more important.

STUTMAN: I will comment on the effect of antigen and of antibody on *in vitro* and *in vivo* immune reactions to mouse mammary tumors. As already described, the antigens in the mammary tumor system are complex, but some are defined. This heterogeneity makes the problem of antigen–antibody complexes too involved right now; I can give some opinions, but there are few facts on this subject. The generation of immune lymphocytes used in the cytotoxicity assay is always by *in vivo* immunization. Animals are injected with syngeneic tumor, the tumor is surgically resected, and the lymphocytes are obtained from

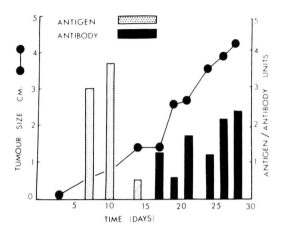

Fig. 31. Serum levels of hepatoma D23 specific antigen and antibody. Serum taken from rats at intervals after subcutaneous implantation of hepatoma D23 were assayed for the presence of tumor-specific antigen and antibody. Tumor-specific antibody was determined by the membrane immuno-fluorescence staining of tumor-bearer serum with hepatoma D23 cells. Tumor-specific antigen was assayed by the capacity of tumor-bearer serum to neutralize antibody in a reference D23 serum, again using membrane immunofluorescence (*Brit. J. Cancer*, in press, 1974).

different sources (i.e., lymph nodes, thoracic duct, spleen, etc.). The assay system is a T-dependent cytotoxic assay *in vitro* using prelabelled adherent target cells. The first set of experiments are related to the effect of solubilized tumor antigens (mainly ML and some MTV antigens, whether obtained by $3M$ KCl treatment or released spontaneously from tumor cells grown in protein-free medium) on the cytotoxic capacity of immune lymphocytes.

The experiments consisted of incubating immune lymphocytes with antigen, washing 6 times, then adding those lymphocytes to prelabeled target cells. The results obtained (Tables 29 and 30) depend on two variables: One is the amount of antigen to which the lymphocytes are exposed, and the other is the time, at a constant antigen dose, during which they were exposed. Table 29 shows the effect of incubating 1×10^6 immune lymphocytes with different concentrations of antigen for 30 min. The incubation mixture volume was one ml. When cells were used at a 100:1 ratio, the cells alone would destroy 33% of the target.

After incubation with low doses of antigen (from 10–50 μg, we observed activation and more efficient killing (Table 31). But when we increased the antigen dose to 300 μg, net inhibition of cytotoxicity occurred. This is not a toxic effect because antigen from other tumors (MC) was ineffective. It is inhibition of the magnitude we produced *in vitro* when we add blocking serum.

Table 31 shows the effect of duration of incubation (at a constant rate of 30 μg of protein) on lymphocyte cytotoxicity. After 30 min or 6 hr, there was clear activation. As in the previous experiments, after the different incubations

TABLE 29
Effect of Preincubation of Immune Lymphocytes with Varying Amounts of Ag

L/T ratio	Antigen[a]	Target loss %
100:1	none	33
100:1	MT: 10 μg	78
100:1	MT: 20 μg	88
100:1	MT: 30 μg	79
100:1	MT: 50 μg	67
100:1	MT: 100 μg	59
100:1	MT: 300 μg	16
100:1	MC: 30 μg	37
100:1	MC: 300μg	20

[a] Antigen incubated with immune lymph node lymphocytes at the indicated concentrations (per ml and per 1×10^6 cells) for 30 min, washed 6 times, and added to target cells (prelabeled with 3H-thymidine or proline). Antigen solubilized from mammary tumor (MT) or methylcholanthrene sarcoma cells grown in tissue culture (MC) by $3M$ KCl.

TABLE 30
Effect of Incubation Conditions on Reactivity of Immune Lymphocytes with Ag

L/T ratio	Duration of incubation[a]	Target loss %
100:1	30 min	77
100:1	6 hr	85
100:1	12 hr	57
100:1	18 hr	48
100:1	24 hr	30
100:	none (no Ag)	33
500:1	24 hr	44
500:1	none (no Ag)	69

[a] Antigen at concentrations of 30 μg protein/ml/10 $\times$ 10^6 (see footnote, Table 29).

TABLE 31
Blocking Serum: Activity of Ig Digests

Type of "serum"	Target loss %
No serum	79
Whole serum	10
IgG (DEAE chrom)	12
F(ab)2 (pepsin + Sephadex G-150)	13
Fab (Papain + cysteine, 1 hr)	13
Fab (same, 4 hr)	16
Fab (same, 4 hr + Sephadex G-100)	13
Fab (same, 18 hr)	14
Fc	75

Separation of Fab digest: starch gel (45×30 cm), 17 hr at 400 V in the cold; Fab: 2 to 4 cm; Fc: 8 to 10 cm cuts. Protein concentration adjusted to 0.5 to 1.1 mg/ml. Prelabeled target was incubated with antibody fragments for 30 min washed 3 times, and then immune lymphocytes at 500:1 ratio were added. The incubation was continued for 36 hr.

the lymphocytes were washed and then added to the target, usually at 100:1 lymphocyte–target ratios. As the duration of incubation increased the response constantly decreased. At 24 hr, the levels were comparable to those obtained by immune lymphocytes at the ratio 100:1 not exposed to antigen. Thus, we do not call this real inhibition. Apparently, the effect of antigen alone on immune T lymphocytes is complex.

The next problem was the effect of antibody at target cell level. In this particular experiment (Table 31), we incubated the target for 30 min with purified immunoglobulin from serum with blocking activity derived from immune mice, or with Ig digests prepared from such serum. The cells were washed 3 times and the immune lymphocytes were added—in this case, at an optimal killing ratio of 500:1. The antibodies are derived from immunized animals. The lymphocytes are also derived from immunized animals, and the hosts for this experiment were MTV-negative animals, so that they can technically react with every antigen in the mammary tumor. Lymphocytes alone kill 79% of target, which is a very consistent response in this system. The whole serum completely blocked cytotoxicity. Ten percent target loss is the maximum level of negativity that we accept. IgG blocked, and, in fact, all IgG subclasses block (not shown in the table). IgM does not block, and we have not tested IgA yet. Table 31 also shows that monovalent Fab fragments from IgG also had the ability to block lymphocyte cytotoxicity. This suggests that, because the effect is specific and there is only one combining site left, the effect is probably the result of action of the antibody, or the half molecule of antibody on the target cell.

As I outlined earlier, one of the antigens involved in the system, ML, is readily modulated. The antibody used in this particular set of experiments has a very powerful anti-ML activity. We know from the TL data that monovalent Fab fragments are capable of modulating such antigen, so I think that this example of blocking at the target cell level by antibody may be related to modulation.

CHAIRMAN KLEIN: Does Stutman think that his system is really quite exceptional? Could this be related to the modulation effect described? Is it also possible that the lymphocytes are not properly activated *in vivo* because the antigen modulates away, and this is why they would be better available to activation *in vitro* than in other, less modulatable systems?

PERNIS: Stutman stated that IgM does not block, but, perhaps, that is not a fair statement. The simple fact is that there are no IgM antibodies in this hyperimmune serum because all of the antibody is IgG. Perhaps, if he had used antibodies earlier in immunization than IgM would block. It will be important to decide this.

STUTMAN: I realize that, and it is a valid argument. Immunized animals were animals that had tumors growing for ten days, and then the tumor was amputated; there are limitations on how we immunize the animals. Perhaps, if we use irradiated cells for immunization, we could shift towards different Ig classes and have a better answer. Regarding immunoglobulin class, it is important to remember that the concentration of the different immunoglobulins in serum varies. The catabolic rate is different, and actually the amount of specific antibody of a certain Ig class that the mouse can produce after antigenic stimulation, as well as the rate of production, are also different.

PERNIS: I found Stutman's data on the effects of monomeric Fab in modulation troublesome. It has, in fact, been stated by Boyse that monomeric Fab would modulate. However, one must be very careful that, in the Fab preparation used, a small amount of aggregates, which are, in fact, polymeric, do not remain as this would establish the cross linking, which is likely to be an essential factor in modulating events.

STUTMAN: We were aware of that and tested several Fab preparations trying to get as clean a preparation as possible. If one does the same experiment *in vivo*, using preimmunized animals injected with small numbers of tumor cells known to be rejected, blocking occurs if tumor cells were incubated with antibody before injection. Under those conditions, cells pretreated with blocking serum produce 30% growing tumors, while cells incubated with irrelevant serum are rejected. This effect is not seen when a Fab fragment of IgG, having demonstrable *in vitro* blocking activity, is used.

HALL: Is complement provided?

STUTMAN: No complement is added. The mixture contains inactivated serum, lymphocytes, and target, but not added complement.

TERRY: The clearance of Fab is very different from that of intact IgG, so I do not think that your experiment is a fair negative test of the biologic effect of Fab.

STUTMAN: It is stuck to antigen.

TERRY: Yes, but that binding presumably reflects an equilibrium reaction, and once dissociated, the Fab will disappear in hours, while intact IgG will remain in the circulation for days.

MARTIN: The assumption that, in this system, high antigen concentration is directly inhibitory to cytotoxic T lymphocytes contrasts with other studies which indicate the difficulty of direct inactivation of cytotoxic cells with antigen. Possibly, therefore, some form of indirect suppression occurs. Lymphocyte populations in Stutman's work would probably contain lymphoid cells which can respond to antigen by blast transformation or by the elaboration of MIF, lymphotoxin, etc. These factors may nonspecifically suppress the activity of cytotoxic lymphocytes. Has Stutman tested a cell population immune to two cellular antigens to see whether the addition of one antigen will interfere with the cytotoxic activity of cells responsive to another antigen?

STUTMAN: We have not done that type of experiment. In the short incubation period used (30 min), blast transformation is minimal. After longer incubation, we tried to separate blasts by velocity flotation at unit gravity. Indeed, purified blasts were not very good killers. Some of these results may be explained by blast formation and also by unfavorable culture conditions for blast survival. We may be selecting against blasts. I agree that there are problems in this model, but we have heard of the problems in practically every model.

The type of response obtained in the mammary tumor system depends on the host used for immunization. Here we are concerned with what antigens the host can recognize and what responses it can produce. In Table 32, cytotoxic lymphocyte and cytotoxic antibody activities, and whether blocking occurs, are charted. Depending upon the type of lymphocyte donor used for immunization, different responses are obtained. If the MTV animal is immunized or hyperimmunized with mammary tumor (Group 1, Table 32), a good cytotoxic lympho-

TABLE 32

The Complexities of the Immune Response to Mammary Tumors in Mice

Type of donor of lymphocytes or antibodies	Cytotoxic lymphocytes	Antibodies in serum	
		Cytotoxic	Blocking
1. MTV − immunized with MT (MTV+)	+++	++	+
2. MTV + immunized with MT (MTV+)	+	+	+
3. MTV + with spontaneous growing MT	+	±	±
4. MTV + normal (at least 3 months old)	+	−	+
5. MTV − normal (any age)	−	−	−

1.   In group 1, blocking antibody (b1.Ab) blocks mainly type 1 cytotoxic lymphocytes (ly) and acts on target, probably through modulation.

2.   b1.Ab. from group 2 blocks LY from groups 2, 3 and 4.

3.   b1.Ab. from group 2 blocks LY from groups 2, 3, and 4. B and C are most probably immune complexes.

4.   Cytotoxic Ab from groups 2 and 3 usually potentiates Ly from that group, but not from group 1. Cytotoxic Ab from group 1 potentiates or blocks (depending on concentration) Ly only from group 1.

5.   b1.Ab from group 4 blocks mainly Ly from group 4 and, to a lesser extent, from group 3.

6.   Group 5 represents the C3Hf-virus-free strain. In DBA/2 and in Balb/c, cytotoxic lymphocytes can be detected in old (more than 6 months old) animals and, in some cases, blocking antibodies, which are apparently directed against a different antigen from those above. These strains are infected with MTV-L.

7.   Both the antigen detected by the type 1 system as well as the antigens detected by the 3–2 and the 4 groups are cross reacting *within* groups.

cyte response results, which is mediated mainly by T cells. This animal responds to the three main antigens, ML, MTV, and P. MTV-mice also produce cytotoxic antibodies, even complement dependent and blocking factors.

We observe two types of blocking effects. These experiments were done by adding the serum first, washing gently, and then adding the immune lymphocytes, similar to Sjögren's report, but using prelabeled adherent cells at 500:1 lymphocyte–tumor ratios. With serum that has only blocking activity, we get simple dilution curves, and usually the titer is about 1:16. At high concentration, it blocks, and, with dilution of the serum, no more blocking is detected. This is understandable. With sera containing the complement-dependent cytotoxic antibody, we get a different dilution curve. At high concentration of antibody, potentiation is seen from approximately 70% target loss for cells alone, to approximately 90% at low dilutions (1:4 to 1:16). At intermediate levels (1:32 to 1:128), a certain degree of blocking occurs, which is never of the level of the "pure" blocking. The blocking obtained with "pure" blocking serum completely protects the target (10–16% target loss), while the blocking produced by dilution of serum containing cytotoxic antibodies is of the order of 30–35% target loss (versus 70–75% for the cells alone, in absence of blocking). Upon further dilution, the effect is lost.

When MTV-positive animals are used (Group 2, Table 32) which react against ML and the private antigens, the magnitude of cytotoxic-lymphocyte response observed is much less (30–40% target loss at 500:1 ratios). In this instance, antibody-dependent lymphocyte cytotoxicity is responsible for approximately half of the cytotoxicity, the other half being mediated by T cells. We cannot find conventional cytotoxic antibodies, but we do find blocking factors in serum. The picture is somewhat similar in an MTV-positive animal with its own growing mammary tumor (Group 3, Table 32). Cytotoxic lymphocytes are present, but blocking is not easy to detect in serum (approximately 40% of the tumor-bearing mice have no blocking factors in their serum). We still do not know what this means.

Normal animals (Groups 4 and 5, Table 32), whether MTV-infected, infected only with the low pathogen MTV, or completely virus free, show spontaneous age-dependent activity of their lymphocytes, either as blast response toward soluble antigen or cytotoxicity on target tumor cells. It should be stressed that such animals have *no* tumors. It probably represents the response of the animal to his own virus. We can also detect in its serum factors that block cytotoxic lymphocytes. In mice—free of conventional, milk-borne MTV, but infected with MTV-L—the low pathogenic virus gives results similar to those in the MTV-positive mice. Here, we find something in serum that can be detected by immunofluorescence on target cells and has blocking activity against cytotoxic lymphocytes. None of these "spontaneous" activities in cells or serum are detected at any age in virus-free mice (Group 5, Table 32). Using these different possibilities, we can analyze the interaction of serum factors and cells on target cell destruction *in vitro* and *in vivo*. We are finding some puzzling responses, but we believe that it is a valid model.

ALEXANDER: I would like to describe some work by Thomson and Currie on interference by circulating antigen with the efferent arm of the immune response to tumors, emphasizing particularly its relationship to metastatic spread.

The first indication that antigen shed by a growing tumor may assist in "escape" came from studies which showed that the nodes draining a tumor, although highly stimulated, did not function normally. The observed impairment was ascribed to the combination of stimulated lymphocytes with antigen, which was continually being released from the tumor (Alexander, et al., (Proc. Roy. Soc. B., **174**, 237, 1969). Since then, evidence has been accumulating that tumor-specific membrane antigens which constitute the point of attack by the host on the autochthonous tumor are present in a soluble form in body fluids (e.g., blood, lymph, and urine) of the tumor bearer (see Table 33). They are effective in providing escape because they combine with the effector arms (antibodies as well as some types of specifically cytotoxic cells) and thereby neutralize them. Moreover, in a soluble form, the tumor antigens are very poor immunogens, at least in the absence of adjuvants. In other words, when soluble these antigens do not stimulate the immune defenses but, nonetheless, inhibit the antibodies and cytotoxic cells that are produced when the same antigens are presented to the host as part of a plasma membrane.

Table 33 summarizes the methods that have been used to demonstrate the presence of soluble substances in the molecular weight range of 50,000 daltons in the blood, lymph, and urine of both man and rats with tumors, and which have the immunological properties to be expected of tumor antigens. Materials with the same immunological properties as these serum components have been isolated by papain digestion of membranes derived from melanomas and hypernephromas (Currie, unpublished). From a rat sarcoma, one of the tumor antigens was obtained in a high state of purity by affinity chromatography (Thomson, Sellens, Eccles, and Alexander, *Brit. J. Cancer,* **28,** 377, 1973). By radioimmunoassay criteria, the antigen isolated from the tumor could not be dis-

TABLE 33

Methods for Detecting Soluble Tumor-Specific Transplantation
Antigen (TSTA) in Body Fluids

I. Inhibition of cytotoxicity of mononuclear cells from blood or lymph nodes of tumor bearers:

in man (Currie and Basham, *Brit. J. Cancer,* 26, 427, 1972)

in rats (Currie and Gage, *Brit. J. Cancer,* 28, 136, 1973)

II. Serological:

Neutralization of syngeneic antiserum obtained from rats after excision of tumor (Thomson, Steele, and Alexander, *Brit. J. Cancer,* 27, 27, 1973).

Radioimmunoassay using ^{125}I-labeled TSTA isolated from tumor by affinity chromatography (Thomson, Sellens, Eccles, and Alexander, *Brit. J. Cancer,* 28, 377, 1973).

---

tinguished from the circulating antigen found in the serum of tumor-bearing rats.

Detailed studies showed that there are three distinct mechanisms by which antigen gains access to the circulation in a soluble form:

1. *By autolysis of tumor cells:* When tumor cells are injected s.c. into nonimmune rats, circulating antigens appear within 24 hr in the blood of both normal and immunosuppressed rats. It is well established that the majority of cells administered as s.c. inoculum undergo rapid autolysis and that only a minority survive to give rise to the transplantable tumor. Antigen introduced in this way is cleared within a few days.

2. *As a consequence of immune attack:* With some tumors, like the MC-1 rat sarcoma, soluble antigen cannot be detected in the serum of immunosuppressed (i.e., after whole-body X-irradiation) tumor-bearing rats. We interpret these data to show that the soluble antigens appear because tumor cells are being lysed by the immune reactions of the host. However, in the case of another chemically induced rat tumor, the MC-3 sarcoma, circulating antigen can be detected in the serum of immunosuppressed rats bearing this tumor (Currie, unpublished).

TABLE 34

Detection of Soluble TSTA in Tumor-Bearing
Serum and in Tissue Culture Supernatant of
Sarcoma Cell Cultures by Inhibition of Specific
Cytotoxicity of Lymph Node Cells

Test system[a]	Inhibitor added from either tumor-bearing serum or tissue culture supernatant	Target cells killed %	Inhibition of killing %
MC-1 tumor cells con-	None	65	—
fronted with lymph-	MC-1 serum	0(−3)	100
node cells from rats	MC-3 serum	68	0
with MC-1 tumor	HSN serum	63	2
	MC-1 supernatant	59	9.5
	MC-3 supernatant	67	0
	HSN supernatant	60	9.0
MC-3 tumor cells	None	47	—
confronted with lymph-	MC-3 serum	8	84
node cells from rats	MC-1 serum	44	6
with MC-3 tumor	HSN serum	45	5
	MC-3 supernatant	1	98
	HSN supernatant	41	12
	MC-1 supernatant	39	17

[a]The tumors used were transplantable rat sarcomas syngeneic to the hooded strain. The MC-1 and MC-3 tumors were induced by methylcholanthrene and the HSN by benzpyrene. In these three tumors, individually specific transplantation antigens were demonstrated by grafting techniques.

3. *By spontaneous release:* Table 34 illustrates a series of experiments in which the presence of soluble antigen in serum and tissue culture supernatants was determined by measuring the capacity of these fluids to inhibit the cytotoxic action of immune lymph node cells to specific tumor cells *in vitro*, as described by Currie and Gage (*Brit. J. Cancer,* **28,** 136, 1973). The immune lymphoid cells were obtained from nodes draining growing tumors. It is evident that the serum of tumor-bearing rats exerts a specific inhibitory activity towards cells cytotoxic to either the MC-1 or MC-3 sarcoma cells. However, while the supernatant from tissue cultures of the MC-3 sarcoma had a similar inhibitory activity on the serum from MC-3 tumor bearers, only minimal activity was found in the supernatant of MC-1 sarcoma cultures. We conclude that the rate of spontaneous shedding of tumor antigens by growing tumor cells is much higher for the MC-3 than the MC-1 sarcoma.

We also examined the relationship between the rate of spontaneous shedding of surface antigen and the capacity to metastasize. The MC-1 and MC-3 sarcomas differ not only in the rate which they shed antigen *in vitro*, but they also have quite diverse growth patterns *in vivo* (see Table 35). The MC-1 tumor does not metastasize spontaneously in normal (i.e., not immunosuppressed rats), and rats can be cured of both i.m. and s.c. tumors by surgical excision, even when these are quite large. The MC-3 tumor, however, metastasizes rapidly both by blood-borne and lymphatic spread, and local surgery as early as seven days after an i.m. implant of tumor is unsuccessful. All the rats so treated die of distant metastases. Initially, we were inclined to attribute the metastatic

TABLE 35
Comparison of Two Chemically Induced
Transplantable Rat Sarcomas

Property	MC-1 sarcoma	MC-3 sarcoma
Growth pattern *in vivo*	Local only, curable by surgery	Metastasizes to nodes and lung
Resistance to challenge following hyper-immunization with irradiated sarcoma cells	Powerful protection	No protection
Specific *in vitro* cytotoxicity lymphoid cells from nodes draining the tumor	+++	+ + +
Soluble TSTA in serum of tumor-bearers		
a) Normal	+ +	+ +
b) Immunosuppressed	−	+ +
Soluble TSTA detected in tissue culture supernatant	−	+ +

behavior of the MC-3 to its being nonimmunogenic, because it proved impossible to immunize rats even against a challenge with as few as 10^2 cells by repeated immunization with irradiated MC-3 cells. Immunity to the MC-1 sarcoma on the other hand could readily be induced by this immunization procedure. This is not, however, the correct interpretation, because *in vitro* tests showed that the growing MC-3 tumor evokes a powerful immune response when measured by the *in vitro* cytotoxic activity of the cells in the draining node. Indeed, by this test the antigenicity of the MC-3 is not markedly inferior to or quantitatively different from that of the MC-1 tumor (see Table 34). The fact that the growing MC-3 sarcoma elicits an immune response in the syngeneic host is further demonstrated by the fact that a rat with a growing MC-3 tumor shows specific concomitant immunity if challenged at a distant site with MC-3 cells.

The capacity of the MC-3 sarcoma to metastasize and the failure to induce immunity to it with irradiated cells cannot, therefore, be attributed to the absence of tumor-specific antigens. It is tempting to associate these properties of MC-3 sarcoma cells with their ability to shed antigens in a soluble form. A metastatic deposit of MC-3 cells may avoid destruction by the host because it is enveloped by soluble antigen which intercepts the host's defenses. The rate of shedding of antigen may determine the size of the tumor that can escape from the immune defenses. If the amount of antigen that is shed is low, then only relatively large tumor masses will be protected and metastases will be eliminated by the host—this is presumed to be the case for the MC-1 sarcoma. If shedding is intense, then even small tumor foci will escape—hence, the high rate of spontaneous metastatic spread of the MC-3, and its capacity to be transplanted with a very few cells.*

CHAIRMAN KLEIN: This brings us back to the discussions in the first session about the differences between lysis, shedding and ligand-induced shedding. Of course, if *in vivo* correlations can be shown between any of these phenomena and ability to metastasize or grow on a large number of tumors, this would be of extraordinary importance.

Until now, we have had several demonstrations of blocking by antigen-antibody complexes and by antigen alone. We heard some evidence of antibody blocking, but it was my impression that those who were testifying about it did

---

Editors' comment: These data, and the interpretation Alexander gives them, have one important ramification not brought out clearly at the time of the Conference. Nonimmunogenicity of tumors is herein defined in terms of *in vitro* reactivity and elicitation of concomitant immunity *in vivo*, rather than in terms of the usual model, in which failure to immunize to retransplanted tumor is the end point. As pointed out by several conferees earlier and in a prior footnote, *in vitro* reactions are universally detected in cells responding to so-called nonimmunogenic tumors. This emphasis broadens our concept of tumor immunogenicity and focuses attention on the factors which prevent or repress the immunogenic potential of tumors by transplantation criteria.

not emphasize it, and they also emphasized antigen-antibody complexes, rather than antibody. One very definite exception is in the data of Stutman, suggesting that antigen can lead to activation, rather than blocking, as long as it is present in small doses, and it is rather important to underline the dosage dependence of this phenomenon.

SHELLAM: In this context, I shall discuss some preliminary evidence for blocking in a strongly immunogenic system, that of the immune response of rats to a Gross virus-induced lymphoma (C 58NT).

With Knight, I have studied the effect of either serum from tumor-bearing rats or of virus alone on cell-mediated immunity, measured *in vitro* using a four hour ^{51}Cr-release assay. In the majority of rats injected with 10^8 cells, tumor growth is abrupt and rejection follows in about 9 or 10 days. Only a small percentage of injected rats show progressive growth of tumors; in immunosuppressed rats, progressive growth is the rule.

First, we investigated the mechanism of the cellular immune response *in vitro*, using spleen cells from rats injected 10 days previously with 10^8 (C 58NT) D cells, and ^{51}Cr-labeled lymphoma target cells. The cytotoxic activity in the spleen peaked at 10 days. The response was specifically directed towards tumors induced by viruses of the MuLV complex. When macrophages are removed with silica for 24 hr *in vitro*, or adherence to plastic prior to assay, we find no discernible effect on cell-mediated ^{51}Cr release.

When one specifically depletes the T lymphocytes by thymectomy plus irradiation and marrow reconstitution, such animals have no cell-mediated response to the tumor, and the deficiency is corrected by the injection of T cells. The treatment of immune cells with a specific anti-T serum also abrogates cytotoxic activity. This anti-T serum was made by absorption of ALS with erythrocytes and bone marrow, and it showed no cytotoxicity for lymph node cells from B rats, nor did it affect plaque formation to SRBC *in vitro*. It was presumed, therefore, to be specific for T cells. Finally, when B cells and macrophages were removed on nylon columns and the eluate tested, cytotoxic activity was not lost. In fact, the activity was increased due presumably to enrichment for effector cells. In this case, B cell contamination is between 1 and 4%, and macrophage contamination is between ½ and 1%. We believe that this is good evidence for T-cell killing in this assay.

We have examined the serum of tumor-bearing rats for blocking factors. For this, we tested that small percentage of rats which show progressive growth (5%) and rats immunosuppressed by irradiation or ALS treatment. Serum from these tumor-bearing rats, when added directly to the reaction mixture of immune spleen cells and target cells at a final dilution of 1:5, markedly blocked cell-mediated release of ^{51}Cr from target cells. Immune cells were used at a ratio of 100:1 with target cells. Sera from rats in which tumors have regressed exert

TABLE 36
Blocking Effect of Serum Factors on a Lymphoma
Cell-Mediated Immunity

Status of serum donors	Reduction in specific lysis by immune spleen cells of (C58NT)D target cells (ratio 100:1)	
	%	Experimental Values[a]
Hyperimmune	−7.8	15.2/14.1
Regressor	5.0	22/23
	4.3	13.5/14.1
	13.5	12.2/14.1
	17.0	11.7/14.1
Progressor	28.8	9.9/14.1
Intact animals	35.5	9.1/14.1
	46.8	7.5/14.1
	48.2	7.3/14.1
	83.0	2.3/14.1
Immunosuppressed	52.1	11/23
800R	34.8	15/23
ALS	36.2	14.7/23

[a] $\dfrac{\% \text{ specific } ^{51}\text{Cr release with test serum}}{\% \text{ specific } ^{51}\text{Cr release without test serum}}$

only a small blocking effect, but this difference is statistically significant. Results are shown in Table 36. Sera from animals repeatedly injected with tumor and which never become progressors did not exhibit blocking in this assay; in fact, such sera, even at high dilutions, augmented cell-mediated cytotoxicity. We have not observed this with progressor sera. Sera having these effects are heat inactivated so we are not dealing with complement-dependent effects.

COHN: Do regressor animals show an increase in cell-mediated immunity during and after the time the tumor is regressing?

SHELLAM: We have not yet examined that. We have found a reasonable correlation between tumor size and blocking effect of serum, when sera are examined sequentially from rats during the growth or rejection of a tumor. Lastly, since this is a virus-releasing tumor we have investigated directly the effect of virus itself on the cytotoxic *in vitro* response by testing purified viruses of the MuLV complex and soluble extracts of lymphoma cells. These reagents were added directly, in graded doses, to the mixture of immune cells and labeled cells *in vitro* at a ratio of 100:1. The results are shown in Table 37. The concentrations shown refer to the amount, in μg of virus or membrane protein

TABLE 37
Blocking Effect of Purified Viruses on a Lymphoma
Cell-Mediated Immunity

Viral antigens	Dose μg	Reduction in specific lysis by immune spleen cells of (C58NT)D target cells (ratio 100:1) %
Soluble papain digest of	400	73
(C58NT)D cells	100	35
	100	44
MuLV-G[a]	10	3
	1	5
MuLV-M[b]	25	31
	100	44
MSV-M[c]	10	14
	1	6
	400	−6
Newcastle disease virus	100	−5
	10	−4
	1	2

[a]Gross pseudotype of murine leukemia virus (MLV).

[b]Moloney pseudotype of murine leukemia virus (MLV).

[c]Moloney pseudotype of murine sarcoma virus (MSV).

in ml, of the reaction mixture. We found that extracts of the tumor cell exert a very marked blocking effect and that viruses of the MuLV complex also exhibit a blocking effect. However, an unrelated virus did not block the response. We can conclude that the cytotoxicity of T cells can be inhibited in the chromium-release assay *in vitro*, either by one of the tumor-associated antigens, the virus, or by serum factors from rats with progressively growing tumors. We have not yet gone on to examine whether the factors are antigen–antibody complexes or antibody, or antigen alone. The fact that sera from irradiated rats bearing tumors show blocking may constitute a clue that antigen alone could block in that situation, since the presence of antibody should be minimal. We have also tested formalized preparations of these viruses to exclude blocking as a functional inactivation of effector cells by virus; formalized virus exerts just the same blocking effect, although the infectivity of that virus has been completely nullified by formalization.

CHAIRMAN KLEIN: There is a remarkable contrast between what Shellam and Stutman have told us. May this be related to the nature of the target cells? Stutman was using a mammary tumor. Weiss showed years ago that immunization of MTV-negative mice against MTV-positive mammary tumors often leads to enhancement. Rejection is not as regular or as frequent as in other systems. This is, in other words, a relatively easily enhanced system.

WEISS: There is also strong evidence of a tendency towards enhancement when one uses mammary tumors and hosts devoid of the two recognized mammary tumor viruses (Weiss *et al.*, *Israel J. Med. Sci.*, **7**, 187, 1971; Jacobs and Kripke, *J. Nat. Cancer Inst.*, submitted for publication). In contrast, if one tests MTV-infected tumors in MTV-free hosts, the tendency is overwhelmingly towards resistance (Weiss, *Cancer Res.*, **29**, 2368, 1969).

CHIECO-BIANCHI: Tumor cells may also escape host control because of a deficiency in the immune system. First, let me illustrate what we believe is an example of genetically controlled immune depression in the mouse. The AKR mouse, a natural carrier of the Gross leukemia virus, develops spontaneous lymphomas in high incidence at 7–9 months of age. In almost all cases, the T lymphocytes are affected by the neoplastic transformation as revealed by the θ-antigenicity of the lymphoma cells. Therefore, we investigated the function of peripheral blood and spleen lymphocytes of AKR mice at different ages before lymphoma appearance. Because stimulation by PHA is a property of at least one subpopulation of T cells, we used the PHA responsiveness of blood and spleen cultures, evaluated by ^{3}HTdR uptake, as a tool to determine the functional state of the T cells. The results obtained (Biasi *et al.*, *Proc. First Intern. Symposium on Standardization of Human Tumors*, Bologna, 1973, in press) indicated that, in preleukemic, 6-month-old mice, no decrease occurs in the number of PHA responsive lymphocytes, as compared to 1 or 2–3-month-old donors. However, when 2–3-month-old AKR mice were studied in comparison with low-leukemia CBA mice, they exhibited a marked reduction in PHA reactivity of blood and spleen lymphocytes. Moreover, AKR mice had a significant decrease of spleen-direct PFC after immunization with SRBC or LPS-coated SRBC, in comparison to other strains (Collavo *et al.*, in preparation).

Because CBA mice injected at birth with Passage A Gross virus did not show any changes in PHA reactivity of spleen cultures or in the direct spleen PFC, we drew the conclusion that the Gross virus infection cannot account for the immune depression observed in AKR mice. Thus, impairment in immune reactivity may represent a genetically determined property of the AKR strain, which might, in turn, allow a full expression throughout life of endogenous leukemia virus resulting in high percentage of lymphoid malignancies.

The state of environmental (generalized) immune deficiency in the host as a cause of tumor cell escape from surveillance is well exemplified by the following experiments (Collavo *et al.*, *Nature*, in press). CBA mice were thymectomized, lethally X-irradiated, and injected i.v. with syngeneic bone marrow cells. These mice, markedly depleted in T cells ("deprived"), were then in-

TABLE 38
Oncogenesis by M-MSV in Deprived or
Reconstituted CBA Mice[a]

	Total no. mice	No. mice with tumor (%)[b]		No. mice with regressed tumor (%)[c]		No. mice dead with tumor (%)[d]	
Normal	30	0	(0)	0	(0)	0	(0)
Deprived	30	27	(90)	3	(11)	24	(89)
Reconstituted (days ± M-MSV)							
−30	14	0	(0)	0	(0)	0	(0)
+ 1	8	7	(87.5)	7	(100)	0	(0)
+ 5	13	9	(69.2)	9	(100)	0	(0)
+25	6	6	(100)	0	(0)	6	(100)

[a]All mice were injected i.m. with 0.05 ml of M-MSV cell-free tumor extract diluted 10^{-2} w/v. (*Nature*, **249**, 169, 1974).
[b]Percentage of mice with tumor evaluated from total number of mice.
[c]Percentage of mice with regressed tumor calculated from number of mice developing tumor.
[d]Percentage of mice dead with tumor calculated from number of mice developing tumor.

jected i.m. with Moloney murine sarcoma virus (M-MSV). As shown in Table 38, 90% of deprived mice developed tumors, the great majority of which grew progressively and killed the host. On the contrary, no tumors were observed in MSV-injected control mice.

To better evaluate whether restoration of T cell function could reverse the oncogenic response, deprived mice were grafted under the kidney capsule with syngeneic neonatal thymus at different time intervals before or after M-MSV injection. These mice were considered "reconstituted" for T cell function. As seen in Table 38, mice receiving the thymus graft 30 days before M-MSV injection did not develop tumors, while mice which were grafted 1, 5, or 25 days after M-MSV injection presented a tumor incidence of 87, 69, and 100%, respectively, with a latency of 15–19 days.

Furthermore, the mice reconstituted 1 or 5 days following M-MSV injection presented 100% regression, while the mice—thymus grafted 25 days after M-MSV injection—had tumors which progressed until death. Because thymus graft in deprived mice produced a gradual restoration of T cell functions, which is accomplished in about 30 days (Davies, *Transplantation Rev.*, **1**, 43, 1969), these results may be easily explained in terms of complete or partial restoration of T cell activity at the time of M-MSV injection. Now, the question arises whether T cells operate through a cooperation with B cells in producing antibody against M-MSV. In fact, there is good evidence indicating that in this particular system, tumorigenesis is greatly inhibited by humoral antibodies.

243

Therefore, the sera of deprived and reconstituted mice were tested for M-MSV neutralizing antibody, making use of the *in vitro* focus reduction on 3T3FL cells. It was found that mice of both groups produced neutralizing antibody, although the former had a somewhat lower titer. Obviously, this observation does not exclude the possibility that the synthesis of other types of antibody, more efficient in causing tumor destruction, requires the cooperation of B and T cells and, consequently, does not take place in deprived mice. As an alternative explanation, it is also plausible that T cells operate directly *in vivo* by a cytotoxic effect on tumor cells.

The last point in discussion is related to the problem of specific unresponsiveness to leukemia virus-coded antigens. Following the studies of Axelrad, Eva and George Klein, and also our own, it has long been accepted that mice neonatally infected with certain murine leukemia viruses become immunologically tolerant to the same viral antigens later in life. In fact, these mice show persistent viremia and are unable to produce humoral antibody or transplantation resistance even after repeated immunizations. Recent observations indicate, however, that such tolerance is by no means complete. Immune complexes, consisting of virus antigens and specific antibodies together with C', have been detected in the kidney glomeruli of leukemia virus-infected mice. Furthermore, Hellström's finding of blocking serum factors from donors bearing progressive tumors made it possible to formulate the hypothesis that antibodies, either alone or bound to antigen, can interfere with the destruction of tumor so as to mimic *in vivo* a state of immunological tolerance.

In collaboration with Sendo and Aoki (*J. Nat. Cancer Inst.*, in press), we have recently performed some experiments with the aim of testing whether mice neonatally infected with Moloney leukemia virus possess lymphocytes which react specifically with virus-induced cell surface antigens. In Fig. 32, the exper-

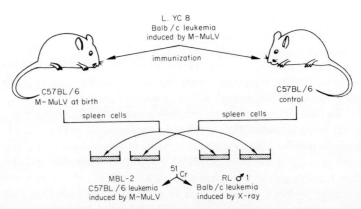

Fig. 32. Experimental model employed for study of immune tolerance to M–MuLV-induced cellular antigens.

imental procedures used are schematically illustrated. Briefly, C57BL/6 mice, neonatally infected with Moloney leukemia virus, were immunized as adults with allogeneic Balb/c Moloney leukemia cells. Their spleen lymphocytes were then assayed at various intervals following immunization against syngeneic Moloney or allogeneic radiation-induced leukemia cells (no cross reactivity between these two transplanted leukemias has been detected). As shown in Fig. 33, in contrast with similarly immunized control mice, spleen lymphocytes from neonatally virus-infected mice showed no cytotoxic activity (as evaluated by the ^{51}Cr releasing test) on syngeneic Moloney leukemia cells.

However in Fig. 34, spleen lymphocytes from the same virus-infected mice were fully reactive against allogeneic radiation-induced leukemia cells, thus proving that the lack of responsiveness was specific. I might add that no blocking activity was found in the sera of Moloney leukemia virus-infected mice, even when the donors were frankly leukemic. Moreover, the neonatally virus-infected mice did not produce virus-neutralizing antibody and did not develop transplantation resistance. On the other hand, these mice contained immune complexes in their kidneys. These results, on the whole, suggest that in mice infected at birth with Moloney leukemia virus, a state of tolerance to Moloney virus-induced cell surface antigens may develop. This tolerance is, however, only partial and involves the T lymphocyte subpopulation responsible for

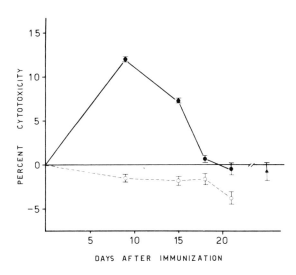

Fig. 33. Cytotoxic activity of spleen lymphocytes from M–MuLV neonatally infected and immunized mice to syngeneic Moloney leukemia MBL-2 cells (*J. Nat. Cancer Inst.*, in press, 1974).

●—● Immunized mice
○----○ M–MuLV neonatally infected and immunized mice
▲ M–MuLV neonatally infected mice

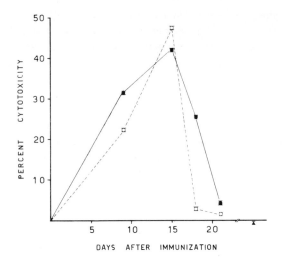

Fig. 34. Cytotoxic activity of spleen lymphocytes from M–MuLV neonatally infected and immunized mice to allogeneic BALB.RL ♂ 1 leukemia cells (*J. Nat. Cancer Inst.*, in press, 1974).

●—● Immunized mice

○----○ M–MuLV neonatally infected and immunized mice

▲ M–MuLV neonatally infected mice

the *in vitro* cytotoxicity. The B cells, on the contrary, respond to virus-specified antigens as shown by the presence of renal immunocomplexes.

CHAIRMAN KLEIN: May we consider the difference (if any) between tolerance and antigen-induced inhibition of the lymphocyte? The only conceptual difference that I see lies in the apparent irreversibility of tolerance. Could it be that the lymphocyte is reversibly blocked? Neonatally virus-inoculated animals have viremia, which is an extreme form of antigen excess. I wonder whether Chieco-Bianchi has tried to incubate and/or wash the lymphocytes to see whether they could be free from antigen and then become cytotoxic?

CHIECO-BIANCHI: No, we have just followed the usual procedure in the chromium test, that is wash twice, sometimes three times, but not more.

KOURILSKY: A problem raised earlier was that of the specific inhibition of the T-cell-mediated cytotoxicity in the chromium-release assay. It is clear that the reaction is blocked by intact cold cells bearing the relevant antigen. The question asked here is whether T-cell-mediated cytolysis can be blocked *in vitro* by soluble antigen. It should be so, since immune cytolytic T cells bear specific

246

receptors for target cell surface antigens, and, therefore, the saturation of these receptors by an excess of soluble antigen should prevent the initial recognition step and hamper subsequent specific cytolysis. However, unsuccessful attempts have been reported, and it is worthwhile to come back to this problem: first in the H-2 system and then in the tumor systems.

Bach recalled earlier experiments suggesting that antigens defined by the SD regions of H-2 are targets for cell-mediated cytotoxity. Neauport-Sautes recently attempted to inhibit cell-mediated cytotoxicity with papain-solubilized H-2 antigens provided by Nathenson. These preparations are far from pure, but they contain H-2 antigens corresponding to the definition of ''serologically defined,'' since they specifically absorb anti-H-2 antibodies.

Briefly, effector cells were spleen cells from Balb/c mice immunized against C57BL/6. [51]Cr target cells were GIL-4 lymphoma cells of C57BL/6. The assay was performed in microplates using 5×10^5 effector cells for 2×10^4 target cells in triplicate wells with a short incubation period (4 hr). In order to prevent renewal of T cell receptor sites during this period, effector lymphocytes were pretreated with puromycin (2.4 µg/ml for 30 min) in conditions defined to prevent synthesis of a T cell product (Fridman and Golstein, *Cell. Immunol.,* in press). In such conditions, inhibition of cytotoxic effects was obtained upon addition of 2.4 to 5×10^5 cold C57BL/6 spleen cells in the assay, but not obtained using cold Balb/c cells. Attempts to prevent cytolysis with soluble C57BL/6 antigen were performed by preincubating effector lymphocytes with the antigen for 30 min at 37°C before the addition of chromium-labeled target cells.

Three different soluble antigenic preparations were used and carefully assayed for their serologically defined antigenic content by quantitative absorption of a cytotoxic Balb/c anti-C57BL/6 cytotoxic antiserum, as compared to the absorbing capacity of intact C57BL/6 spleen cells. One microgram of the more active preparation of antigen had an absorbing activity equivalent to that of 1.5×10^6 cells. However, it failed to induce *any* reduction of the cytoxicity of immune effector cells in our assay, even at a dose of 300 µg (4.5×10^8 cell equivalent), whereas 2.5×10^5 intact C57BL/6 cells were inhibitory. Crude, insoluble C57BL/6 membrane extracts prepared by hypotonic salt extraction also failed to give specific inhibition of cell-mediated cytotoxicity in our experimental conditions. In order to try to circumvent the problem of antigenic monovalence, soluble antigens were polymerized using a mild treatment with glutaraldehyde. Two Sephadex-isolated polymers retained a sufficient, although reduced, antigenic activity. They also failed to inhibit the cytotoxic effector cells at doses equivalent to 3×10^7 intact cells.

Although I know that the interpretation of negative results is always difficult and rarely conclusive, at least it raises the question whether anybody ever inhibited cell-mediated cytolysis in the chromium-release assay, using soluble

H-2 antigens. A few speculations perhaps can be made and also remain relevant for tumor antigens.

One explanation, perhaps the most probable, is that chemical extraction has altered the configuration of surface SD antigens, inducing a decreased affinity for T cell receptors, as compared to native H-2 antigens of the cell membrane. However, it may also be that SD antigenic molecules *per se* are not the proper target for T cell receptors but represent only part of a necessary antigenic configuration. Other alternative explanations, more complicated, imply an additional activation step between the antigen contact with T cell and the killing of the target. At least the immune anti-H-2, T-cell-mediated cytolysis seems remarkably hard to inhibit with soluble antigens *in vitro*, and that may have some bearing on *in vivo* situations.

Now, let us come back to the tumor systems to comment on data from Plata and Levy, in our laboratory, who studied the comparative blocking effect of soluble tumor antigens on syngeneic effector T cells in both chromium-release test (CRT) and microcytotoxicity assay (MA) (Plata and Levy, in press).

In their system (Plata *et al., J. Immunol.,* **112,** 1477, 1974), previously described in the course of this conference, purified T cells and non-T-cell suspensions were prepared from spleens of C57BL/6 mice immunized with MSV and simultaneously assayed in the chromium-release tests (CRT) on syngeneic lymphoma target cells and in a microcytotoxicity assay against adherent, cultured MSV-tumor cells. Between day 14 and 25, following MSV inoculation, both T and non-T cells displayed activity in MA, and only T cell suspensions were cytotoxic in CRT. The blocking capacity of antigen, solubilized by KCl from syngeneic tumors, was comparatively tested in both assays on T- and non-T effector cell suspensions, with appropriate controls. Briefly, serum from tumor-bearing mice blocked MA but not CRT reactions. Soluble antigen preparations suppressed the growth-inhibiting suspensions in the same assay. In contrast, they had no inhibiting effect on T-cell-mediated cytolysis in CRT.

The fact that one T cell effect, e.g., tumor growth inhibition in MA, is inhibited by antigen, whereas another T cell effect, e.g., direct cytolysis in the CRT, is unaffected strongly supports the concept that two different, immune, T-cell-mediated mechanisms of cell damage may be involved in MA and CRT. These can be independently inhibited and can be evidenced in this MSV system because of the different effector pathways in MA and CRT, or if different T effector cells are involved in the two assays. It is possible that different antigens are acting as targets in the MA and CRT, although no evidence for such an antigenic diversity was found so far. The possibility of cooperation between effector T lymphocytes and another subpopulation of cells is not totally ruled out in MA.

In any case, the interpretation of these data requires us to introduce the concept that T-cell-mediated target cell damage may involve different mechanisms in the chromium-release assay and in the microcytotoxicity assay, at least in the systems used here.

CHAIRMAN KLEIN: This brings us back to our earlier discussions (Session II) of the two assays. I think that this is an extraordinary demonstration of the differences between them. The main problem is which, if either, is relevant to what happens *in vivo*.

HOWARD: Referring to Kourilsky's first case, in which he used solubilized antigen in an attempt to inhibit an H-2 killing system, a recent experiment reported by Edidin and Henney *Nature New Biology*, **246,** 47, 1973), using the P-815 mastocytoma is relevant. They capped the SD determinant from the surface of the target and apparently eliminated it, in the sense that the cell was no longer susceptible to the toxic action of alloantisera with specificity for the serological determinants of the H-2^d chromosome. Nevertheless, these capped cells were still susceptible to the toxic action of alloimmune lymphocytes.

I suggest to Kourilsky, following Edidin and Henney, that the elementary explanation for their failure to find inhibition is that the SD antigens are the wrong antigens.

CEROTTINI: I have a word of caution about the interpretation of the results reported by Edidin and Henney. What they have shown is that antibody, bound to H-2 alloantigens, is no longer able to activate the complement system once the antigen–antibody complex has been capped on the cell surface in an appropriate way. As a matter of fact, by using another source of complement, such as rabbit serum, it is possible to induce lysis of cells after capping of H-2 with antibodies and anti-immunoglobulin serum. Therefore, since the serologically defined H-2 antigens are still present on the cell surface, it is impossible to rule out the possibility that specificity of the receptors of the cytotoxic lymphocytes is not directed against them. Of course, this does not mean that the determinants recognized by antibodies and cytotoxic lymphocytes are identical.

COHN: I would like to clarify this discussion of blocking mechanisms, as much for myself as for conferees, by restating it in more general terms.

Consider two cells, a T killer and a target cell, that are interacting via receptor recognition of a surface determinant (Figs. 35 and 36). When two cells interact in this way, there is cooperative binding between them, so that the energy of the interaction is some exponential function of the number of receptor–surface determinant interactions between them.

To take these two cells apart by adding excess free antibody (receptor) or free antigen (surface determinant), the concentration of the excess antigen or

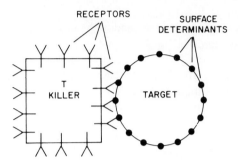

Fig. 35. Interaction between T killer cell and target surface determinant via the T killer receptor.

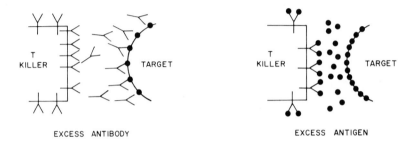

Fig. 36. Blocking of the interaction between T killer and target by excess antibody or excess antigen (concentration must be tenfold above the binding constant).

antibody would have to be roughly tenfold above the binding, constant, receptor–surface determinant. In other words, when a receptor–surface determinant interaction opens or breathes, the probability of its reclosing must be low because of the competing interaction with excess antibody or antigen. The two cells will then unzip anticooperatively.

If an average protein–antiprotein interaction has a binding constant $10^{-6}M$, then the unzipping of two cells will require added concentrations of antibody or antigen of the order of $10^{-5}M$. Consequently, the negative experiments we have heard discussed are meaningless unless it is shown that the added antibody or antigen is $10^{-5}M$. This was certainly not the case in most negative experiments.

The situation I have described is idealized because the specific binding together of two cells via receptor–determinant interactions is certainly accompanied by weak, nonspecific ones (Fig. 37). The interaction between the cells then becomes irreversible, because these nonspecific interactions are also cooperative. However, if excess antibody or antigen is added before the T killer and target are mixed, then what one might find as a function of time is an initial inhibition of interaction followed by a gradual escape from the inhibition (Fig. 38).

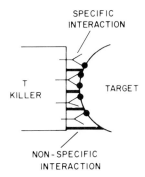

Fig. 37. Nonspecific (charge) interaction between T killer and target, preventing blockage by excess antigen or antibody.

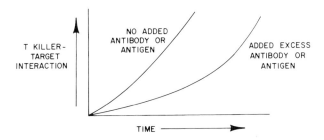

Fig. 38. Kinetics of the escape from inhibition by excess antibody or antigen, when nonspecific interaction obtains.

Given this background argument, examples have been presented to us in which added excess antigen or antibody seem to be acting at very low concentrations to block a cell–cell interaction. In order to explain this, some other mechanism of blocking must be operating, unless by chance the receptor–determinant interactions under analysis have binding constants of $10^{-10}M$, which is unlikely. Two mechanisms come to mind immediately:

1. The determinants or receptors are being modulated, shed, or inactivated by the added antibody.

2. The added antigen or antibody is polymeric or aggregated, and the binding constant in question is now very low.

CHAIRMAN KLEIN: To amplify what Cohn said, we should be reminded of the cases of T cell inhibition we have heard about earlier from Shellam and Chieco-Bianchi. These are situations involving viremia. Is there any evidence concerning the question whether T lymphocytes can be inhibited with soluble antigen derived from solid tumors?

STJERNSWÄRD: Yes, with other tests like lymphocyte stimulation, we have demonstrated inhibition with increased doses of KCl-soluble antigen extracts. Compare also the data presented by Stutman and by Smith—they all have a bell-shaped stimulation–inhibition curve. Whether this is a pure dose–response relationship or whether we interpret it as T cell blocking is open for discussion. But we prefer to interpret it as representing a dose–response phenomenon, rather than specify it as blocking of T cells by soluble antigen.

UHR: In the experiment of Edidin and Henney, in which H-2 was capped, it was assumed that all the H-2 on the surface was in the cap. Vitetta, in my laboratory, has iodinated immunoglobulin on the cell surface and aggregated it on cells with rabbit antimouse immunoglobulin. The aggregate was removed completely after detergent lysis of cells by a combination of high speed centrifugation and immunoprecipitation of soluble complexes by antibody to the rabbit immunoglobulin. No matter how the aggregation is performed, there is always left in the supernatant approximately 15% of iodinated cell surface immunoglobulin which has not been bound by rabbit antimouse Ig. For example, one can allow the surface immunoglobulin to cap at 37° C, using a sandwich precipitation, and then again treat the capped cells with antimouse Ig. Fifteen percent of cell surface immunoglobulin still remains unbound by antibody. Hence, in the H-2 experiment, there may be cell surface H-2 antigens that are not capped and later become available to react with H-2 antibodies.

In reference to Cohn's generalizations, the critical difference between the capacity of free antigen and antigen–antibody complexes to block is probably explained by energetic considerations. Most likely, antibody bridging antigenic determinants is responsible for the efficacy of immune complexes in blocking. Two studies, in which the difference in energy of binding between univalent and polyvalent ligands with immune cells was explored, are those of Davie and Paul (*J. Exp. Med.*, **135**, 643, 1972) and those of Bystryn, Siskind, and myself (*J. Exp. Med.*, **137**, 301, 1973). We found that the difference in binding constant of a polyvalent DNP ligand to the surface of a MOPC 315 cell is a hundredfold greater than that of a univalent ligand.

The possibility that bridging of antigen is the key variable could be easily tested. "Free" antigen, from serum in which blocking complexes have been precipitated by ammonium sulfate, could be mildly aggregated by cross-linking agents such as glutaraldehyde, as Kourilsky described. There are problems with such an experiment. One has to do the cross linking so that antigenicity is not lost and the aggregates are small enough to circulate. With a little work, however, I think one could prove that the key point here is the polyvalency of the antigen–antibody complex.

COHN: In a competing polyvalent interaction, the binding constant to consider might be $10^{-10}M$. In this case, the concentration of the complex required to unzip the cooperative cell–cell interaction would be $10^{-9}M$. However, a piece of membrane would be a large particle, and I am not certain whether, in terms of quantity of material in the extracts we have discussed, this would make very much difference.

UHR: We cannot assume that *in vivo,* all immune reactions reach equilibrium. There may not be time for that. Perhaps, one should look at these events as rates of association and dissociation. For example, a cell may not have the opportunity to achieve equilibrium with antigen or another cell if the interaction alters the cell, e.g., it might emigrate to another compartment. These reactions *in vivo* are more complicated than test tube phenomena in which cells and antigen are in equilibrium.

COHN: It is because of the problem of nonequilibrium conditions that I discussed the time kinetics of the inhibition by added excess antigen or antibody. If one had a nonspecific, nonequilibrium interaction in addition to the specific one, one would expect escape from the inhibition with time.

TERRY: With reference to Howard's original question, when comparing the various *in vitro* assays, it is necessary to examine them at a level of detail that would be inappropriate for a conference such as this. For example, in considering the experiments of Kourilsky, one has to be concerned with the number of target cells, the number of attacker cells, duration of incubation, assay volume, viability of cells in culture, and so on. Experimental differences may not really imply differences in cell function but rather differences in assays and assay techniques.

A specific question for Kourilsky: Was the H-2 antigen reassayed after incubation with the cells to be sure that antigen was not inactivated or destroyed by the cells in the incubation mixture? If the antigen was degraded, it might not block.

KOURILSKY: H-2 antigen was still present in the supernatant following incubation with effector cells.

SMITH: Terry's admonition is quite important, I believe. Blackstock and Forbes in our laboratory find that the average MW of KCl-solubilized MCA-membrane material that stimulates lymphoid cells from draining lymph nodes is somewhat lower than that which stimulates spleen cells from the same animal. We have no satisfactory explanation, but it could be attributed to a different proportion of B or T lymphocytes in the draining lymph node compared with the spleen. This adds to the variables one must account for in all cell systems assessing *in vitro* effects.

253

MARTIN: I would like to bring up the issue of nonspecific inhibition of T cell function. Gorginsky, Smith, and others in our laboratory have investigated the PHA, Con A, and LPS proliferative responses of spleen cells from tumor-bearing mice. They have observed a depressed proliferative response by spleen cells of tumor-bearing mice to the mitogens PHA and Con A, but not to LPS—a B cell mitogen. The impaired T cell response is not due simply to a lack of responsive T cells—by velocity sedimentation it is possible to isolate a rapidly sedimenting population which shows nearly normal levels of proliferative response to PHA and Con A. The less rapidly sedimenting cellular fraction does not respond to these mitogens. Furthermore, when cells of this fraction are mixed with normal spleen cells, the PHA and Con A response of the normal cells is impaired. A similar "suppressive" lymphocyte population cannot be detected in fractionated normal spleen cells. These findings argue for a nonspecific regulation of T cell activity—at least as discerned in the *in vitro* assay.*

HALL: The blocking of the activity of cytotoxic lymphoid cells by circulating antigen implies that there is a primed lymphocyte which meets small fragments of its target antigen and is, thereby, "blocked" or, more properly, inhibited. It would seem to me that, in some of these systems, if lymphocytes which are allegedly "blocked" *in vivo* were simply cultured in a suitable medium, some of them, if they have indeed united with their specific antigen, should go into blast transformation. Does this in fact happen? Does it happen *in vivo?* In the vascular compartment, we know that the circulating half-life of a blast cell is extremely short, and, as Cohn has just suggested, the activated cell is thus removed from the circulation very quickly. Although this concept of inhibition by specific antigen blocking is very nice up to a point, it has serious physiological implications, and it does present the physiologist with even more problems to sort out from the point of view of cellular ecology.

STUTMAN: Hall has made an interesting point. In virus-infected C3H mice between 3 and 5 months of age and before tumors appear, lymphocytes can respond by blast transformation *in vitro* to soluble antigen. Approximately 60% of tested mice show this reactivity. The soluble antigen used contains ML and MTV antigens. Once the animal develops a tumor, and, presumably antigen excess, cells that can be stimulated by this antigen totally disappear. Our interpretation of this experiment is that the blasts are short lived in the animal.

HALL: Stutman's is almost an essential prediction.

Editors' note: Other interpretations of the data Martin describes are possible. See Konda, *et al.*, (*Cancer Research,* **33,** 1878, 1973; **33,** 2000, 1973) and the discussion by Smith in Session V.

NOTKINS: Whether or not antibody can block the cellular immune response to viral antigens seems to depend on at least two factors: One is the way in which the antigen is presented to immune lymphocytes, and the other is related to the properties of the particular antibody.

If lymphocytes from animals immunized with HSV are exposed to UV-inactivated HSV, these lymphocytes are readily stimulated, as reflected by the incorporation of ^{3}HTdR. If the virions are exposed to antiviral antibody in concentration sufficient to neutralize 100% of the virus, lymphocyte stimulation still occurs. If virus is allowed to absorb to the surface of cells and the cell-bound virus is incubated with immune lymphocytes, lymphocyte stimulation also will occur. However, if the cell-bound virus is exposed to antiviral antibody prior to incubation with immune lymphocytes, lymphocyte stimulation is inhibited. These data may be tabulated as follows:

Combination	Stimulation
Immune lymphocytes + virus alone	+
Immune lymphocytes + virus neutralized with Ab	+
Immune lymphocytes + virus absorbed on cells	+
Immune lymphocytes + virus absorbed on cells first + Ab	−

In these experiments, the same antigen is presented to lymphocytes, but in different ways. Our explanation is that antibody interacting with antigens on a cell surface blocks contact with immune lymphocytes or macrophages. However, if the virus–antibody complex exists in the fluid phase, the smaller "soluble" complexes can be processed by macrophages or lymphocytes and are still antigenic.

This may be extremely important in regard to the host's response to virus-infected cells. On the one hand, antibody attached to the surface of infected cells may block the action of lymphocytes, while on the other hand virions or viral antigens released or shed from infected cells can combine with antiviral antibody, and these complexes may still be effective in stimulating immune lymphocytes. In turn, the stimulated lymphocytes could produce lymphokines. Thus, viral antigens released from infected cells may be the driving force *in vivo* in triggering the cellular immune response. Similarly, one wonders whether antigens released from tumor cells, and not just antigens on the surface of cells, may be important in attracting inflammatory cells to the site of the tumor.

Recently, Sigel and his colleagues at the University of Miami showed that lymphocyte stimulation was affected by the class of the immunoglobulin. Sigel found that rubella virus incubated with antirubella antibody of the IgG class could stimulate immune lymphocytes, while rubella virus incubated with antiviral antibody of the IgM class did not stimulate immune lymphocytes. There are several explanations: First, IgM was reacting with different determinants on the virion than IgG; second, the larger IgM molecules were sterically blocking the lymphocytes from reaching free antigenic determinants on the virion. They also showed that the rubella-IgM complexes could block stimulation of normal (i.e., nonimmune) lymphocytes by PHA. They suggested that the virus–IgM complexes had adsorbed to the lymphocytes and were blocking PHA receptors.

I stress that in all these studies it was lymphocyte stimulation and not cytotoxicity that was measured, but I believe it has relevance to the tumor problem.

WEISS: With regard to the question of shedding, or liberation, or peeling off of cell surface antigens, Doljanski and her associates determined whether there is a greater degree of shedding by transformed neoplastic, than by analogous normal cells. They introduced, into the culture medium, cells labeled with glucosamine and choline and followed the appearance of macromolecules containing the label in fresh medium. In Rous sarcoma of chickens and in several other tumors, a consistently more rapid liberation of cell surface substances by the transformed cells could be established. The shed, labeled macromolecules from transformed cells, attach with a high degree of specificity to sensitized lymphoid cells of autochthonous and allogeneic origin.

If one speculates, as have Feldman and Cohen, that self-tolerance may be dependent, at least in part, on the elaboration in soluble form of organ-specific and other cell antigens leading to blocking of effector cells, then what we may be seeing is a preemption by neoplastic cells of a vital physiological mechanism making for self-tolerance.

The material that comes off living "healthy" cells *in vitro,* in the Rous sarcoma of chickens, seems to be different from that shed by cells of actively growing tumors *in vivo.* What peels off damaged or actually lysing cells may be a still different entity. We measure this difference by affinity and biological consequences of binding of these cell surface materials to sensitized lymphocytes. It would appear from experiments, thus far, that the material coming off living tumor cells *in vivo* binds more firmly, the material coming off apparently healthy cells *in vitro* is next in order of affinity or full steric complimentarity, and the material coming off "unhappy" or lysing cells binds with the least avidity.

Sulitzeanu examined the pleural and ascitic effusions of patients with bronchogenic, ovarian, and other cancers and found in raw pathological material, untreated in any way, what seems to be typical "rosettes" of tumor cells surrounded by lymphoid cells and macrophages (Fig. 39). In many of these rosettes, the tumor cells in the center seem to be damaged. The rosettes show an intimate interaction between lymphoid cells and cancer cells, damaging to the neoplastic variants, and it may be that what one sees here is an *in vivo* defense reaction which could be blocked by free antigen in the fluids or tissues.

256

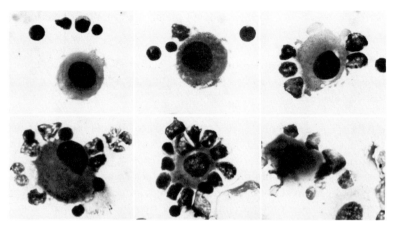

Fig. 39. Association between tumor cells and a variety of normal host cells in the pleural effusion of a patient with endothelioma. The clusters consist of a central neoplastic cell surrounded by a variety of host-cell types: lymphocytes, blast cells, macrophages, and eosinophilic cells. The cells forming the clusters were tightly held together, as evidenced by the fact that they did not disrupt even after five successive washings. In some clusters, the neoplastic cell is seen completely surrounded ("rosettes"), and, in some instances, both the neoplastic cell and the surrounding host cells show clear evidence of damage.

We tend to think of cell damage almost exclusively in terms of lysis or very severe damage, as indicated by a significant release of chromium or other labels from target cells. One should remember that there may be far more sensitive indicators of cell damage, such as inhibition of metabolic capacity.

In our laboratory, Steinitz has just completed a systematic study on inhibition of protein, RNA, and DNA synthesis by plasmacytoma cells of Balb/c mice in contact with either allogeneic or syngeneic splenocytes. It appears that there is a sequence of inhibition of such synthetic ability, as measured by inhibition of uptake almost instantaneously upon contact, RNA synthesis some time later, and protein synthesis after that (Steinitz and Weiss, submitted for publication). In some instances, the damage caused is irreversible very shortly after contact, although the manifestation of such damage becomes obvious only after some hours. In some cases, damage to metabolic pathways is reversible. Antigens, which make for lymphoid cell attachment and which cause this inhibition of synthesis, may be distinct from antigens that facilitate the attachment of lymphoid cells manifested by lysis or chromium release.

The technology of measuring damage occurring before, or short of, gross lysis may contribute a great deal to the field. It should be taken into account that inhibition or interference with synthetic pathways may result from cell–cell interaction. Sublethal damage to neoplastic cells may also alter the host–tumor interaction in terms of changes in the nature of substances peeling off the membrane of the injured cell.

MANNINO: I assume that the shedding of the antigen Weiss referred to involves only *in vitro* events.

WEISS: We place the cells in tissue culture and examine for shedding either in primary cultures, very early after the cultures are established, or in long established cultures.

HOWARD: The third point Weiss raised is especially important. For a long time, we have considered that the release of macromolecules from target cells was the necessary condition for proving the presence of lymphocytes potentially capable of prejudicing a graft or, presumably, an antigenic tumor. This may not be so. With regard to skin graft rejection, there is no reason to believe that the flagrant disappearance of intracellular protein from the cell, as monitored by chromium release *in vitro,* is actually the event which causes the rejection of the skin graft, that, in fact, it has anything to do with it. For example, chromium release takes place over a matter of hours, while rejection of a graft takes place over a matter of days, even in preimmunized recipients. We should also be interested in effects of the kind that Weiss described, small prejudicial inhibitions of intracellular phenomena caused by adding potentially cytotoxic cells to targets. This is an important advance.

MARTIN: Is the effect Weiss describes on tumor cell DNA metabolism necessarily an indication of an effector cell function? Is it possible that reduced ^{125}IUdR uptake by tumor cells is a reflection of alteration in the culture milieu, brought about by effector-target cell interaction?

WEISS: Inhibition extrapolates virtually to the moment of contact, even in circumstances where there is no cell lysis for many hours to come, or at all. So, damage to synthetic pathways may be precedent to more severe damage, but not necessarily in all cases.

MARTIN: As an example, if two normal fibroblasts make contact, they can switch off DNA synthesis, and yet one would not necessarily extrapolate that to immunological, destructive events.

WEISS: In all of these experiments, we have a variety of specificity controls, including lymphoid cells from normal donors of the same age against the same target cells, and both normal and sensitized lymphoid cells reacting with a variety of normal and other neoplastic target cells. Inhibition of DNA, RNA, or protein synthesis by sensitized effector cells, as we have described, is against a background of these controls.

VAAGE: We have data of interest from kinetic studies of the development of an immune resistance response during progressive growth of a sensitizing primary tumor implant. The system is syngeneic MCA-induced fibrosarcomas in pathogen-free C3H mice. The sensitization method is by implantation of a primary tumor. Then, at various times, we challenge the ability to resist the growth of additional subcutaneously implanted tumor cells.

The peak of the curve (Fig. 40) is 100% resistance, i.e., all animals are able to reject 100,000 live tumor cells injected subcutaneously. Immune response develops rapidly, full development requiring about 11 days. It remains maximal for a short period, but, when the tumor reaches a size of about 8 mm in about 18 days, immune resistance declines. Mice begin to lose their ability to reject challenge implants of tumor cells.

This experiment concerns the concept of concomitant immunity, which is the entire area under the bell-shaped curve, because the assay is done in the presence of a growing tumor. It concerns the concept of blocking or desensitization. Blocking is the term that will survive, and that covers the area to the right of the descending curve, the part of the resistance which is lost. If the tumor is removed at a time when it is 11 mm in size, rapid recovery to full resistance (Fig. 41) occurs and is detectable within 24 hr after surgical removal. If one kills the tumor by a single dose of lethal local radiation, recovery is delayed for as much as 7 days after radiation. The delay is simply a result of the antigen mass continuing to persist, although the tumor is killed. If daily injections of killed tumor tissue (5,000 R) are made from the time of surgical removal, depression is sustained for a long time. I have sustained such tumors in this way for as long as 10 days.

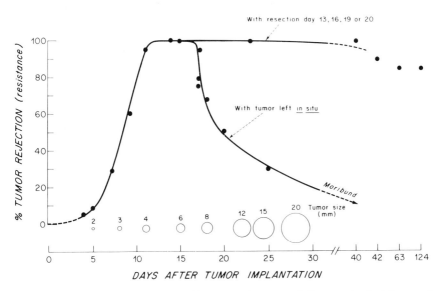

Fig. 40. The development and decline of immune resistance to challenge under the influence of a progressively growing subcutaneous fibrosarcoma (*Cancer Research*, **33**, 493, 1973).

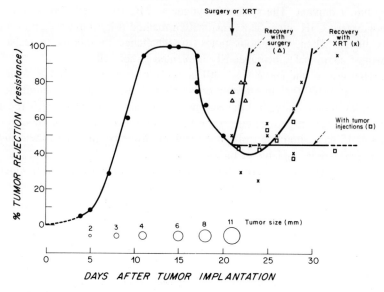

Fig. 41. The recovery of immune resistance following tumor-curative therapy of 11 × 11mm tumors (*Cancer Research*, **33**, 493, 1973).

If one uses this as a model for clinical consideration, immunotherapeutic attempts designed to treat by injection of autologous tumor preparations might have the effect of maintaining depression or blocking, rather than the intended stimulation of resistance.

CHAIRMAN KLEIN: The phenomenon, in which Vaage has protection against the new implantation of a tumor and yet no rejection of the established tumor, is interesting. Does it depend on the size of the challenging inoculum?

VAAGE: The type of depression I have described is detected only by challenging subcutaneously, not intravascularly. Immune resistance seems to be so effective that depression is not detectable under conditions which reveal depressed resistance to subcutaneous challenge.

CHAIRMAN KLEIN: Does Vaage mean to say, then, that it is concomitant immunity against circulating tumor cells, no matter how large the tumor is? Is that correct?

VAAGE: Yes, the animals retain considerable concomitant immunity up to the last testable point, the point where the animal becomes moribund.

CHAIRMAN KLEIN: Would you then conclude that whatever kills the circulating tumor cell is not what you are measuring in the *in vitro* system?

VAAGE: I do not know.

STJERNSWÄRD: In the search for a relevant *in vitro* test that may reflect the tumor–host relationship *in vivo*, we worked with a lymphocyte stimulation test adopted for fresh biopsy tumor cells as targets.* The validity of positive stimulation by autochthonous tumor cells as a test reflecting tumor-associated immunity is supported by:

1. Frequency: The frequency of stimulation of autochthonous lymphocytes, by malignant compared to nonmalignant cells of the same origin, differs. Fresh biopsy cells from 31 of 85 tumors induced significant stimulation compared with 3 of 51 nonmalignant cells (Vanky, Stjernswärd, Klein, unpublished).

2. Reproducibility: Using frozen tumor cells, it is now possible to repeat these tests. Stimulating cells remain stimulating and nonstimulating remain nonstimulating.

3. Dose–response kinetics: The stimulating ability of various ratios of lymphocytes to tumor cells has been compared with ratios of control cells. The optimally stimulating lymphocyte–tumor cell ratio was usually 1:1. The curves achieved correspond to those characteristic for the stimulation of lymphocytes by other antigens. Nonmalignant cells were not found to stimulate in any ratio tested.

4. Serum-mediated inhibition: The specificity of serum-mediated inhibition of lymphocyte stimulation by autochthonous tumors further indicates that the stimulation found in the MLTI test reflects a tumor-associated phenomenon. Tumor cells which stimulated autochthonous lymphocytes were incubated with various sera, and the stimulating ability of the tumor cells was assessed. Autochthonous sera and sera from allogeneic tumor patients, with tumors of the same type as the stimulating autochthonous tumor cells, inhibited to a higher frequency (84% and 68% respectively) than sera from healthy controls or from

*Editors' comment: Throughout the conference, as in this exchange, various conferees have expressed concern about the *in vivo* relevance of *in vitro* data. This matter has been resolved as well as the data base permits. A less directly confronted problem is related to the significance of various *in vivo* models in terms of pertinance to clinical cancer problems, and this is the issue Sterjernswärd raises here.

The fact is that few of the models in widespread current use have this transcendental quality. Vaage's experiments with concomitant immunity seem to justify categorization as relevant, for example. New *in vivo* models are, however, badly needed in order to explore many immunobiologic aspects of the human tumor–host relationship. The needed models are not those which test the surveillance mechanism, i.e., prophylactic models involving the prevention of tumor establishment. The needed models are those involving tumors having a range of biological behavior patterns resembling those occurring in humans, and those in which immunotherapeutic modalities can be tested. This means that the models must involve an established tumor–host relationship, with or without interruptions, which leave minimal residues of tumor cells that will emerge again to grow and kill. Models involving long periods of latency between tumor removal and recurrence will be particularly important. While studies in man alone can ultimately give the needed information, major supplementation of the few models meeting the criteria of clinical relevance is vital at this point.

cancer patients with "unrelated" tumors (9% and 15% respectively). (Vanky *et al.*, *J. Nat. Cancer Inst.*, **51**, 75, 1973; Stjernswärd, Vanky, and Klein, *Brit. J. Cancer*, 28, Suppl., 1973)

I will report differences in the tumor-associated reactivity of blood lymphocytes and tumor-draining lymph node cells found in sarcoma patients. The results demonstrate a tumor-specific nonreactivity to tumors by lymph node cells draining large tumors. The material is unique in that the tumor burden is large and that the tumors are of long duration. It consists of 12 patients with various forms of sarcomas (synovial sarcoma, osteosarcoma, chondrosarcoma, neurofibrosarcoma, fibroliposarcoma). Nine of the 12 patients had some reactivity between their first or sixth local reoccurrance of tumor with an average size, at time of testing, of about 10 × 10 cm. In the lymphocyte-stimulation tests, the capacity of circulating blood lymphocytes to be stimulated was compared with that of tumor-draining lymph node cells against the same autochthonous tumor cells. We also tested the ability of the local lymph node cells to stimulate autochthonous blood lymphocytes and vice versa, and both lymphocyte compartments were tested for their ability to be stimulated by allogeneic cells as well as by PHA. To make a positive or negative conclusion possible, we were careful to include adequate controls. Negative controls consisted of a combination of cells alone, treated with mitomycin-C, and also of lymphocytes and lymph node cells tested from healthy controls.

Circulating blood lymphocytes were stimulated to increase DNA synthesis by autochthonous tumor cells in 7 of 12 patients tested. The second finding was that lymph node cells were not stimulated by the same tumor cells. Thus, the same tumor cell that stimulated circulating blood lymphocytes did not stimulate the local lymph node cells. The third finding was that local lymph node cells stimulated circulating blood lymphocytes in autochthonous combination to increased DNA synthesis, but not the opposite. Circulating blood lymphocytes did not stimulate autochthonous lymph node cells to increase DNA synthesis. We included positive controls establishing stimulability by PHA, for both circulating blood lymphocytes and lymph node cells. This finding also argues against differences in viability. We also included, as controls of stimulability, lymph node cells and circulating blood lymphocytes from 13 non-tumor-bearing "normal" donors. Local lymph node cells in this combination only stimulated in 1 out of 13 patients tested, as compared to 7 out of 12 when testing lymph node cells from tumor-bearing hosts against autochthonous circulating blood lymphocytes.

The conclusion that we draw is that the results demonstrate a tumor-specific nonreactivity to tumors in lymph node cells draining large tumors. At present, however, this explanation cannot be differentiated from the interpretation that the clones' ability to respond to the tumor is exhausted, and all the cells capable of responding to the tumor-specific stimulus already have been transformed. The second point would be that the stimulation of circulating blood lymphocytes, by cells from the lymph nodes draining large tumors in a higher frequency than found in the same test combination from healthy controls, may reflect a tumor-specific tumor product of either whole tumor cells or membranes of tumors in the local lymph node cells.

CHAIRMAN KLEIN: You also have serum blocking data that suggest the presence of tumor-derived antigen in the lymph nodes.

STJERNSWÄRD: Yes, we do.

CHAIRMAN KLEIN: Is this not the strongest evidence that you are really dealing with tumor-derived antigen?

STJERNSWÄRD: Exactly, this is not the occasion to review the data in detail, but your conclusion is correct. The specificity of a serum-mediated inhibition of lymphocyte stimulation by autochthonous tumor cells has been investigated in detail in autochthonous stimulating lymphocyte–tumor cell combinations.

CHIECO-BIANCHI: How pure are those lymph node cell preparations from contamination by macrophages?

STJERNSWÄRD: There is no selection of cells. We make a mechanical suspension of the lymph nodes which may well contain both macrophages and tumor cells. Microscopically, these lymph nodes are without tumor invasion. The details have just been published (Vanky, et al., J. Nat. Cancer Inst., **51,** 17, 1973).

WEISS: Some eight years ago, Vaage conducted experiments in our laboratories analyzing acquired immunity to autochthonous and isogeneic spontaneous mouse mammary tumors. We used, very naively, liver tissue from the tumor-bearing animals as one of several tissues which we could get very easily without sacrificing the animal. The observations which came from this work were that liver from autochthonous or allogeneic mice bearing actively growing tumors was a better immunogen against that tumor than the tumor tissue itself (Vaage and Weiss, Cancer Res., **29,** 1920, 1969)! Liver tissue from animals not carrying a tumor, and liver from animals carrying non-cross-reactive tumors, were without effect. It seemed that there was something in the liver of an animal carrying a tumor mass—some would like to think that this is activated antigen—which stimulates heightened specific tumor resistance.

STUTMAN: In experiments with BSA–anti-BSA complexes on lymphocytes, using ^{125}I labeled BSA, we injected the ^{51}Cr-labeled thoracic duct lymphocytes into syngeneic animals and recovered labeled antigen in the liver at 24, 48, and 72 hr after injection. At these times, the labeled lymphocytes could be detected no longer. Thus, the lymphocytes may be cleaned up, and the antigen retained by the liver.

WEISS: Judging from the work of Askonas and others, such antigen taken up by liver phagocytic cells could indeed be highly immunogeneic.

MARTIN: We have been shown that for an immune response to be maximally effective against a tumor *in vivo*, the response should be against many tumor antigens. Because it is easier to examine a positive rather than a negative phenomenon, much of the present discussion has centered on the analysis of the immune response discernible in the tumor-bearing host. Possibly, not enough attention has been given to the lack of specific immune responses in certain tumor-bearing hosts. Accordingly, I would like to present a model which illustrates that not all antigens on a tumor are necessarily immunogenic. With Esber, I have compared the specificity of the immune response of C57BL/6 mice to irradiated EL-4 leukemia cells with that of C57BL/6 mice to irradiated RBL-5 leukemia cells. EL-4 and RBL-5 are syngeneic with C57BL/6 mice, in terms of the H-2 locus. Mice injected with irradiated EL-4 developed lymphoid cells active in the colony-inhibition assay against EL-4, but not against RBL-5. Similarly, cytotoxic lymphoid cells, generated *in vitro* from spleen cells of mice preimmunized with EL-4, were specifically lytic for EL-4 in a 4 hr ^{51}Cr-release assay. Mice immunized with RBL-5 developed lymphoid cells active in the CI assay against both RBL-5 and EL-4 cells. *In vitro* generated cytotoxic lymphoid cells from RBL-5 immunized mice were lytic for both RBL-5 and EL-4 cells. It, therefore, appears that RBL-5 and EL-4 share a common antigen. EL-4 appears, in addition, to express an antigen not present on RBL-5. In EL-4 immunized mice, it appears that the common antigen does not evoke a detectable immune response, i.e., it is nonimmunogenic. We have similar evidence for nonimmunogenic antigens in several other tumor systems. The point I want to make is that evidence for such tumor antigens will not be forthcoming if investigators limit their analyses to the preexisting antitumor response.

CHAIRMAN KLEIN: What is the quantity of this component when you do quantitative absorption in the two cell lines?

MARTIN: EL-4 and RBL-5 show a similar susceptibility to lysis by serum and cells of Balb/c mice immunized against the H-2^b histocompatibility anti-

264

gen. The similar levels of lysis of both target cells, achieved by sera and cytotoxic lymphoid cells of C57BL/6 mice immunized with RBL-5, suggests that the tumor component which lacks detectable immunogenicity on EL-4 is expressed in comparable amounts on EL-4 and RBL-5. Quantitative absorptions with the two tumor cell lines have not been performed.

ALEXANDER: What radiation does Martin apply to the cells used for immunization? Did he study the fate of the sterilized cells, as some cells lyse quickly following radiation?

MARTIN: The dose of radiation is 2000 R.

ALEXANDER: Did you ascertain how long the cells survived after radiation?

MARTIN: I did not.

ALEXANDER: I suggest that there could be a different explanation if, for example, EL-4 cells happened to behave like small lymphocytes and lysed within 4 hr, whereas the sarcoma cells did not lyse even in 2 months.

MARTIN: Spleen cells from an RBL-5 preimmunized animal can be boosted *in vitro* with irradiated EL-4. The antigen would, therefore, not appear to be completely destroyed by irradiation. This finding may also indicate that requirements for a secondary immune response may be less strict than those for a primacy response against a given antigen.

ALEXANDER: In the one case, where Martin is seeking to use the primary immune response, it is well known that antigen presented on a membrane is particularly effective; for a secondary type response, there may be no need to present the antigen on an intact membrane. I am not saying it is necessarily so. I only seek to emphasize that care must be taken with some of the lymphoma cells after irradiation to make sure that they do not break up quickly.

CHIECO-BIANCHI: Did Martin check EL-4 for virus contamination?

MARTIN: EL-4 has a type A, type C and probably other viruses. In fact, most transplantable cell lines have type C viruses and are known from other studies to share certain viral-related antigens. The finding of specificity in syngeneic immunization really indicates lack of significant response to the common, viral-determined antigens on the various laboratory cell lines, such as EL-4, P815, L1210, etc.

BACH: This is a general set of remarks, concerning genetic aspects of the blocking of whatever recognition function is involved in MLC, with reference to a special strain combination. H-2 complex has four regions, K, I, S, and D. Bailey found a spontaneous mutation in the C57BL/6 mice H-2 complex, which he mapped to the left of S. This is the H(z1) strain.

In all probability, this mutation is within the I region. We were perplexed by Widmer's observation that there were elements of the H-2 complex, other than the H-2K and H-2D serologically-defined antigens, whose products could be recognized in MLC. The mouse sero-immunogeneticists told us that this central region did not determine any products which were recognized serologically. On extensive cross immunization, and other protocols, Bailey *et al.* could find no cytotoxic or agglutinating acitivity against H-2K or H-2D antigens. Bailey's finding, that these strains reject skin grafts and the aforementioned findings, were the first evidence that factors other than H-2K and H-2D SD antigens of the H-2 region may be important in skin graft rejection. Despite the apparent SD identity, the LD difference in this case results in MLC activation and skin graft rejection, and we obtained cytotoxicity in CML. This is the one strain combination which argues that the target for CML maps in the SD region.

Several years ago, Ceppellini got everybody excited about blocking antisera related to HL-A. We all thought that these antisera were anti-SD. We have recently become more and more aware of LD, and the question arose of whether one could get blocking antisera in an LD different combination by cross immunization, despite the fact that one could not generate cytotoxic sera. Peck has cross immunized the strains C57BL/6 and H(z1) extensively, and he finds good blocking antisera. C57BL/6-H(z1) "antiserum" blocks the reaction of C57BL/6 to H(z1), or the reaction of H(z1) to C57BL/6. Likewise, H(z1) and C57BL/6 antiserum will block both one-way MLC reactions but not third-party combinations, in the same way. Despite the fact that there are presumably no anti-H-2K and anti-H-2D antibodies in this particular combination, we must recognize, as Terry, Klein, Shreffler, and their associates have found, that in the "I" region there are genes which determine serologically-defined antigens. These antigens, as Terry told us, are probably on B cells. B cells are also the prime stimulating cells in the MLC.

Despite the findings which seem to fit together so well, I would warn that we do not know whether the antisera to the Ia antigens in the I region, or what Terry calls the β-antigen, are detecting LD. There could be many genes in this area and, thus, many products. Clearly, we would like to define the membrane products which are involved in this particular mutation.

During the past two years, Ballou, Sundharadas, and Bach have worked to develop a method of solubilizing lymphocyte membranes which would, hopefully, allow their display in a gel based on charge separation, in the absence of SDS or other detergents. Membranes are isolated by nitrogen cavitation and dissolved in 100%, weight per volume, chloral hydrate. This allows the virtually complete solubilization of membranes and separation on what appears to be a charge difference. Ribosomal proteins, made in this way and tested for their functional properties in the Nomura ribosomal reassembly system, showed retention of activity. C57BL/6 and H(z1) membranes analyzed in this system give about 25 bands visible in the gel. One major banding difference is seen, but the rest of the bands are identical. We hope that this approach will allow us not only to say that there are differences but to get enough product to test for function.

ALEXANDER: Are these antisera cytotoxic to the respective cells? How did Bach solubilize the nitrogen-cavitated membrane preparations?

BACH: No antibody activity against H-2K or H-2D was obtained by Bailey, Cherry, and Snell. Chloral hydrate is the solubilizing agent, and the antigen preparations are run on acrylamide, not SDS.

CHAIRMAN KLEIN: I take it you find no link between antigenic activity and the bands that you are seeing?

BACH: The only link is the genetic link. We presume that with a spontaneous mutation we are dealing with something fairly restrictive; however, we do not know this.

CEROTTINI: How do you explain that a given serum is able to inhibit stimulation of MLC in both directions, if the antigenic determinants are carried by B cells only, as has been suggested?

BACH: Several possibilities exist. First, the serum may recognize not only the receptor site on the allogeneic cell but also the foreign LD antigen, whatever that is. Second, if the Ir product is a receptor site and if LD is identical with Ir, then having antibody to LD also gives an antibody to the receptor site. We may be dealing with a receptor site antiserum here, and the idiotype of the receptor is LD.

CEROTTINI: In that case, the antigens should be present on both T and B cells?

BACH: Yes, they should.

GOOD: What is Bach's evidence that B cells are the primary stimulating cells in MLC?

BACH: I was quoting Terry; I have no evidence for it.

UHR: Two studies are interesting in terms of Bach's comments on the role of B cells in MLC. Vitetta and I collaborated with Jan Klein in the analysis of the antigens recognized by the antisera raised between strains congenic in the I region *(Immunogenetics, 1, 82, 1974)*. We used two methods to label the antigens: tritiated precursors or enzymatic surface radioiodination. The results of these studies indicate that there is a molecule with MW of approximately 30,000 daltons which is the dominant antigen recognized by the antibody raised in these animals. This antigen appears to be synthesized primarily by B lymphocytes. There also are some antigens synthesized by lymphoid cells and present on the cell surface, which were recognized by autoantibodies in the sera used. Nathenson, Cullen, and their coworkers have performed similar studies using the antisera raised by Schreffler *(Proc. Natl. Acad. Sci.,* in press); their results are essentially analogous to our own.

It is important to emphasize that the I region contains hundreds of genes. Thus, there may be several dozen different kinds of proteins coded for this region. We have described one of them. Its function can be elucidated by the kind of studies Bach has suggested. Our results fit together nicely with those described by Terry.

BACH: Yes, I believe they do.

COHN: As we approach the end of this session, I shall present a framework within which we might consider the immune response to transformed cells. In the prior sessions, we have been presented with a myriad of examples of different types of immune response to tumors, without taking fully into account how the immune system functions normally. Without facing the fundamentals of the system, we cannot hope to integrate all the phenomena presented to us.

As I see it, there are three issues:

1. How is the normal self–nonself distinction made?
2. What normally determines the class of the response—cell mediated or humoral?
3. How does this normal response get sabotaged by the cancer?

In order to discuss them, I make the following assumptions:

1. Antigen- sensitive cells of all categories and with receptors which interact with self- and nonself-determinants are generated continuously.

2. Each antigen-sensitive cell, upon interacting via its receptors with antigen, has two pathways open to it, paralysis or induction.

3. Paralysis, which is likely the death of the cell, results when its receptors, upon interacting with antigen, trigger intracellular signal 1, which is cAMP mediated.

4. Induction results when antigen is associatively recognized by two specific systems: the receptor on the antigen-sensitive cell leading to signal 1 and the associative antibody system leading to signal 2, which is cGMP mediated intracellularly.

For our discussion, I need only symbolize the associative antibody system as diagrammed in Fig. 42, but it is well to point out that associative antibody is expressed on thymus-derived cooperating cells, is coded at least in part by the histocompatibility linked Ir-1 locus, and might function as cytophilic antibody on a third-party cooperating cell.

The four assumptions are illustrated in the two diagrams (Figs. 42 and 43).

There are several explanatory comments to make:

1. Signal 1 is common to the paralytic and inductive pathways. No cell can be induced which is not paralyzable.

2. The inducible and paralyzable antigen-sensitive cell upon induction differentiates to a noninducible and nonparalyzable effector end cell. This effector cell might act as such (T^c or T^k) or might secrete its antibody product [plasmacyte (P)], which acts in conjunction with another nonspecific system (macrophages, basophils, monocytes, complement).

3. Induction also leads to the production of more antigen-sensitive cells.

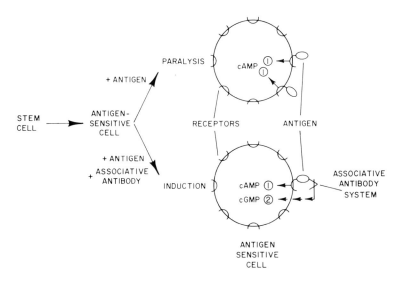

Fig. 42. Two-signal (associative recognition) model for the induction and paralysis of antigen-sensitive cells.

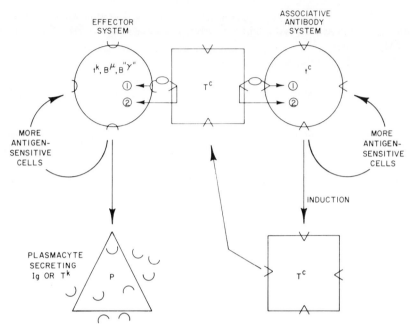

Fig. 43. Illustration of the asymmetry between the induction of the associative antibody system and the effector system; t^c: thymus-derived, antigen-sensitive cooperating cell; T^c: induced functioning, cooperating end cell. This cell could secrete its associative antibody which acts cytophilically (see text); t^k: antigen sensitive, thymus-derived killer cell; T^k: induced-functioning, thymus-derived, killer end cell; B^μ: antigen-sensitive, bone-marrow–derived precursor for IgM synthesis; $B^{"\gamma"}$ antigen-sensitive, bone marrow–derived precursor for all other immunoglobulin classes.

It is possible to create conditions which favor one pathway or the other; that leading to end cells or to more antigen-sensitive cells. The function of the end cell is X-ray (or mitomycin) resistant, whereas the induction of the antigen-sensitive cell which involves replication, as diagrammed, is X-ray sensitive.

4. The associative antibody system regulates self-nonself discrimination (paralysis versus induction) whereas the effector system carries out the usual protective functions of the immune system.

5. The relationship between the associative antibody and the effector system is asymmetric in that the former is required for the induction of the latter, not vice versa. Failure to recognize this has led to mistaken interpretations of experiments on the specificity, induction, and paralysis of T and B cells.

The self–nonself distinction arises according to this model as follows:

The immune system arises during fetal development, at a point in time and at a rate which is optimized between making the self-nonself discrimination and defending the organism. This means that if it arises too early, the later appearance of adult antigens would present a problem of autoimmunity, whereas if it

270

arises too late there would be no protection against neonatally encountered pathogens. Further, if antigen-sensitive cells, antiself and antinonself, were generated too rapidly (e.g., as an extreme case) autoimmunity would instantaneously result. In the absence of the associative antibody system, antiself antigen-sensitive cells interacting with self components are paralyzed, whereas the antinonself cells accumulate. As long as the self-component is present, tolerance to that component is maintained. If the self-component disappears, e.g., a fetal antigen, the immune system then recovers recognition of it, and the adult treats it as foreign. This, presumably, is the origin of the immune response to tumor-specific antigens of fetal origin. The key point here is that associative recognition of at least two determinants on an antigen is obligatory for induction (signal 1 plus signal 2), whereas an interaction between antigen and the receptor on the antigen-sensitive cell leads to paralysis (signal 1). In the absence of associative antibody, the interaction of the receptors on an antigen-sensitive cell and antigen can only lead to paralysis.

The associative antibody system also regulates the class of the response, cell mediated or humoral. I realize that there are several types of both cell-mediated and humoral response, but, for the moment, it is simplest to do some grouping and refer to the behavior of the thymus-derived antigen-sensitive killer cell (t^k) as an example of the cell-mediated system and the behavior of the bone-marrow-derived antigen-sensitive E and B^γ cells as an example of the humoral response. The nature of this regulation is illustrated in Fig. 44.

What this graph shows is the following:

1.   As the effective level of the associative antibody system rises, the response to antigen is different.

2.   At "zero" levels of associative antibody, receptor interaction with antigen leads to paralysis.

3.   At very low levels (to high levels) of associative antibody, the antigen-sensitive cooperating thymus-derived cell (t) is induced.

4.   At low effective levels the antigen-sensitive cell-mediated killer cell (t) is induced.

5.   At intermediate effective levels, induction of the antigen-sensitive cell-mediated killer cell (t^k) is inhibited but the antigen-sensitive IgM bone-marrow-derived cell (B^μ) is induced.

6.   At high levels the induction of B^μ is inhibited, but the antigen-sensitive IgG bone-marrow-derived cell (B^γ) is induced.

This describes the phenomenology but does not give the mechanism. Bretscher has proposed that the different classes of antigen-sensitive cells, t^c, t^k, B^μ, B^γ, respond to different levels of signal 2. For example, t^k is induced but B^μ is not at low levels of signal 2, whereas at intermediate levels, induction of t^k is inhibited whereas B^μ is induced. This seems an eminently reasonable idea.

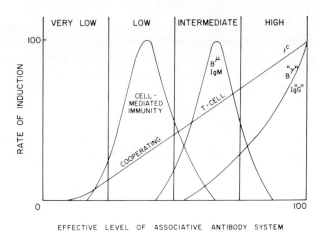

Fig. 44. Responsiveness of various cell types as a function of the effective level of the associative antibody system.

The effective level of the associative antibody system depends upon several factors: concentration of antigen, level of the associative antibody, binding constant of antigen to associative antibody. A more rigorous, but correspondingly lengthy, analysis would require substituting the number of inductive signals per receptor for the effective level of the associative antibody system in the abscissa. This can be illustrated using one variable, the effect of concentration of antigen on the response (see Bretscher, 1974 for detailed analysis).

At either low or high concentrations of antigen, the effective level of the associative antibody system is low and a cell-mediated (t) response is induced. At optimal concentrations of antigen, the effective level of associative antibody is too high for induction of t^k (it is inhibitory) and the humoral response is induced.

To clarify this, consider examples in which the effective level of associative antibody would be low, favoring a cell-mediated immune response:

1. antigens close to self-components, e.g., fetal antigens, tumor-specific antigens, histocompatibility antigens, modified self-components (DCNB-painted skin)

2. antigens which have few foreign surface determinants, derived either by chemical modification or incurring naturally, e.g., aceto-acetylated flagellin, or SRBC, mycobacteria coated with nonimmunogenic lipid, schistosoma coated with glycolipids from host erythrocytes, neoplastic cells which escape complement-dependent humoral-killing mechanisms, virus-infected cells.

3. low and high concentrations of antigens, e.g., SRBC (Mackaness, this conference; McCullagh, *Transplantation Reviews,* **12,** 180, 1972).

4. Thymus-depleted animals (Bretscher, *Cell. Immunol.,* in press; Gershon and Kondo, *Immunology,* **18,** 723, 1970).

The next point to be made follows from the requirement that induction of cell-mediated and humoral immunity be, in large measure, mutually exclusive, i.e., the immune system can under certain conditions lock into a cell-mediated response. This would not be possible if there were no inhibitory feedback mechanism, whereby the cell-mediated system itself (or a parallel-induced system) inhibited the induction of the associative antibody system. This is symbolized in Fig. 45 and includes Bretscher's specific proposal as to mechanism (in press).

The specific comments to be made about this are:

1. The inhibition of induction of t^c could be carried out by the effector cell, T^k itself, or by another cell (T^S) which is induced under the conditions described earlier for the induction of cell-mediated immunity.

2. An inhibitory signal 3 is postulated—delivered by the T^k cell. This implies competition between induction via signal 2 and inhibition via signal 3. Conditions for switching in and out of a cell-mediated response are now predictable.

3. The model is minimal in that inhibition via signal 3 might also act on B cells, but there is no need to suppose that at the moment. Regulation of induction of B cells can be carried out uniquely on the level of the associative antibody system.

This formulation puts the whole problem of "T cell suppression," as it is colloquially termed, into proper context, not as a mechanism of the normal self–nonself discrimination but as a regulatory mechanism for the class of re-

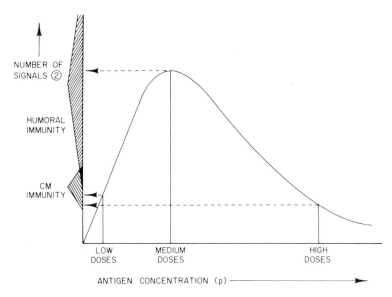

Fig. 45. Concept for the regulation of class of response as a function of antigen concentration, i.e., *effective* associative antibody level.

sponse. So-called ''T cell suppression'' has two regulatory components: (1) the effective level of the associative antibody system, and (2) the ''cell-mediated'' inhibition of the induction of associative antibody.

The last point deals with one way in which a normal immune response could be sabotaged by a tumor. We have termed this abnormal induction. Normally, two determinants are associatively recognized by the antigen-sensitive and associative antibody system because they are on one antigen. The self–nonself discrimination depends upon this fact. However, the antigen-sensitive cell cannot tell whether or not another determinant on the antigen is being recognized by the associative antibody system. It only knows that it is receiving signal 2. Consequently, any cell receiving signal 1 via a receptor–antigen interaction will be induced by signal 2, which might be delivered via associative antibody recognition of a cell-surface determinant which is not on the antigen. This is diagrammed in Fig. 46.

The surface determinant in question might be a histocompatibility antigen, a virus, a lectin (Con A, PHA, PWM, etc.), lipopolysaccharide, or a piece of foreign membrane. The abnormal delivery of signal 2 sabotages the immune system in two ways:

1. The self –nonself discrimination cannot be made because the interaction between a self-component (to which there is no associative antibody) and an antigen-sensitive cell, which would ordinarily lead to paralysis, is converted into an inductive stimulus by associative antibody recognition of the unrelated foreign surface determinant. This leads to selection for autoimmune reactivity, e.g., NZB mice, and decreases the number of cells capable of recognizing foreign determinants. It might be well to recall here that there is a relatively high incidence of autoimmune disorder in patients with Hodgkin's disease and other lymphomas.

2. Low levels of associative antibody, which might permit induction of a purely cell-mediated response only, are made more effective by polymerizing foreign determinants on the surface of the antigen-sensitive cell. This leads to induction of a humoral response, which is enhancing because it blocks effective killing by the cell-mediated system. Such a situation might arise if tumor-specific antigens (membrane fragments) are shed and, like LPS, are bound to other cells, in particular antigen-sensitive cells. These foreign determinants put on the surface of the antigen-sensitive cell could increase the effective level of associative antibody and lead to enhancing humoral antibody formation.

Another way in which enhancing humoral antibody could be induced, instead of a cell-mediated response, would be a two-step process involving normal induction (Fig. 47). The transformed cell might express tumor-specific surface determinants at such a density that humoral antibody would be induced. The complement-dependent killing reaction would select for a variant tumor cell which reduced its level of surface antigen to a point where complement lysis

IV. INTERFERENCE WITH IMMUNE DESTRUCTION OF TUMORS

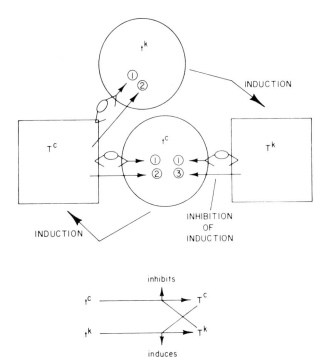

Fig. 46. The Bretscher hypothesis for the regulation of cooperating cells by T killer or suppressor cells.

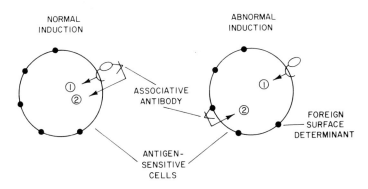

Fig. 47. Comparison between normal and abnormal induction illustrating the uncoupling of associative recognition for induction.

was ineffective, thus converting the humoral killing response into a protective one. The resistant variant with surface antigen at low density would, ordinarily, induce a cell-mediated primary response which might even be stabilized by feedback, as discussed earlier. However, in the preimmunized animal, the high levels of associative antibody permit effective induction of humoral antibody by concentrations of antigen too low to induce, if a primary response were involved.

These thoughts are offered in the search for some kind of conceptual background, of which this is but one example, to guide the next and final session in which we consider responsiveness to tumors and ways of manipulating the immune system.*

*Editors footnote: The following references also apply to Cohn's discussion in pp. 268-275 of this session. In them, the reader can trace the development of Cohn and Bretscher's conceptual analysis of induction and cell cooperation and can examine the data which underlie their assumptions. "A Theory of Self–Nonself Discrimination," Bretscher and Cohn, Science, 169, 1042, 1970; "A Model for Generalized Autoimmunity," Bretscher, Cell. Immunol., 6, 1, 1973; "The Control of Humoral and Associative Antibody Synthesis," Bretscher, Transplantation Rev., 11, 217, 1972; "On the Control between Cell-Mediated, IgM and IgG Immunity, and its Relevance to Cancer," Bretscher, Cell. Immunol., in press; "Immunology: What Are the Rules of the Game?" Cohn, Cell. Immunol., 5, 1, 1972; Cohn, "Comment on Abnormal Induction," in Uhr and Landy (Eds.), Immunologic intervention, New York: Academic Press, 1971, pp. 72–73; Cohn, "Conference Evaluation and Commentary," in McDevitt and Landy (Eds.), Genetic control of immune responsiveness, New York: Academic Press, 1972, pp. 367–448.

SESSION V

CLINICAL IMPLICATIONS OF THE DATA BASE CONCERNING THE TUMOR–HOST RELATIONSHIP

Malignancy in immunodeficiency diseases—Immunodeficiency in cancer patients—The nude mouse as a model for immune surveillance—Reevaluation of the immune surveillance concept—Immune facilitation of tumor growth (immunostimulation)—Assessment of immune function in cancer patients—Immunosuppressive effects of radiation therapy—Correlation of *in vitro* tests of specific immunity with clinical status—Immunotherapeutic approaches to cancer in man—Clinical studies on effect of immunopotentiating agents such as BCG, MER, *C. parvum,* mixed bacterial vaccine—Mechanism of BCG antitumor action—Tumor immunotherapy via immune reconstitution.

CHAIRMAN GOOD: The purpose of this session is to consider the inter-locked subjects of malignancy in patients with immunodeficiency, immunodeficiency in patients with malignancy, and the experimental and clinical concepts of immunopotentiation and immunotherapy in patients with cancer. My brief contribution is in two parts: (1) the occurrence of cancer in patients with the primary immunodeficiencies, and (2) immunodeficiencies in patients with cancer. We will then turn to the consideration of the rationale for immunotherapy both in model systems and in the clinic. Here we need to discuss in depth the concept of immunodeficiency in cancer and the evidence underlying immunopotentiation, immunotherapy with BCG, *Corynebacterium parvum*, and mixed bacterial vaccines. Finally, we should consider cellular and macromolecular engineering as possible approaches to improvement of management and treatment of cancer.

The primary immunodeficiency diseases are associated with malignancy both in the dramatic experience of individual cases and the compelling observations made in several small series of patients. More recently, efforts to survey populations of children and adults with primary immunodeficiency disease for the incidence of cancer has been attempted through an international registry operated under the auspices of the World Health Organization and the support of the National Cancer Institute. This registry is headquartered in Minneapolis and New York and run by Kersey, Spector, and myself. The data linking primary immunodeficiency with malignancy are recorded in Table 39. These data show that between 2 and 10% of patients having each of several different forms of primary immunodeficiency have developed malignancies. This incidence of about 7/100,000 per year is clearly in excess of the incidence of cancer in the general population of children. Leukemias and lymphomas occur in about 3 per 100,000 children per year, and solid tissue malignancies occur with an incidence of approximately 4/100,000 per year. Children and young adults having primary immunodeficiencies, therefore, experience a frequency of cancer 100–1000 times the incidence in the general population. As is shown in Table 40, children from the general population have different types of malignancy than those who also have primary immunodeficiency. Primary cancers of bone, central nervous sytem, and other sites like kidney and rhabdomyosarcomas make up a substantial proportion of fatal malignancies in children of an unselected population. By contrast, lymphomas and especially reticulum cell sarcomas are of inordinate frequency in children having primary immunodeficiency. In certain forms of primary immunodeficiency, such as the common variable form, epithelial malignancies as well as lymphoreticular cancers also seem to occur at excess frequency.

Table 41 shows that epithelial tumors are confined to the common variable form of immunodeficiency and ataxia telangiectasia. Patients with x-linked infantile agammaglobulinemia, severe combined immunodeficiency, Wiskott–

279

TABLE 39
Incidence of Malignancy in Primary Immunodeficiency Syndromes

Disease	Approx. no. patients with immuno- deficiency disease	No. patients with malignancy	Estimated risk
Congenital X-linked immunodeficiency	100	6	6%
Severe combined system immunodeficiency	400	9	2%
IgM deficiency	70	6	8%
Wiskott-Aldrich syndrome	300	24	8%
Ataxia telangiectasia	500	52	10%
Common variable immunodeficiency	500	41	8%
Total	1870	138	7%

TABLE 40
Mortality from Cancer of Various Types
in Children under 15 Years of Age

Type of cancer	Incidence in children		
	Unselected population[a]	With primary immunodeficiency[b]	
	%	All areas %	U.S. Only %
Leukemia	48	25	25
CNS	16	4	3
Lymphoreticular RCS, lymphosarcoma	8	67	69
Bone	4	2	0
Other	24	2	3

[a]Death certificates of 29,457 children in U.S. (*J. Pediatrics,* 75, 685, 1969).
[b]From Immunodeficiency-Cancer Registry.

Aldrich syndrome, and isolated absence of IgG and IgA with increased levels of IgM, leukemia, lymphoma, lymphosarcoma and especially reticulum cell sarcoma are more common.

The epithelial malignancies that occur in patients with the variable immunodeficiency syndromes require special comment. The cases reported have frequently been carcinomas of the stomach. In this context, it is of interest that a high frequency of histamine-fast achlorhydria, atrophic gastritis, and pernicious anemia also occur in conjunction with this form of immunodeficiency.

The registry lists more than 185 occurrences of cancer as having been re-

TABLE 41

Types of Malignancy Reported in Primary Immunodeficiency Diseases

Disease		Histologic types of tumors				
	Epithelial %	Lymphoreticular %	Leukemia %	Mesenchymal %	Nervous system %	Total
Congenital X-linked immuno-deficiency	0[a]	1 (17)[b]	5 (83)	0	0	6
Severe combined system immuno-deficiency	0	6 (67)	3 (33)	0	0	9
IgM deficiency	0	5 (83)	0	0	1 (17)	6
Wiskott–Aldrich syndrome	0	19 (79)	3 (13)	1 (4)	1 (4)	24
Ataxia-telangiectasia	6 (11)	32 (62)	11 (21)	1 (2)	2 (4)	52
Common variable immuno-deficiency	12 (29)	23 (56)	4 (10)	1 (2)	1 (2)	41
IgA deficiency	9 (69)	2 (15)	0	1 (8)	1 (8)	13[c]
Total	27 (18%)	88 (58%)	26 (17%)	4 (3%)	6 (4%)	151

[a]Number of individuals reported to May, 1973.
[b]Malignancy type for each primary immunodeficiency disease.
[c]Occurring in 7 individuals.

corded in patients receiving immunosuppressive therapy for organ transplantation. The frequency of lymphoreticular cancers and especially reticulum cell sarcomas is 6–100 times more frequent than expected in immunosuppressed patients. The frequency of all cancer in these patients is also significantly greater than in members of the general population. Why these malignancies occur is not clear. Proposals have been made that such cancer is linked to the immunodepressive drugs *per se*, to immunosuppressive agents such as potential chemical oncogens, and to host versus graft or graft versus host reactions.

Early in the course of establishing the practice of kidney transplantation, 17 patients were known to be inadvertantly transplanted with cancer cells present in the transplanted organ. In five, widely disseminated epithelial malignancies were studied and treated. In four of these five patients, successful treatment resulted simply from stoppping immunosuppressive therapy. Metastatic malignancy could, therefore, be treated effectively by simply permitting the immunological system to express itself in those individuals in whom a cancer had been transplanted inadvertantly. This represents a special case, of course, because such malignant cells have strong transplantation alloantigens. These findings, however, *do* reveal the potentiality of the immunological system for eliminating cancer if the host treats the tumor cells as though they have strong transplantation antigens.

Table 42 shows that in the cases of primary immunodeficiency involving multiple malignancies in a single family, the type of tumor tends to be similar in other involved members of the family. In one notable family studied by Haerer *et al.*, two teen-agers developed carcinoma of the stomach. Five primary malignancies occurred in another immunodeficient patient who lacked IgA. In that same family, another member also had a primary immunodeficiency and multiple cancers. In patients lacking both IgG and IgA, IgM may be greatly increased as Rosen and Gitlin have described. In such patients, lymphoid malignancy is very frequent. Almost all such children who have been followed for a number of years have died with what seems best defined as B cell type of lymphomas.

Other familial diseases in which malignancy occurs in high frequency include Fanconi's hematologic syndrome, Bloom's syndrome, and Down's syndrome. In some such patients, chromosomal breaks occur with high frequency, in addition to numerical abnormalities of chromosomes and other defects. These patients and children with familial myelogenous leukemia and Kleinfelter's syndrome show an additional abnormality that could be important in their susceptibility to cancer. Cultures of fibroblasts from their subcutaneous tissues are approximately ten times more susceptible to transformation by SV40 virus than are fibroblasts cultured from normal persons. This abnormality was not found with fibroblasts cultured from the connective tissues of patients with different forms of primary immunodeficiency disease.

TABLE 42
Immunodeficiency and Malignancy in Sibling Pairs

Age	Sex	Primary immunodeficiency disease	Malignancy
6	M	AT[a]	Acute lymphoblastic leukemia
5	F	AT	Acute lymphoblastic leukemia
3	M	AT	Acute lymphoblastic leukemia
15	M	AT	Acute lymphoblastic leukemia
21	F	AT	Adenocarcinoma of stomach
19	F	AT	Adenocarcinoma of stomach
12	M	AT	Lymphoblastic leukemia
6	M	AT	Acute leukemia
		AT	Lymphoma
		AT	Lymphoma
		AT	Lymphoma
14	M	AT	"Malign lymphosarcomatoses"
10+	M	AT	"Histiocytosarcoma"
4	M	AT	Lymphosarcoma
6	M	AT	Lymphosarcoma
12	M	CV[b]	Lymphosarcoma
3	F	aplastic thymus	Lymphosarcoma
19	F	CV	Reticulum cell sarcoma
11	F	CV	Reticulum cell sarcoma
58	M	CV	Chronic lymphatic leukemia
60	M	CV	Chronic lymphatic leukemia
21	M	CV	Lymphosarcoma
5	M	CV	Lymphosarcoma
6	M	Wiskott-Aldrich	Malignant reticuloendotheliosis
3-1/2	M	Wiskott-Aldrich	Myelogenous leukemia
21	F	IgA	Multiple primaries
16	M	IgA	Reticulum cell sarcoma
	M	IgM	Lymphoreticular
	M	IgM	Lymphoreticular
	M	IgM	Lymphoreticular

[a]AT: ataxia-telangiectasia.
[b]CV: common variable.

Now let us go to my second point—the other side of the coin. Immunodeficiency occurs in many, if not all, patients with malignancy. For example, in Hodgkin's disease anergy is often present. Careful studies have revealed this to occur early in the course of the malignancy and to progress as the disease advances. A very poor prognosis is associated with the lymphocyte-depleted form of the disease. The confusion about the immunodeficiency of Hodgkin's disease seems to be settled now, and our earlier studies linking Hodgkin's disease to anergy, to relative unresponsiveness to sensitization, to susceptibility to skin allotransplantation, and to resistance to passive transfer of cell-mediated immunity, are supported by the recent definitive studies of the Stanford group, led by Kaplan and his associates, and by the studies of Eltringham and Levey.

Counterpoint to Hodgkin's disease is the immunodeficiency associated with multiple myeloma. Here a defect in production of circulating antibodies is characteristic. By contrast, cell-mediated immunity is usually intact. In Hodgkin's disease, antibody formation is well preserved while cell-mediated functions are severely deficient. In multiple myeloma, antibody formation and normal immunoglobulin synthesis are compromised. In chronic lymphatic leukemia, the malignant cell is usually an IgM-producing B lymphocyte, but less frequently it produces IgG, IgA, or IgE. It is associated with progressive deficiency of normal antibody production.

Over 70% of solid tissue non-Hodgkin's lymphoma is of the B lymphocyte class. When these patients are carefully studied, immunodeficiencies can frequently be shown. A small proportion of the solid tissue non-Hodgkin's lymphomas are T cell or are histiocytic malignancies. In the Sezary syndrome and its nonleukemic counterpart, mycosis fungoides, the malignant cells seem to have markers suggesting the T lymphocyte class.

Immunodeficiency is not only encountered in patients in whom malignancy involves the lymphoid apparatus. Immunodeficiency may also be encountered in patients with various kinds of epithelial malignancies. For example, even early in the course of their disease, patients with head and neck cancers may have profound defects in ability to develop and express delayed hypersensitivity responses. Little information is yet available as to the basis for such deficiency in immune function. Nonetheless, this phenomenon deserves analysis for many reasons. If such deficits can be understood and corrected, patients with advanced cancer may be able to cope better with intercurrent infections. Further, if immunity plays any role in resisting cancer, understanding and correcting these defects may form the basis of all adjuncts to therapy.

To illustrate what may be learned by relatively simple studies in this direction, I shall describe briefly efforts of my two associates, the Tsakraklides, to relate the morphology of the draining regional lymph nodes to prognosis in cancer of uterus, breast, and colon. The morphologic patterns of lymph nodes draining cancer of these organs may be classified as follows:

1. lymphocyte-predominant patterns in which the lymph node has been clearly stimulated and in which the response has occurred primarily in the deep cortical regions where T lymphocytes abound;

2. germinal-center-predominant pattern in which the regional lymph nodes also have been stimulated and in which germinal centers are most abundant;

3. unstimulated pattern in which the lymph nodes show little or no evidence of stimulation, proliferation, or accumulation of lymphoid cells;

4. the lymphocyte-depleted pattern in which depletion of lymphocytes from both T and B areas and fibrosis of the node are characteristic.

In general, the lymphocyte-predominant and germinal-center-predominant patterns are associated with better prognosis than are the unstimulated and lymphocyte-depleted patterns. Tables 43 and 44 illustrate these relations in breast cancer. The relationship holds whether or not metastasis to the nodes has already occurred. The lymphocyte-predominant pattern is associated with a predominance of T cells and more vigorous T cell responses, and germinal-center predominance with excesses of B cell numbers (data not shown). Whether or not these interesting associations can be used predictively or in planning reconstructive therapy will only be determined by future studies and therapeutic efforts. All of the initial morphologic studies were done in double blind retrospective analyses. Prospective studies are underway and already tend to confirm evidence for association of the morphological patterns with the distribution of the different lymphocyte classes and functions mentioned.

These findings in both primary immunodeficiency disease and cancer can-

TABLE 43

Correlates between Histologic Pattern and Five-Year Survival

	Number of cases		
Histologic pattern	Total	Alive	Surviving
Lymphocyte predominance	149	125	84% (77-89%)[a]
Germinal center predominance	47	34	72% (57-83%)
Lymphocyte depletion	11	4	36% (11-68%)
Unstimulated	70	44	63% (51-74%)
Total	277	207	75% (69-80%)

[a]Confidence limits.

TABLE 44

Correlates between Lymph Node Histology and Ten-Year Survival

	Number of cases		
Histologic pattern	Total	Alive	Surviving
Lymphocyte predominance	83	57	69% (58-78%)[a]
Germinal center predominance	23	10	43% (36-76%)
Lymphocyte depletion	8	2	25% (13-65%)
Unstimulated	44	22	50% (35-65%)
Total	158	91	58% (29-66%)

[a]Confidence limits.

not be taken as unequivocal support for an unmodified concept of immunosurveillance. They do, however, continue to speak for an important and, perhaps, essential relationship between immunity and malignancy. There continues to be hope that these studies may lead to understanding of the scientific basis for immunologic contributions toward prevention and treatment of cancer.

COHN: In Table 42 you show that morphologically-identical cancers arise with higher than random frequency in immunodeficient sibs. Is immunodeficiency the cause, or is immunodeficiency simply revealing a phenomenon which we would not ordinarily see because it occurs with too low frequency? As an example of the latter, if one injects inbred Balb/c mice with mineral oil, over 80% of the tumors so induced are plasmacytomas.

CHAIRMAN GOOD: There must be an interaction of the two processes, the one inducing the malignant state and the other permitting its full expression. We have now observed multiple cases from about 20 families, and the pattern of cancer reported by the pathologists is consistent.

COHN: The data needed do not involve frequencies of immunodeficiency in sibs but the frequency of identical cancers in otherwise normal sibs.

CHAIRMAN GOOD: We have this abundant data from Fraumeni's studies, which show patterns of cancer in families and a predominance of certain forms of cancer, such as breast or colon.

COHN: I am trying to ascertain if the identity of cancers in sibs is related to immunodeficiency or to an independent phenomenon.

CHAIRMAN GOOD: One pattern is of reticulum cell malignancies in certain families with immunodeficiency and of gastric cancers in another family with immunodeficiency. This patterning in families is not yet understood. In contradistinction to what we originally thought from inadequate data, our data now argue that a particular population of malignancies occurs in patients having primary immunodeficiency disease. The door is open to malignancy as we originally concluded, but I no longer interpret these data as strongly supporting the concept of immune surveillance against cancer.

COHN: Still pursuing my point, does an individual who has cancer and is, as a consequence, anergic have a higher probability of getting a second tumor? Or is it impossible to gather these kind of data because the first cancer kills before a second can arise?

CHAIRMAN GOOD: These data are gathered, but they are hard to interpret because of the influences of treatment. There is no question that second primaries occur more frequently, but why they occur is unclear. Second primaries could have the same cause as the initial cancer, and this might not be attributable to the immunodeficiency state but rather to the persistent oncogenic agent or even to an oncogenic effect of therapy, such as X-irriation, alkylating agents, or immunosuppressive drugs.

STJERNSWÄRD: Good's data show that the dominant tumors originate in lymphoid organs. These data have also been quoted for some years as support for the existence of an immunologic surveillance mechanism. They could also be interpreted in exactly the opposite way. It is a valid interpretation that tumors arise by two different mechanisms—chronic immunostimulation and immunosuppression?

My interpretation is that the high frequency of lymphoreticular tumors is not directly due to immunodeficiency but to chronic antigenic stimulation in an immunodeficient host. I gather that many such patients have chronic infections, virus and bacterial, which in the old days was the cause of their death. This interpretation is supported by experimental data demonstrating increased incidence of lymphoid tumors after chronic antigenic stimulation of mice (Metcalf, *Brit. J. Cancer*, **15**,769, 1961; Schwartz and Beldotti, *Science*, **149**,1511, 1965; Walford, *Science*, **152**,78, 1966). Clinical data, demonstrating an increased frequency of reticulum cell sarcoma in patients immunosuppressed but stimulated by an antigenic transplant, could also be interpreted as supporting the idea (Stjernswärd, *J. Nat. Cancer Inst. Monograph*, **35**,149, 1972).

CHAIRMAN GOOD: There is no question that deficient patients are exposed to excessive antigenic stimulation. When the IgA system is lacking, excessive stimulation from antigens absorbed from the intestinal tract can be expected. Patients with selective IgA deficiency will often have specific antibody directed against IgA in the circulation. Over one-half have precipitating antibody to BSA. A variety of autoimmune diseases occurs frequently. My interpretation is that the latter reflects excessive antigenic stimulation, by a wide variety of organisms and antigens which stimulate the intact immunologic functions. Whether excessive stimulation of lymphoid cells is associated with malignant change in these patients remains an open question.

STJERNSWÄRD: The increased risk of lymphoid tumors after chronic antigenic stimulation, borne out both in experimental and existing clinical data, may temper the present enthusiasm for uncritical stimulation of various types of cancer patients by nonspecific immunostimulants, such as BCG. In our experiments, BCG given prophylactically against ^{90}Sr-induced sarcomas in the primary host did lead to a decreased frequency of osteogenic sarcoma but an increased frequency of leukemia (Nilsson, Revesz, and Stjernswärd, *Rad. Res.*, **26**,378, 1965).

CHAIRMAN GOOD: The reason we are discussing this is to force us to think about what we are doing when we use immunotherapy.

LANDY: I would like to come back to an issue relating to Cohn's query. What information has thus far been derived from the study of malignancies that occur in identical twins?

CHAIRMAN GOOD: With some malignancies, there is striking concordance in identical twins; in others, such as chronic myeloid leukemia, there is discordance. In the acute myeloid leukemia, in acute lymphoid leukemia, and in melanoma, we see striking concordance. Even identical twins who have been geographically separated from early childhood may develop melanomas at the same site at approximately the same time in life.

SMITH: Good must have looked at the studies of Berg, Black, and the Japanese workers on lymphoid responses in breast and gastric cancer. They made the same essential conclusion but in a much less sophisticated way with respect to dissecting the morphologic changes in terms of T and B cell representation.

CHAIRMAN GOOD: Yes, Black was investigating this question in the early 1950s, but, because of lack of knowledge of the distribution of different lymphoid cells in lymph nodes, he could not describe the lymph nodes in such a way that would make it possible for others to follow up his work and establish its reproducibility. When several pathologists, including those at Memorial Hospital, tried to confirm Black's findings in respect to his emphasis on sinus histiocytosis, they could not reproduce his findings. But, when I talk to Black and go over his papers now, I realize that the sinus histiocytosis pattern he described is similar to what the Tsakraklides and I now describe as the lymphocyte-predominant pattern. We do not find that sinus histiocytosis itself is very helpful. Black's emphasis on sinus histiocytosis was unfortunate. Black was right, however, and the Japanese workers who described stimulated and depleted patterns were observing relationships similar to those we now emphasize.

BACH: In the lymphocyte-depleted pattern, Good found the histologic patterns consistent with both T and B cell suppression. What about the percentage of T and B cells in the peripheral blood?

CHAIRMAN GOOD: We are now correlating the percentage and absolute numbers of T and B lymphocytes, since these have not been well defined in any of these diseases. The lymphocyte-depleted pattern is an infrequent pattern, and we do not have a lot of material yet, but we will attempt to answer this question.

CHIECO-BIANCHI: I prefer to be somewhat more cautious in interpreting the histological pattern of lymph nodes draining the cancer area. A number of variables, not strictly connected with the tumor status, may actually alter the picture. For instance, a biopsy very often precedes mastectomy. In these cases, the granulomatous reaction present in the surrounding mammary tissues may influence the node structure. Also, in elderly persons, the pattern Good describes as lymphocyte depletion is frequently observed even if the tumor mass is located in the internal quadrants of the breast.

CHAIRMAN GOOD: Despite real efforts, we have been unable to correlate the findings with anything except the ultimate prognosis. We find no correlation with age, sex, previous biopsies, or other factors. I am aware of the general decline in the lymphoid structural apparatus with age, but it has not yet been well studied in the regional nodes of man.

PREHN: We may have a model in nude mice of what Good has been seeing. Our nude mice are in a germ-free state and many of them are now over a year old. Curiously enough, we have seen five or six reticulum cell sarcomas in these animals. The ultimate incidence is probably going to be very high, just as it is in these immunodeficiency patients. At the same time, we have observed no other spontaneous malignancies of any kind, which reinforces Good's statement that perhaps these immunodeficiency states do not provide good evidence to support the general surveillance idea.

CHAIRMAN GOOD: We may have overinterpreted the data on these patients to be supportive of the concept of surveillance in the past. They may support the existence of immunologic surveillance against certain forms of cancer. I feel quite certain that the general view of immunologic surveillance against cancer is neither supported nor rejected by these observations.

Stutman has also been working with nude mice and, like several others now, does not observe malignancies—especially epithelial malignancies. But nude mice are an imperfect model in a number of ways. They do have adequate B cell immunity, at least with respect to IgM, and they may have immunologic defense against many things on that basis alone.

TERRY: Regarding nude mice, are they really totally T-cell deficient?

CHAIRMAN GOOD: Whether nude mice have any T lymphocytes depends much on their genetic background. However, MLC responsiveness alone is a treacherous indicator. With Bach, we have described patients with severe, combined immunodeficiency disease who seem to have MLC reactivity but no other evidence of T lymphocytes. Gatti and I described this situation in a patient with a DiGeorge snydrome. Stites and Fudenberg found that early fetal liver cells can show this effect, presumably before the development of any thymus or T lymphocytes.

In light of the observations coming from Lafferty and his associates, we think that MLC reactivity, in this circumstance, may be evidence of allogeneic stimulation rather than, as Bach contends, due to liberation of blastogenic factor. Lafferty found that the proliferative stimulus to mesenchymal cells by allogeneic T cells acts before any development of the thymus in chick embryos.

One has, therefore, to be very careful in using MLC data itself as evidence of immunocompetence. I have now encountered incontrovertible evidence that proliferative responses may occur with peripheral blood cells in the absence of a thymus. Further, severe GVH reactions occur in recipients of marrow transplants who have had positive MLC reactions. Even if mitomycin at maximal dose is used to inhibit the proliferation of the stimulating cells, allogeneic stimulation can be effected. I submit that this may be the explanation of data indicating strong MLC reactions occurring where weak ones are really appropriate—the so-called paradoxical MLC reactions may be due to this allogeneic effect.*

PREHN: It should be pointed out that if the nude mouse is an imperfect model of surveillance, then there is no relationship between ordinary transplantation

*Editors' note: A list of references to data in this section was requested from Good and is as follows: Good, "Relations between Immunity and Malignancy," Proc. Nat. Acad. Sci., 69, 1026, 1972; Gatti and Good, "Occurrence of Malignancy in Immunodeficiency Diseases," Cancer, 28, 89, 1971; Kersey, Spector, and Good, "Primary Immunodeficiency Diseases and Cancer: The Immunodeficiency Cancer Registry," Int. J. Cancer, 12, 333, 1973;Tsakraklides, Olson, Kersey, and Good, "Prognostic Significance of the Regional Lymph Node Histology in Cancer of the Breast," Cancer, in press; Lafferty, Walker, Scollay, and Killby, "Allogeneic Interactions Provide Evidence for a Novel Class of Immunological Reactivity," Transpl. Rev., 13, 198, 1972; Stutman, "Tumor Development after 3-Methylcholanthrene in Immunologically Deficient Athymic-Nude Mice," Science, 183, 534, 1974; Black and Speer, "Sinus Histiocytosis of Lymph Nodes in Cancer," Surg. Gynecol. Obstet., 106, 163, 1958; Kelly and Good, "Immunologic Deficiency in Hodgkin's Disease," in Bergsma and Good (Eds), Immunologic deficiency diseases in man, New York: National Foundation Press, 1968, pp 349–356; Levey and Kaplan, "Impaired Lymphocyte Function in Untreated Hodgkin's Disease," New Eng. J. Med., 290, 181, 1974; Seligmann, Preud'-homme, and Brouet, "B and T cell Markers in Human Proliferative Blood Diseases and Primary Immunodeficiencies with Special Reference to Membrane Bound Immunoglobulins," Transpl. Rev., 16, 85, 1973; Preud'homme, Griscelli, and Seligmann, "Immunoglobulins on the Surface of Lymphocytes in Fifty Patients with Primary Immunodeficiency Diseases," Clin. Immunol. Immunopath., 1, 241, 1973; Gajl-Peczalska, Park, Biggar, and Good, "B and T Lymphocytes in Primary Immunodeficiency Disease in Man," J. Clin. Invest., 52, 919, 1973.

immunology and tumor surveillance, because the nude mouse will accept a graft from virtually any source.

CHAIRMAN GOOD: No question about that.

STUTMAN: Our nude mice are on a different inbred background—CBA/H—and are kept pathogen free but not germ free. The mean life span of such mice is a year to a year and a half. The overall incidence of spontaneous tumor observed so far is minimal. CBA has a relatively low incidence of spontaneous lung adenomas, and the nude CBA have the same incidence—20%. No lymphomas have occurred in these mice yet.

When exposed to chemical carcinogens, MCA injected at birth or urethane given in four doses starting at birth or as adults, the overall incidence of tumors of any type was comparable between the immune-deficient homozygote nudes and the immunologically-normal nude heterozygotes. The only malignancies that did not develop in the homozygous nudes after exposure to urethane were, of course, thymomas and thymus-derived lymphomas. All other tumors (lung adenomas, hepatomas, hemangiomas, etc.) had exactly the same incidence in the immune-deficient nudes and in the immunocompetent heterozygotes. Tumor incidence was similar in homozygous athymic nudes and in the normal heterozygote siblings. No differences were found in overall latent period in the metastasizing ability of the MCA sarcomas, between the homozygote (nu/nu) and the heterozygote (nu/+). We actually inserted a dominant gene (viable yellow) that favors spontaneous tumor development (lung adenomas, hepatomas, and lymphomas) on the nu/nu background. In these experiments, still in progress, the overall incidence of spontaneous tumors within 9–12 months of age is exactly the same in the immunologically deficient nu/nu and in the immunologically competent nu/+.

CHIECO-BIANCHI: Was carcinogen injected in adult or newborn animals? In newborns the optimal oncogenic response may exist both in nude and in normal mice.

STUTMAN: Adults were injected. Since there are no differences between the two groups, and the carcinogen doses were adjusted to body weight, such experiments seemed unnecessary. Urethane was also administered to adults.

WEISS: What is known of the ability of nude mice to effect antibody-dependent lymphocytotoxic activity, as in the Perlmann system? What is known of the ability of their B or K cells to attack target cells in the presence of antibody?

E. KLEIN: Cells taken from nude mice exert killing effects when antibody is present.

WEISS: In that case, in the absence of T surveillance mechanisms, this could be compensated for by other cellular systems.

PREHN: Perhaps human tumors are rejected in nude mice by a B cell response. We have also observed that human tumors do not grow as well as expected in nude mice, though if the nude mice are kept warm, they grow better. We have observed, however, in some instances at least (and we have not yet done a systematic analysis of this), that the human tumors that do not grow do not appear to be rejected. They just do not grow. You can see them there a long time after inoculation, just sitting there, apparently viable but not doing anything. It may be a lack of a proper environment for growth, rather than an active rejection process.

CHAIRMAN GOOD: We hope Prehn will elaborate on that later. Mosche Schmidt and I have observed nude mice to grow huge tumors, localized tumors, from inocula of human malignant cells. These tumors may get up to nearly one-third the size of the mice without metastasizing. All you have to do to get these huge human tumors to melt away is to give the nude mouse a thymus—and wham!

COHN: Aside from the possibility that the nude mutation is not all or none but leaky, experimentally studied nude mice could not be blank because the animals result from a cross between male nu/nu and a female nu/+. The offspring are being fed by the thymus of the mother. Further, even if one thymectomizes the mother, the two fetuses, nu/nu and nu/+ are living together in the uterus, and cross feeding each other.

STUTMAN: It is now easy to breed females with nu/nu males, since both are fertile when kept in pathogen-free conditions.

COHN: Were all of the experiments Stutman described carried out with offspring of nu/nu male x nu/nu female crosses?

STUTMAN: We started using heterozygote carriers for breeding, and the majority of the experiments were done with their offspring. The nude females do not feed their young because they have a displasia of the mammary gland; consequently, they have to be fosternursed in normal females.

COHN: Just answer my question. Were the data Stutman presented gathered by using nude mice derived from a homozygous male by homozygous female cross?

STUTMAN: The MCA experiment was done using nudes derived from mating heterozygote carriers (*Science*, **183**, 534, 1974). The rest of the experiments have been done with two sets of animals, the ones derived from heterozygote as well as from homozygote matings, without obvious differences in the results.

PREHN: We can certainly raise nu/nu mice. Unfortunately, our experiments with the nu/nu mice are still incomplete, but I would point out, in that connection, that there is a big problem in continuing to keep nudes or grow nudes in this manner. I think there will be a very strong pressure for developing nude mice that actually have thymus function and thymus activity. So for safety's sake, I think we have to keep breeding them from heterozygotes.

CHAIRMAN GOOD: Immunosurveillance as originally divined by Ehrlich, formulated in terms of allograft immunity by Thomas, and restated by Burnet and by me, is indeed assaulted by the information on nude mice. However, nude mice still have considerable immunologic capacity, especially in regard to B cells and humoral immunity. We, therefore, have much to learn about how to interpret data from these animals as supporting or disproving the surveillance concept.

LANDY: In a sense, Good's comments are relevant to the overall experience in human tissue transplantation. I remind him that, at the Brook Lodge conference on immune surveillance (1970), he attributed the clinical emergence of tumors in organ-transplanted patients to the immunosuppression applied. However, in the light of present knowledge would that not more likely be due to an effect by allogeneic tissue?

CHAIRMAN GOOD: It very well could. At the time of that Brook Lodge conference (1970) Lafferty had just come out with his report and it was not discussed. The implications of his work have really become apparent more recently, and have influenced my thinking a great deal.

HALL: The broad issue of immune surveillance in normal animals must be considered in terms of what goes on in the peripheral tissues where the first malignant transformation takes place. It has been known since the early 1930s that the number of mononuclear cells in peripheral tissue fluid of the sheep is extremely low, perhaps about 500/mm^3, only half of which are lymphocytes, the rest probably being monocytes. Apparently, there is the same ratio of T cells to B cells in the periphery as elsewhere. Of course, in the sheep this is a bit difficult to interpret. The number of immunoglobulin-bearing cells may be taken as indicating the number of so-called B cells. We have no positive markers for T cells. The other fact was developed recently by Scollay. With great effort, he collected the peripheral lymphocytes and showed that, although they had the same distribution of immunoglobulin markers as lymphocytes in the blood and efferent lymph, they were quite incapable of responding in MLC or in carrying out the normal lymphocyte transfer test in the skin.

Here we have two rather awkward pieces of evidence. There are very few lymphocytes in the peripheral tissues of the normal animal, and those we do find show a totally different pattern of reactivity: really, no reactivity at all, when compared with the lymphocytes with which we commonly deal in peripheral blood or efferent lymph. In other words, there is, as yet, no firm physiological basis for peripheral sensitization and immune surveillance.

KLEIN: We cannot really discuss the question of whether the nude mouse shows evidence for or against immunological surveillance without defining the surveillance hypothesis more critically. If it is implied that all tissues are in a "hyper-excited" state with regard to the generation of potentially malignant cells and that these cells are eliminated all the time by T cell killing, the experience with nude mice certainly argues against this. However, this is, admittedly, a highly artificial model.

The evidence for immune surveillance is rather good for most virus-induced tumors, whereas it is poor or nonexistent for carcinogen-induced tumors and many of the so-called spontaneous tumors. As discussed in the preceding session, this may be related to the selection of Ir genes during the evolution of each species, highly competent to recognize tumor-associated antigens induced by ubiquitous viruses that infect most members of the species during the reproductive age. If, therefore, one wishes to test the role of surveillance in nude mice, one would have to expose the animals to some of these viruses, such as polyoma or MLV and then study whether their residual immune system can deal with the transformations efficiently or not. Actually, we have heard that MSV-induced tumors do not regress in nude mice, in contrast to their behavior in hosts with an intact T cell system. Much more needs to be done on this question, however, since nude mice have a considerable immune potential, as has been pointed out by several conferees. Although it is said to accept hetero-transplanted tumors rather indiscriminately, the figures show that the incidence of takes is actually far from 100%; many implanted biopsies or culture lines are rejected. Presumably, this rejection occurs via humoral antibody and complement, with or without the cooperation of non-T lymphocytes.

COHN: Klein has brought us back to the fundamental point, namely, the problem of immune surveillance. However, he introduced the element of efficiency into the immune-surveillance hypothesis by stressing that it was a little too naive to think that T killer cells would wipe out *de novo* arising cancers. Consequently, I would like Klein to define what *he* thinks the immune surveillance hypothesis is, and now that we have been through several sessions discussing this problem, what experiments would convince any of us that immune surveillance does or does not exist.

KLEIN: In response to Cohn, one could perhaps redefine immune surveillance as the genetically determined ability to deal with neoplastic transformants induced by potentially oncogenic viruses of ubiquitous occurrence in a given species. If one restricts the concept this way and starts looking at the genetics of susceptibility, e.g., to polyoma or other natually occurring viruses in a given species, a great deal of new information may emerge concerning the role of the Ir genes in the recognition of tumor-associated antigens.

However, remember that other genetic influences can profoundly modify tumor incidence. Genetic differences exist in the ability of normal tissues of different strains to undergo the same kind of neoplastic transformation, when placed in the same host environment. Kirschbaum, Heston, Prehn, and others implanted tissues of high and low tumor strains into a common F_1 hybrid host, and tumor incidence was recorded. This included such cells as the mammary glands, the adrenals, ovary, thymus, and lung. The carcinogenic agents varied from viral through hormonal to chemical carcinogens and also included some cases of spontaneous malignant transformation. In every case, the normal tissue of the high tumor-incidence strain gave rise to a larger number of tumors than the normal tissue of the low-incidence strain. This showed that genetic factors, fixed by inbreeding, influence the probability of neoplastic transformation at the level of the target tissue itself. This is certainly a nonimmunological mechanism. It would be interesting to see what happens if the different tissue susceptibility genes are introduced into nude mice by appropriate intercrossing and backcrossing and what the tumor incidence would be in the presence and absence of the thymus, in cases where a given target tissue has a high inherent susceptibility to neoplastic transformation.

COHN: We have introduced another kind of surveillance mechanism which is nonimmune in origin. Certainly, there are mechanisms which operate to correct faulty replication of DNA, for example, and others are imaginable. This might, in part, explain why the incidence of cancer in long-lived (elephants) or short-lived (mice) animals is the same per animal. However, if this is the surveillance hypothesis under analysis, then both our discussion and the data that has been presented here are not relevant. I want to remind you that we are discussing *immune* surveillance.

Let us try to define immune surveillance in terms of two components: the transformed cell and the immune recognition of it. The hypothesis is that a normal cell, when it is transformed to neoplastic, will grow as a tumor in the absence of an immune system. The definition of a neoplastic cell is that it grows as a cancer in an animal which has no effective immune system. The first assumption of the immune-surveillance hypothesis is that every time a normal cell is transformed it expresses a new determinant, which because it is foreign to that immune system, will be immunogenic. The second assumption is that a properly functioning immune system will, in general, reject the newly arisen neoplasia.

The way in which transformed cells escape or sabotage the immune system is another question of great importance which follows our clarification of the immune-surveillance hypothesis. If this is not the immune-surveillance hypothesis under discussion, then I do not understand the relevance of data we are discussing.

KLEIN: The immune system reacts, provided it has been selected to do so, by the fixation of appropriate Ir genes.

COHN: There is no objection to proposing that germ-line genes code for the recognition of tumors, although I think it is unlikely.

KLEIN: If the appropriate Ir gene has not been selected for, the probability is that it will be absent with nonrecognition i.e., absence of surveillance, as the result.

COHN: That is one possible mechanism, all right.

KLEIN: Yes, I believe it is.

CHAIRMAN GOOD: A clinical situation which seems to run parallel to the hybrid experiments may be hereditary xeroderma pigmentosa. Here increased susceptibility to malignancy has no apparent relationship to immune deficiency.

Could Prehn present his cogent arguments against the concept that immunodeficiency is associated with malignancy, that the immune system may actually be necessary to provoke tumors?

PREHN: Surveillance has been defined in the past to encompass the idea that as soon as, or very shortly after, transformation of a cell takes place, the immune reaction comes along and kills it off. We have rather good evidence that the weak, early immune response does not do this, but, quite the contrary, that it makes the tumor grow better.

The most recent evidence for this comes from my colleague, Jeejeebhoy. He has analyzed the capacity of peripheral lymphoid cells to produce colony inhibition at varying intervals after they have been stimulated by implantation of tumor. He put three different MCA sarcomas into isogeneic animals and at 5 days and at 12 days harvested the peripheral lymphocytes. He then did a colony inhibition assay in soft agar, a modification of the Heppner technique, with a ratio of 100:1 lymphoid cells to target cells. He found that, at 5 days, there seemed indeed to be a stimulation of colony formation by these lymphoid cells, as compared with normal cells. At 12 days, the same experiment yielded mostly inhibition. In a couple of cases, there apparently was still stimulation.

The reaction apparently had specificity, in as much as there was only a small degree of cross reactivity between 2 of the sarcomas in the stimulation at the 5-day period. Serum from the 5-day animals combined with the 5-day lymphocytes potentiated the stimulation effect. That is, the stimulation was more marked in the presence of noninactivated mouse serum. At 12 days, serum combined with lymphocytes apparently produced an inhibition of what stimulation remained. It also produced an inhibition of the inhibitory reaction. So, whatever was going on was inhibited by serum at 12 days.

Past experiments, from my own and other laboratories, show that there is a marked dose dependency in this sort of reaction, i.e., that the fewer the lymphocytes one added, the more likely stimulation rather than inhibition of target cells occurred.

In passing, it is a rather common observation that completely normal lymphocytes sometimes produce a vast amount of stimulation. The immunostimulation of target cells demonstrated by Jeejeebhoy is over and above the stimulation produced by normal lymphocytes.

It stands to reason that the immune response to any nascent tumor has to go through a weak phase before it gets strong. I postulate that it has to go through a stimulatory phase before it can become inhibitory. Consequently, when we talk about immunotherapy, we have to worry not only about producing blocking factors that may interfere with the immune response, but also about the stage or level of immunity.

ALEXANDER: Lymphoid cells actually raise the cloning efficiency of fibroblasts. It may, therefore, be inappropriate to use cells from the unstimulated nodes of normal mice as a control for the effect of "immune" lymphoid cells. I say this because, at 5 days after immunization, the draining nodes will be especially rich in immunoblasts (by 12 days this response will have died down). Such blast cells may provide more nutritional support than ordinary lymphoid cells. I would be more convinced by the experiments of Jeejeebhoy and Prehn, if lymph nodes stimulated by some antigen were used as the control, rather than cells from unstimulated nodes.

PREHN: I have no comment other than that it did appear to have speci*ⁱ*

CEPPELLINI: Is there information about the incidence of either spontaneous or induced tumors in allophenic mice?

KLEIN: Mintz has shown that in the allophenic C3H/C57BL mice, most of the mammary tumors arise from C3H cells. This is another demonstration of a genetic determination mechanism where the susceptibility to undergo a neo-plastic change is fixed at the target tissue level.

MARTIN: Mintz and her colleagues have also examined the incidence of lung and liver tumors in allophenic mice derived from genetically-susceptible and genetically-resistant mouse strains. Her data suggest that cellular genotype, rather than an immunologic mechanism, determines tumor development. The majority of tumors are composed of cells derived from the susceptible parental strain. However, her data do not exclude a surveillance mechanism.

STJERNSWÄRD: Prehn brought out a very important point, and that is a con-structive scepticism to the relevance of our *in vitro* tests. We may just be confirming our prejudices. A lymphocyte–tumor cell ratio of 500:1 may be ideal to produce inhibition of tumor growth, but does this ratio actually occur *in vivo?* One who wants to find stimulation of tumor growth makes all his ex-periments with a different lymphocyte–tumor cell ratio.

So far, we have neglected the population *not* killed *in vitro*. What is im-portant is not the number killed, but the cells remaining with the possibility of later multiplication. Do the cells not killed represent a different tumor subpop-ulation? Another problem is in the effector cells used. Repeatedly, one hears the statement of "nonspecific" cytotoxic effects if cells are not purified in a certain way. Is it not so that only tests using whole blood give a meaningful correlation reflecting the *in vivo* situation?

PREHN: Regarding immunostimulation of tumors, it seems to me that we can consider as established the fact that the immune mechanism can stimulate the growth of target tumor cells. The question is what role, if any, it may have in *in vivo* oncogenesis. We really do not know. However, immunostimulation very satisfactorily explains why tumors are immunogenic in the first place. We can take Baldwin's evidence that they are not necessarily immunogenic, i.e., they have the "option" of not being so, and then ask the question why are most of them immunogenic. I suggest that, in fact, it may be due to immuno-selection. The immune mechanism may select for immunogenic tumors.

The mechanisms of stimulation are unknown. There is some evidence from other laboratories that it can be mediated by T cells and other evidence that it cannot be mediated by macrophages. Stimulation can be produced by low levels of specific antibody as well as by low levels of lymphotoxin. The fact that the immune response can be either stimulatory or inhibitory to target cells, depending upon circumstances, suggests that it plays a regulatory rather than a merely defensive role. It certainly did not evolve in order to stimulate tumor growth; this must be a perversion of some related normal activity. The recently developing evidence that lymphoid cells have the potential to react against "self" as well as "nonself" suggests a role for the lymphoid system in normal growth regulation—certainly a very old idea.* One of my students, Pliskin, has been gathering evidence that the lymphoid system may play a role in liver regeneration. I think that this sort of investigation will prove very instructive in the years to come.

When I discuss immunostimulation, I am often accused of undermining the immunological approach to the cancer problem. Nothing could be further from the truth. The very fact that immunosurveillance may be less effective than was generally believed offers an opportunity that would not otherwise have existed. A highly efficient surveillance mechanism would mean that there was little hope of improving the situation by any type of immunotherapy, but an inefficient mechanism may possibly be augmented. However, the existence of immunostimulation as well as immunoinhibition of target tumor cells means that attempts at immunotherapy may be even more hazardous than was already apparent. The possibility of doing harm by altering the immune mechanism to a stimulatory level of activity is very real, and I am quite sure that this has already occurred in some instances. It seems to me that a much better methodology for assessing the level of the host's immune responsiveness to his tumor is required before immunotherapy can be put on a rational scientific basis.

VAAGE: In response to the contention that all tumors are or should be antigenic, I have found, in about 100 spontaneous C3H mammary carcinomas tested, that only 25–30% induce immune-resistance response to challenge in syngeneic animals. In the C3Hf strain, in which the tumors are much delayed, they appear on the average of 24 months of age. In the syngeneic C3Hf strain, about 6% of 36 tumors induced immune-resistance responses.

CHAIRMAN GOOD: Isn't there a problem there with respect to overcoming the tolerant state when you test a resistant animal?

VAAGE: I have met that objection before. It seems to me that overcoming tolerance would be a random phenomenon, while immunogenicity or nonimmuno-

---

*Afterthought by Smith: It occurred to me, at the time of Prehn's statement, how close this concept fits into the data Martin has presented, and those presented in Session I regarding detection of stimulatory effects of multiple self-antigens on lymphoid cell subsets taken from tumor-bearing animals. Perhaps, the reactions observed are reflective of this normal process rather than an expression of neo-antigens on tumor cells.

genicity is always clearly defined for each individual tumor in repeated experiments.

BALDWIN: With respect to Vaage's statement and the issue Prehn just raised, we must consider whether a tumor expresses antigens in a much different light. Vaage has just been reporting on whether spontaneous tumors express rejection antigens and, as we found in many spontaneous tumors, this is not the case. These are not the same tumors Prehn was talking about. If one looks at all of the tumors that are not immunogenic, an embryonic antigen will generally be demonstrable on their cell surface.

COHN: We are losing track of the argument. If the immune-surveillance hypothesis is as I defined it, and we start with the assumption that a normal cell when it is transformed to a neoplastic cell possesses an altered surface, then there is the question of whether or not this changed surface is immunogenic. If the transformation from normal to neoplastic does not change the surface in a way that can be recognized by the immune system, then no immune-surveillance mechanism can operate. Either we simply put that class of tumors aside and do not deal with them at this conference, or we deal with them in terms of other possible non-immune-surveillance mechanisms.

    Even if we consider only those tumors which, when they arise, do express a new surface component recognized by the immune system, we have been confusing the question of whether or not the immune system is *efficient* in rejecting the tumor with whether or not the immune system is *recognizing* the tumor-specific determinant as immunogenic.

WEISS: We have found that tumors such as spontaneous mammary carcinomas of mice which do not seem to trigger protective immune reactions in the host are still recognized by lymphoid cells with a high degree of specificity *in vitro*. In some instances, the cells are damaged, if damage is measured by various changes in metabolic patterns. Therefore, inadequacy of surveillance in terms of gross destruction of the tumor cell, as assayed *in vitro,* must not be equated automatically.

TERRY: Cohn is oversimplifying the situation, and I wonder if, within his formulation, it is even possible to test the hypothesis. The spontaneous tumors that Vaage and Baldwin are talking about, which do not give challenge protection and, therefore, appear to be nonimmunogenic, represent the end point of a long selective process *in vivo*. We have no way of determining the immunogenic characteristics of the spontaneous tumor at the time of initiation, or when very few cells were present, by analyzing the immunogenic potential of the tumor when it is fully grown, so to speak.

PREHN: Somebody needs to point out what is obvious to many people. We get so intrigued by the surveillance hypothesis that whenever data of this sort are presented we immediately rationalize and say that this means that the immune defense has broken down. It is just as likely, in a formal sense, that malignant tumors cause a breakdown of the immune response as the breakdown of the immune response causing a malignant tumor.

KLEIN: This is to respond to some of the points made by Vaage, Alexander, and Cohn in regard to surveillance.

If we start by asking whether any tumor cell has a changed membrane, compared with the normal cell from which it has been derived, and whether such changes appear regularly in the course of neoplastic transformation, there is no compelling evidence for this. It seems a reasonable hypothesis to me, however, particularly when considering that growth control receptors must be localized on the cell surface.

The next question is whether this change is necessarily recognized by the host as an antigenic change or not. Here I am somewhat worried about the argument that the *in vitro* lymphocytotoxicity experiments have answered this question in the affirmative. As Weiss mentioned at an earlier session, Cohen and his associates have evidence that the lymphocyte is capable of recognizing normal fibroblasts *in vitro*. This shows, in other words, that under the conditions of the *in vitro* system, antigens can be recognized that may have no significance as rejection-inducing antigens *in vivo*. We also heard, particularly from Baldwin, that tumor cells can express fetal antigen *in vitro* that do not appear to serve as targets for rejection response *in vivo*. For these reasons, I would be hesitant to take the results of *in vitro* cytotoxicity alone as evidence for tumor recognition *in vivo*.*

CHAIRMAN GOOD: Can Pinsky now tell us something about the testing of immunological function in various kinds of cancer in man.

PINSKY: This is a brief distillate of extensive studies we have carried out in over 1000 patients with cancer. My colleagues are Old, Oettgen, Hirshaut, Wanebo, and Lunday.

Editors' comment: Somewhere between the rigorous logical constraints imposed by Cohn, the facts provided by the nu/nu mouse, and Prehn's immunostimulation data, old immune surveillance *(circa* 1970) came a cropper. It has been replaced by nothing so easily defined or widely supported. New surveillance is, apparently, a multi-factorial system involving not only immune elements, both inhibitory and stimulating, and both T and B cell components, but also genetically determined factors, allogeneic effects (can there be a compatible syngeneic effect?) of local effector cells, and variable expression of surface antigens. This lacks both the attractive simplicity of the old surveillance and its inviting possibility of a clean experimental testing in relatively defined systems. Perhaps the new surveillance should never have emerged from this cocoon—but it holds promise of becoming a very interesting and complex butterfly.

The patients were studied for their ability to develop delayed cutaneous hypersensitivity to 2,4-dinitrochlorobenzene (DNCB). Our aim was to use a technique which differentiates the patient population from the normal population and, at the same time, generate responders and nonresponders in order to correlate responsiveness with factors in the clinical course. The inner aspect of the upper arm was sensitized with 2000 μg of DNCB dissolved in 0.1 ml of acetone. Test sites of 100 and 25 μg are applied to the ipsilateral forearm at the same time. The liquid was confined within a plastic ring measuring 2 cm in diameter. (Recently, we have used an aerosol spray which delivers the appropriate dose to the skin.) The solution then evaporates, and the area is covered with bandaids for two days.

The 100 μg site is considered the test site, and reactions there within 2 days are considered evidence of preexisting immunity to this chemical. Although it is not widely distributed, a very small percentage of patients have preexisting immunity, and, in that case, this is not a test for *de novo* immunity. At 14–21 days after sensitization, challenge doses are applied if the patient has not reacted already at one of the test sites. Most of the patients were challenged with 200 and 50 g, as well. The test is then read at 48 hr for induration and erythema; only the presence of induration is counted as a positive test. Equivocal reactions with erythema but no induration are extremely rare, however, and often the patient can be trained to read the test himself. Over 95–96% of normal individuals will develop induration at the 100 μg test site within 48 hr of challenge. This was chosen as the cutoff for DNCB positivity.

In patients with cancer, as disease progresses, the probability of reacting in this way diminishes. Of patients with no known metastases (NKM), 83% react, contrasted with positive responses in 67% of patients with regional metastases (RM), and only 41% in patients with distant metastases (DM). Of perhaps even more significance (Table 45), the pattern of DNCB reactivity depends not only on the extent of disease, but on which particular cancer is present. Patients with localized epidermoid carcinoma of the head and neck region have lower incidence of reactivity than patients with advanced cancers such as melanoma, sarcoma, and carcinoma of the lung. The explanation for this finding is not clear but could be a reflection of the fact that immunologic reactivity and susceptibility to certain cancers may both be the result of some preexisting factor.

Despite these differences, in patients who have had definitive surgery (i.e., success in removing all known tumor) DNCB reactivity at that time correlates very well with a good short-term prognosis (Table 46). This confirms the observations made by Morton several years ago. We have also found that when we perform a battery of intradermal skin tests for preexisting immunity to common antigens (candida, mumps, tuberculin, and streptokinase/dornase), the ability to react to any one of these does not correlate as well. This suggests that responsiveness to a new antigen may be more important for a patient's

302

TABLE 45

Incidence of DNCB Reactivity in Patients with
Different Types of Cancer

Diagnosis	Localized		Generalized	
	Patients no. tested	positive %	Patients no. tested	positive %
Carcinoma of:				
Lung	10	100	10	80
Cervix	6	100	4	25
Breast	21	90	3	0
Colon and rectum	30	80	0	–
Head and neck	19	42	6	33
Sarcoma	5	100	15	73
Melanoma	11	91	19	74

TABLE 46

Correlation of DNCB Reactivity at the Time of
Definitive Surgery with the Incidence of Recurrence
Six Months after Surgery

	DNCB +	DNCB –	Total
No recurrence	54	9	63
Recurrence	3	7	10
Total	57	16	73

$\chi^2 = 12.5$, $p < 0.001$.

prognosis than the ability to maintain immunologic memory to some previously encountered antigen.

In expanding these studies, we were looking for a group of patients who would not respond to DNCB, in order to test a new immunopotentiating agent. These patients were challenged with 200, 100, 50, and 25 μg. In a group of 172 patients who failed to respond to 100 μg at 48 hr, 37 responded to 200 μg and 13 responded quite normally at some time after 48 hr without additional antigen application. These delayed responders might be the *in vivo* equivalent of patients with cancer whose lymphocytes seem defective in dose-response tests measured at a given time *in vitro*, but whose lymphocytes respond quite well after more prolonged exposure to antigen or mitogen.

Table 47 includes additional patients and more prolonged follow up. Again, all patients are surgically free of disease at the time of DNCB skin testing. While patients without metastases at the time of surgery have a better prognosis if the DNCB skin test is positive, those in whom regional lymph-node metastases have already occurred do not show such a convincing correlation. This may indicate that once metastases have occurred, immunological reactivity is not as important to the patient's outcome as biologic activity of the tumor.

TABLE 47

Correlation of DNCB Reactivity at the Time of Definitive
Surgery with the Incidence of Recurrence or Death at Six,
Twelve or Twenty-four Months after Surgery

Stage of cancer[a]	DNCB result	Total no.	6 months no.		12 months no.			24 months no.		
			Followed	Recurrences	Followed	Recurrences	Dead	Followed	Recurrences	Dead
NKM	+	70	64	1	61	6	1	47	6	4
NKM	−	18	16	4	13	6	2	9	5	4
RM	+	44	42	9	38	15	6	23	18	9
RM	−	15	14	5	14	7	6	13	9	8
NKM and RM	+	114	106	10	99	21	7	70	24	13
NKM and RM	−	33	30	9	27	13	8	22	14	12
NKM and RM	+and−	147	136	19	126	34	15	92	38	25

[a]NKM: Infiltrating cancer, no known metastases.
RM: Infiltrating cancer, regional metastases.

On the other hand, in a group of 23 patients with nonresectable carcinoma of the lung, there was no clinical difference in extent of disease between those who were DNCB positive and those were DNCB negative. But the survival times were twice as long in the group who responded to DNCB. The survival times of the 9 patients who were DNCB negative yielded a median of only 6 months, while the 14 who were DNCB positive lived 12+ months. Hence, in a group of patients with residual cancer, the DNCB test correlates very well with the prognosis.

BACH: Of the 9 patients DNCB negative, is it true that none of them survived more than 6 months?

PINSKY: No, median survival of this group was 6 months.

CHAIRMAN GOOD: There is clear evidence from all the observations that progressive loss of immunologic function occurs in this population.

PINSKY: Yes, within a group of patients the course of any single progressive tumor correlates with decreasing DNCB reactivity. It is also quite clear that patients with sarcoma, melanoma, and carcinoma of the lung, in general, have a worse prognosis than patients with carcinoma of the head and neck. One simply cannot equate bad tumors and poor immunologic reactivity.

CEPPELLINI: Did Pinsky establish a correlation between his tests and the ability of the serum of these patients to block lymphocyte activity?

PINSKY: We have not correlated the *in vivo* results with any *in vitro* tests, as yet.

CEPELLINI: The point is that in our studies there are factors in the serum, very likely immunoglobulins, which react against lymphocytes, and it does not have to do with tumor antigen. One can visualize that tumors stimulate some kind of autoantibody which inhibits.

CHAIRMAN GOOD: We are cognizant of such substances both in transplanted patients and in patients with a variety of malignancies. Some of them are clearly removable with anti-immunoglobulin antisera, and others are not. A whole set of substances that interfere with tumor immunity needs to be sorted out.

COHN: Take the case where you have a patient who is not responding to challenge with DNCB, is that patient not responding to his own tumor?

PINSKY: That is the other side of the coin that Ceppellini referred to, and this is something now being looked at very carefully. In those tumors for which we have *in vitro* tests, we are now trying to make this sort of correlation. Up to now, the number of human tumors for which there are clear-cut tumor-associated mechanisms *in vitro* are very few in number.

COHN: Are serum Ig levels lower?

PINSKY: There has been no correlation between the DNCB results and serum Ig levels. There has also been no correlation between absolute lymphocyte count and the results of this test, except in one situation. Patients with advanced disease, on chemotherapy or radiation therapy, have decreased DNCB reactivity and have lower lymphocyte counts. In the early surgical patients, there is also no correlation.

ALEXANDER: A delayed hypersensitivity skin test can be negative for at least two reasons: The patient has no immune response, or there is a defect in the inflammatory mechanism. I understand that, to some extent, one tests for this capacity by measuring the response to croton oil. Only if this is positive can a negative delayed hypersensitivity test, of the type used by Pinsky, be attributed to a failure of the lymphoid system.

PINSKY: We have not looked specifically at responses to croton oil, although we are aware of a study reported in *The New England Journal of Medicine* some time ago, in which a group of patients with more advanced cancer on adrenocorticosteroid and chemotherapy were examined. Virtually all of the patients negative to DNCB were also nonreactive to croton oil. But in our system we have a very good inflammatory stimulus, the 2000 μg sensitizing dose. That is a very high dose, and it is likely to cause severe inflammation. But the point can be made that practically all of our patients show an inflammatory response at this dose. Also, a significant number of patients who are negative to DNCB are able to react to at least one of the intradermal tests for preexisting immunity; so they can demonstrate delayed cutaneous hypersensitivity reactions under the appropriate stimulus.

While it is perfectly obvious that if someone has absolutely no inflammatory reaction in the skin, he cannot have a positive skin test, it is also obvious that inability to mount an inflammatory skin response cannot be responsible for most negative DNCB skin tests.

ALEXANDER: While I have been delighted at the debunking given to the overemphasis of immune surveillance as a determining factor in carcinogenesis, there is, in fact, recorded in the literature a most impressive experiment by Lurie which is relevant to and supports the concept of immune surveillance. Lurie was a famous investigator in the field of tuberculosis, and, over a lifetime, he built up, by inbreeding, colonies of rabbits which differed markedly in their susceptibility to tuberculosis. Naturally, his interest lay in ascertaining why some strains were susceptible and others were not. He succeeded in resolving this problem. This work is summarized beautifully in his book, *Resistance to Tuberculosis, Experimental Studies in Native and Acquired Defensive Mechanisms* (Cambridge, Harvard University Press, 1964), in which it is conclusively demonstrated that the reason why these rabbit colonies differed in their susceptibility to tuberculosis was due to the level of activity of their mononuclear phagocytes. The monocytes and macrophages of all his rabbit lines phagocytosed tubercle bacilli, but only the macrophages of the lines resistant to the disease killed the ingested Mycobacteria.

At the time of Lurie's retirement in the early 1960s, local circumstances required him to destroy most of these carefully built up rabbit colonies. However, as a first-rate pathologist he performed careful post mortems on all these animals, in the course of which he made a most remarkable observation that the age-related spontaneous cancer incidence (this involved rabbits of all ages) was correlated with their resistance to tuberculosis. A graphic summation of Lurie's findings is shown in Fig. 48. The rabbit line that had the highest resistance to tuberculosis had the lowest age-specific incidence of tumors; the rabbit line of intermediate resistance to tuberculosis had a significantly higher incidence of cancer, while the colony that was most susceptible to tuberculosis had the highest incidence of uterine cancer. In my view, it is tempting to link this genetically based high-microbicidal activity of macrophages in certain rabbit lines with their increased resistance to cancer—in contrast to those animals whose monocytes could not kill tubercle bacilli and in whom there was a greater incidence of cancer.

PINSKY: Rokitansky, in "A Manual of Pathological Anatomy" (1855), made the observation that the prevalence of tubercles and cancer in organs were reciprocal. He showed a table of frequency in various organs; those that have high prevalence of tuberculosis had a very low incidence of cancer.

It is very interesting that a century ago tuberculosis of the lung was frequent and cancer rare, and today the situation is reversed.

HOWARD: Animals selected for their general immunological competence is a very loose notion, so perhaps it is worth asking whether tumor incidence or type has been documented for the Biozzi sublines of high and low antibody response mice (*J. Exp. Med.*, **132,** 752, 1970). In this circumstance, the differences appear to have been localized to the differentiation of plasma cells. T cell functions are perfectly normal in both sublines. As with the Lurie rabbits described

307

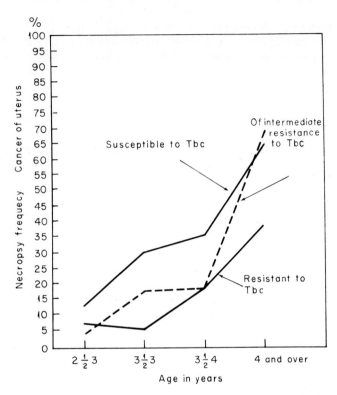

Fig. 48. Relation of cancer of the uterus and native resistance to tuberculosis in the Phipps rabbit colony, 1931–1961.

by Alexander, the lesion apparently is restricted to another immunologically interesting cell class, and here again T cells are normal.

HALL: There is more information about Biozzi's high and low responder lines of mice. As I understand the situation, in the low antibody responder, which, incidentally, is much more resistant than the high responder to facultative intracellular parasites, the macrophages are so active that they destroy most of the antigen almost as soon as it is injected; consequently, it would not be available for inducing antibody formation. As far as I know, tumor incidence has not been established.

BACH: One unfortunate thing about Lurie's experiments is that the rabbit population he had available was not a random breeding population, despite its size. We do not know its exact breeding history, and we do not know its original genetic constitution.

ALEXANDER: Neither do we know that for man.

CHAIRMAN GOOD: Martin used *in utero* carcinogenesis as a model. But *in utero* carcinogenesis may be more than just that. Diethylstilbesterol, given to mothers during pregnancy, has led 20 years later to carcinoma of the vagina in their female offspring. This rare tumor seems to represent an *in utero* carcinogenic influence of this hormone.

What other prenatal carcinogenic influences have a similar end point in some common malignancy? Martin's model also keeps alive the issue whether or not the histocompatibility portion of the genome is involved in creating the tumor-associated transplantation antigens. We know that a virus can turn on expression of the TL alloantigen. Thus, genetically TL-negative mice can have TL-positive tumors because of the depressing influence of a leukemia virus. The question is how often do carcinogenic agents use this avenue to create tumors that will be stimulated enough to grow.

MARTIN: The alloantigen expressed on the transplacentally induced lung tumor is noteworthy because it can serve as a strong transplantation antigen resulting in syngeneic rejection of a large inoculum of tumor. If the immune-surveillance mechanism against lung tumor development in normal C3Hf mice is due to reactivity against the A alloantigen expressed on nascent autochthonous tumors, then, since strain A mice normally express this component, their immune-surveillance potential against lung tumors may be restricted.

In other words, in strain A mice the alloantigen expressed on normal tissues might be regarded as a tumor-susceptibility alloantigen (TSAA). Heubner and his colleagues have demonstrated a close association between inheritance of Gross virus expression and susceptibility to leukemia. Animals which do not express Gross virus antigens may be relatively resistant to leukemia, not because they lack an oncogene (as postulated by Huebner) but, rather, because their immune surveillance may be effective against Gross virus antigens derepressed on autochthonous leukemias. Validation of the concept of TSAA will offer the prospect that appropriate tissue-typing methods may indicate, at least in part, the susceptibility of an individual to particular types of tumors.

The protection afforded a particular mouse strain by the successful repression of the TSAA on the normal tissues of this strain is clearly limited, however, since a particular type of tumor can occasionally arise in all strains of mice. There are a number of possible tumor escape mechanisms. The locus determining the TSAA may not be derepressed in tumor cells. TSAA may be nonimmunogenic. TSAA may be immunogenic but evoke an immune response inappropriate for tumor rejection. If the locus coding for the TSAA is viral in nature, infectious spread of the virus from malignant to normal cells may result in "antigenic conversion" of normal cells, preventing the immunologic distinction between malignant and nonmalignant cells. Experimental evidence for each of these escape mechanisms has been obtained in studies on transplacentally induced and spontaneous murine tumors.

Concerning the mechanism of immune surveillance, the findings of Stutman and of Prehn that tumor incidence is not increased in congenitally athymic (nude) mice, does not necessarily rule out immune surveillance as such. Rather, their evidence can be viewed as favoring a thymus-independent immune-surveillance mechanism.

We have detected IgM antibodies, cytotoxic for a variety of tumors, in sera of both normal and nude mice *(Nature, 249, 564, 1974)*. Some of the specificities recognized by natural antibodies in a given serum can be absorbed by normal tissues of certain allogeneic strains. Detailed studies of the specificity of the antisera may help define the nature and strain distribution of TSAA. In addition, studies of the biologic role of these antibodies may yet provide an important insight into the mechanism of immune surveillance.

NOTKINS: Perhaps we should now question an assumption basic to tumor immunology, that all important antigenic changes occur on the surface of tumor cells and that these are the only ones essential for immune recognition of these cells as foreign, with consequent rejection. Is it really essential that there be antigenic changes only on the cell surface to call immune rejection into play? Could there not be antigenic changes within the cells and maybe strong antigenic changes, as a result of different enzymes being produced, which may not be entirely reflected on the cell surface. Could it not be that such components are secreted locally at the site of the tumor, that there then ensues an immune response to these particular antigens, and that this, in turn, brings in macrophages to act nonspecifically at this site? It may now be timely to look at antigens within the tumor cell as well as those on the membrane.

STJERNSWÄRD: I would direct attention now to mammary carcinoma as a model for determining the possible role of human tumor immunity and exploring the possibility of immunotherapy. Breast cancer has always been considered as a localized disease, treated by intensive and sometimes even nonconstructive local therapeutic approaches. The data show, however, that 50% of patients having tumor classified as less than 5 cm plus local node involvement are dead due to distant metastasis within five years. In this situation, involving minimal residual tumor, postoperative irradiation induces long-lasting lymphopenia. This irradiation-induced lymphopenia is of the same magnitude as that induced by immunosuppressive treatment in kidney transplantation. Such patients have a significantly increased incidence of second spontaneous tumors.

Briefly, some of the details of this ongoing study merit mention. Thirty-four patients have been studied serially. 4500 R irradiation of the mammary lymph-node chain down to the fourth intercostal space results in a reduction of circulating blood lymphocytes to at least 700/mm³; some patients go as low as 400/mm³. After 3 months, 1 year, and 2 years respectively, the lymphocyte levels in peripheral blood average 1000, 1200 and 1600 mm³. Monocytes are not diminished but increase in number immediately after irradiation. Cells that have C'3 receptors, Fc receptors, and ability to phagocytose immunoglobulin-coated erythrocytes are found in increased numbers immediately after irradiation. E-rosette lymphocytes are decreased (Stjernswärd *et al.*, *Lancet,* **1,** 1352, 1972).

In addition to quantitative changes in various leucocyte subpopulations, functional tests are altered, such as decreased ability to be stimulated by PHA. This functional impairment holds even if the data are expressed per 10^6 E-rosette lymphocytes. Irradiation of other major areas, as for bladder carcinoma or uterine cancer, also leads to lymphopenia. The cause of the lymphopenia is irradiation, but we do not know why it is so long lasting, especially considered in terms of the large size of the total lymphocyte reservoir. Three possibilities might explain the effect: (1) direct hit of circulating lymphocytes (most likely), (2) indirect effect of irradiation via the thymus, and (3) a serum-mediated factor which affects lymphocytes.

ALEXANDER: Even local irradiation, given in repeated, fractionated doses, would eventually affect every circulating lymphocyte in the body.

STJERNSWÄRD: We find it difficult to arrive at valid figures. Do we know what proportion of lymphocytes would be hit by 1000 R, fractionated over 20 days, over a skin surface of 70 cm².

CHAIRMAN GOOD: It is clear that not only in this site, but in other areas as well, local irradiation given over a long period will really deplete the lymphocyte population, and it takes them a long time to come back.

HOWARD: There are many aninal models, as you probably know, where local lymph node irradiation fails to cause a continuing lymphocyte deficiency. Only by chronic irradiation of the blood in an extracorporeal circuit or by chronic irradiation of spleen or lymph nodes can a generalized lymphopenia be produced in experimental animals. The property that the successful methods have in common is in providing a continuously high radiation flux in vessels or organs through which recirculating lymphocytes pass continuously. It is virtually impossible that a divided dose of 4500 R to a very restricted area of the body not containing a major lymphocyte traffic organ could provide the necessary conditions. Another curious property of the lymphopenia described by Stjernswärd is that it is marked in the peripheral blood, which usually shows less dramatic effects than the thoracic duct following a chronic local irradiation regime.

311

Presumably, this is because the blood lymphocyte compartment contains cells from proliferating sources, like the thymus and bone marrow, which are not in equilibrium with the main lymphocyte recirculation stream. Furthermore, it has been noted that lymphocyte deficits induced by chronic local irradiation are rapidly reversed when the irradiation is stopped, providing the thymus has not been removed.

Stjernswärd's lymphopenia is maintained for a very long period after radiotherapy is completed. In my view, the lymphopenia described by Stjernswärd has enough anomalous properties, compared with animal models, to merit further investigation.

PREHN: Is the prolonged lymphopenia radiation dose related?

STERNSWÄRD: The decrease in number of circulating lymphocytes comes on rapidly. Maximal depression is often found after one-half or three-fourths of the planned irradiation dose has been given. We do not have sufficient data to establish any dose–response relationship.

In 1959, Paterson and Russell brought attention to a related problem. Their data show an increase of liver metastases during the first and second year in 300 patients who received radiotherapy after radical mastectomy for cancer, as compared to those who got radical mastectomy alone. Bruce compared simple mastectomy and radiotherapy with radical mastectomy only, with about 200 patients in each group, and found increased mortality in the irradiated group. The mortality figures were 6.3% versus 3.4% at 1 year and 8.6% compared to 4.4% at 2 years. In unpublished data involving a large group of patients from Radiumhospitalet, Norway, Host found that distant metastasis in stage II of breast cancer appeared earlier in a group that got radiotherapy after a radical mastectomy. The data were interpreted to indicate that radiotherapy did not increase the total number of metastases but accelerated their appearance.

The large breast cancer trial in the United States has yielded data again indicating the same increase in metastases in irradiated groups (Fischer et al., and Slack, personal communication). We can conclude from all the data that after radical mastectomy patients ended up with about a 10% higher number of distant metastases. The percent survivors also decreased in the irradiated group.

All of these controlled clinical trials indicate the same trend of about 5–10% increase and/or earlier appearance of distant metastasis in certain stages of breast cancer in which patients received postoperative radiotherapy. The figures are indicative but not conclusive. There seems to be a correlation between minimal residual tumor, long-lasting lymphopenia, and a 5–10% earlier appearance of metastases. Early immune surveillance, if it exists, has already been outflanked and failed.

PREHN: Is it possible that 10% of these distant metastases are actually within the radiation field?

STJERNSWÄRD: Tumor recurring at the site of the primary, in the skin around it or in the draining lymph nodes, is classified as a local and regional recurrence. Tumor found in the pulmonary tissue, including that within the postoperative irradiation field, is classified as a distant metastasis. Postoperative irradiation actually diminishes the number of local and regional recurrences. May I emphasize that a careful analysis of large well-defined series of patients is required if small differences are to be meaningful.

The conclusion we draw, based upon available data, is that host immunity in such cancer patients is of marginal effectiveness or limited.

DELLA PORTA: Three or four years ago, we studied the peripheral lympho-cytes of a small series of patients with malignant melanoma using the Takasugi–Klein *in vitro* method (Fossati *et al., Int. J. Cancer*, **8,** 344, 1971). Sixty per-cent of the patients had peripheral lymphocytes reactive against melanoma target cells, using 13 different primary cultures of melanoma cells.

We found no initial correlation with the clinical stage of the disease. Fol-low up of these patients again gave no correlation with the outcome of the dis-ease (Veronesi *et al., Europ. J. Cancer*, in press). We have now extended the study to a larger series of patients, and again we observe no correlation with clinical stages.

My colleagues Fossati and Canevari also have studied complement-dependent cytotoxicity of serum from melanoma patients on one melanoma cell line. A summary of the data obtained is in Table 48. If the sera were tested before surgery, 30% were positive when the tumor was small and localized (Stage 1), 60% were positive if metastases were found in the local lymph nodes (Stage II). Among patients with widespread tumor (Stage III), only one of 13 had a cytotoxic serum.

In clinically tumor-free patients, less than 7-months postoperation, only 1 serum of 7 tested was cytotoxic. One to four years after surgery, 25% of clini-cally tumor-free patients had positive sera. When we retested the sera of the same patients later, none were positive. Controls included sera from patients having unrelated tumors and from healthy donors. Cytotoxicity was found in 5–10% of such sera. We need more follow up data to conclude that any mean-ingful correlation exists between the result of the cytotoxic test and the clinical outcome.

In another small series of malignant melanoma patients, sera harvested within a few days both before and after surgery, was studied the same day and on the same target cell. Before surgery 5 of 7 were negative and after surgery 6 of 7 were positive.

313

TABLE 48

Complement-dependent Cytotoxicity of Cancer Patient Sera
on a Cell Line of Malignant Melanoma

Sera	Stage of disease	Positive cases/ total cases	Positive %
Malignant melanoma			
Before surgery	I	5/17	29
	II	14/24	58
	III	1/13	7
3-7 months after surgery	Clinically tumor free	1/7	14
Between 1-4 years after surgery	Clinically tumor free	4/15	26
Retested 3-12 months later	Clinically tumor free	$0/12^{a}$	–
Controls			
Unrelated tumor	I-II-III	2/20	10
No tumor	–	1/18	5

Three out of the 4 sera previously positive are included. Assay was performed in microplates (Falcon No. 3034). Cells were incubated with serum (dil. ½, ¼, ⅛) for 45 min; the serum was discarded and, as source of complement, guinea pig or rabbit serum was added for 18–24 hr. Cells remaining after exposure to serum and active or inactivated complement were counted. A reduction greater than 25% was taken as positive.

BACH: What percentage of controls were positive in the Takasugi–Klein assay? That is, what was the reactivity of normal lymphocytes from presumably normal patients or patients having other tumors?

DELLA PORTA: At least 20% were positive. This is the reason why I feel that we do not know whether the lack of correlation between clinical stage and outcome truly represents what was going on *in vivo* or is due to a shortcoming of the *in vitro* test. I must emphasize that the patients studied for cell-mediated immunity were different from those involved in the cytotoxicity tests.

BACH: Barbara Alter attempted to follow up the findings of the Hellströms that lymphocytes of blacks were active against melanoma cells. In the Madison population, the lymphocytes of several nonblacks were highly active. We did not use the Takasugi–Klein assay, rather the chromium assay and melanoma cell lines.

PERLMANN: In serological studies of other tumors, it seems difficult to establish tumor specificity of the antibodies. The more investigators have looked, the more they have found reactions with various kinds of target cells. Does Della Porta know how specific the sera of his patients are for melanoma cells? What is the incidence of positive reactions with other target cells?

DELLA PORTA: The test is evaluated by means of an internal comparison between active and inactivated complement. In a number of instances, serum from melanoma patients was tested both on melanoma and breast carcinoma cells. Three of five were positive on melanoma target cells, and zero of five on cells from breast carcinoma. The sera from the breast cancer patients were positive in two of eight instances on the melanoma cells, and four of eight on the breast carcinoma cells.

We realize that extending this type of study gives difficulties as with all *in vitro* tests. So far, the reaction seems to be quite specific, in the sense that a large group of sera from patients with different types of tumor was negative on the same melanoma cell. Specificity is also suggested by the burst of cytotoxicity observed soon after surgery.

PERLMANN: It has also been reported that melanoma target cells of different origin may not respond in the same way to the serum of an individual patient. Do Della Porta's positive sera affect different melanoma target cells in the same way, or does he sometimes find lysis of certain melanoma cells but not of others?

DELLA PORTA: The serological tests have been done so far on only one line. Data on experimental tumors show that the immunosensitivity of a target cell may vary in time depending on growth parameters.

KLEIN: It could be very important to develop such serologic tests. The antigenic mosaic on the tumor cell surface can only be mapped with the help of serology, as Boyse and his coworkers have mapped the lymphocyte surface for a large number of genetically determined, but strictly lymphocyte-specific receptors.

It will be essential to pull out, from the universe of antibodies that react with a given tumor cell surface, those well-defined reference combinations giving reproducible reactions. If melanoma serum could provide this, in relation to melanoma cells, and if this were clearly a tumor-associated or cell-type-associated reaction, one could screen other cells for the presence of the antigen by absorption and other sera for the presence of the same or cross-reactive antibodies by blocking or competition. If a large number of sera are simply screened against a large number of cells, confusion will increase, whereas the testing of sera in relation to particular reference systems can create some kind of order. This approach has been very rewarding in the serological definition of EBV-associated antigens.

DELLA PORTA: I certainly agree with Klein that this is a very important approach. However, we need first to have suitable sera to work with.

COHN: I am interested in mechanisms. Della Porta showed us that seven days before removal of the melanoma, no antibody was detectable in the serum. After removal, there is a burst of antibody activity in the serum. Does he know whether the negative serum is a consequence of the tumor simply acting as an immunoabsorbent soaking up the antibody or is the postoperative appearance of antibody, due to increased synthesis of antibody, as a consequence of removal of the inhibitory tumor? Have you tried to extract antibody from the tumor?

DELLA PORTA: We have not done that analysis on human tumors.*

PERLMANN: Patients with transitional cell carcinoma of the urinary bladder have cytotoxic PBL which can destroy bladder carcinoma cells in tissue culture, using the microcytotoxicity tests as described by Takasugi and Klein. Target cells are cells from three established bladder carcinoma cell lines as well as cells from primary cultures. Control target cells are normal bladder epithelial cells or cells of unrelated tumor or tissue origin. Effector cells are blood lymphocytes, extensively purified according to a standardized protocol. Two or three doses of lymphocytes are used for each test. Using this approach, we have found, a bladder tumor, specific cytotoxic reactivity exhibited by the patients' lymphocytes. So far, the assay has not revealed any individual specificity of the cytotoxic reaction, which, however, does not mean that such a difference could not exist. As far as we can tell now, the antigen involved is not a normal bladder epithelial antigen, and there is, as yet, no evidence that we are dealing with a fetal antigen, but this requires further study.

O'Toole et al. have recently fractionated the purified effector lymphocytes in T and non-T cell fractions. Using two independent methods of separation, it was seen that all cytotoxic reactivity resided in the non-T fraction, while the T cell fraction was consistently nonreactive in this test, although its functional integrity was well preserved. The exact nature of the effector cell is unknown. Although we are working with highly purified lymphocytes, the assay requires 24–48 hr of incubation. The participation in the cytotoxic reaction of a few remaining nonlymphocytic effector cells can, therefore, not be entirely excluded. Nevertheless, since the reactions are specific, we may conclude that somewhere along the line humoral antibody must be involved in the reaction. The antibodies could either be absorbed to some effector cells, perhaps as complexes with antigen, when taken from the blood of the patients, or we might have a few

---

*Afterthought by Della Porta: There are several indirect and direct indications that tumor cells may be coated in vivo by antitumor antibodies (for review: Witz, Current Topics in Microbiology and Immunology, 61, 151, 1973). In addition, the absence of antitumor reactivity of sera of tumor-bearing hosts may be due to an excess of soluble antigen liberated from tumor tissue into the circulation with formation of antigen-antibody complexes. The simplest explanation for cytotoxicity of sera raised after surgery is, therefore, that antibody synthesis goes on for a number of days after removal of the tumor bulk. Perhaps, there is also enough circulating or sequestrated antigen to maintain an active immune response.

antibody-producing cells in the system which release antibody during the incubation period. These antibodies would then mediate the cytotoxic reaction by interacting with effector cells equipped with Fc receptors.

CEPPELLINI: Is this reaction blocked by immune complexes?

PERLMANN: We have seen earlier that some patient sera blocked the reaction, and this could have been due to the presence of complexes. However, we have not as yet studied this systematically. The cytotoxic reactivity of the patients' lymphocytes is well correlated with the course of the disease. All these data are published, and I will, therefore, only summarize them very briefly. About 90% of untreated patients with relatively small and localized tumors, most of them in clinical stage T2, give significant tumor cell destruction in this *in vitro* assay. In the groups with large tumors, clinical stages T3 or T4, the incidence of positive reactors is only 50%. So far, we have not been able to confer reactivity on the lymphocytes of nonreactors by washing the cells extensively or by prolonged preincubation *in vitro* before adding them to the tumor cells.

When patients treated with high doses of local X-irradiation were studied, the following pattern emerged: During therapy, none of the patients gave a cytotoxic reaction. However, very shortly after X-irradiation, a significant and sometimes very strong bladder tumor-specific cytotoxicity was seen in all patients who had no clinically detectable tumor. In contrast, in those patients who after irradiation had residual tumor or who developed distant metastases, cytotoxicity was only very weak or entirely absent. I should point out that all these comparisons were made by adding the same numbers of different effector cells to tumor cells at two or three different lymphocyte–tumor-cell ratios.

The strong cytotoxicity, coming up after radiotherapy in some patients, was transient. It usually waned at about one year after therapy. Patients studied 1–10 years after radiotherapy were negative when tumor free, but cytotoxicity usually reappeared when tumors recurred during this period.

Patients who were treated surgically only, either by local resection or total cystectomy, had a different pattern. When the tumor was successfully removed, cytotoxicity of the blood lymphocytes disappeared briefly after surgery and was absent in tumor-free patients. Patients with residual tumors or recurrences after surgery retained their cytotoxicity. Preoperative radiotherapy gave a pattern of reactivity similar to that seen in patients treated with radiotherapy only.

In summary, the patients with bladder carcinoma have a tumor-specific or tumor-associated cell-mediated cytotoxicity *in vitro*, and this is the expression of an activity of thymus-independent effector cells. It also reflects quite precisely what is going on clinically.

Measurable cytotoxicity is, thus, indicative of the presence of growing tumor, but with increased tumor burden it frequently disappears. X-irradiation may change this pattern insofar as it enhances cytotoxicity transiently in those patients in whom the treatment has apparently been successful. While the mechanisms giving rise to these patterns cannot as yet be adequately explained, these results are at variance with what has been reported for other tumors. The results also do not lend support to the statements, repeatedly made during this conference, that cell-mediated tumor destruction as measured by the microcytotoxicity assay *in vitro* only poorly reflects the clinical course of the disease. On the contrary, in urinary bladder carcinoma, the correlations between the *in vitro* test and the clinical events are remarkably good.

CHAIRMAN GOOD: We will now consider clinical efforts to design immunotherapeutic protocols and experimental models pertinent to development and improving immunotherapy.

The possibility of an immunological approach to treatment of cancer has been suggested by the rare but dramatic instances in which widespread human malignancy has spontaneously regressed. In many instances, this apparently has been associated with ongoing infection. W. B. Coley, a New York surgeon, first attempted to use what we now call immunotherapy when he developed and used mixed bacterial vaccines to produce sometimes dramatic regressions of human cancer. The Coley toxin approach fell into disrepute because of its inconsistency and lack of testing by methodology appropriate in assessing any significant clinical effects.

The independent studies of Old *et al.* and of Halpern and associates showed that BCG could prevent development of a number of different forms of cancer. Then, Edmund Klein presented evidence that skin cancer may regress if contact-type delayed allergy was induced in the vicinity of a skin cancer. The method used by Klein was to immunize repeatedly with skin sensitizing chemicals like DNCB and then apply the material to broad areas of affected skin. Cancerous skin reacted with greater intensity than normal skin, and the tumors dramatically regressed. Klein has now used this approach for about ten years. This selective local reaction has not been explained in fundamental terms. Indeed, the basic phenomenon was hard to accept for immunologists of the establishment type—myself especially. I even referred to this in public as imaginative quackery.* But the observation has stood the test of time, has been confirmed, and it stands as provocative modality of treatment of skin cancer. Klein also observed that patients with xeroderma pigmentosa, who have rejected a tumor through this immunoprovocation technique, may develop a high degree of resistance to the cancer which otherwise occurs with great frequency in their skin. The observations of Old *et al.*, Rapp *et al.*, and Zbar *et al.*, indicating

*Editors' comment: The data are still not in as to whether Edmund Klein's therapeutic approach to actinic and basal cell cancers represents a major *improvement* on techniques involving application of fluorinated pyrimidines, freezing, or other treatment modalities successfully tested in these diseases.

that BCG prevents as well as leads to the regression of certain forms of experimental cancer and those of Edmund Klein set the stage for current efforts to use BCG as a modality of cancer therapy. Of 50 or so major cancer centers in the United States and Canada today, at least 48 are testing protocols in which BCG is used in an effort to prevent recurrence of cancer or leukemia or to treat existing cancer. It may be appropriate for Pinsky to review data from the BCG trials at the Memorial Sloan Kettering Cancer Center.

PINSKY: This study was carried out in a group of 55 patients having metastatic malignant melanoma of the skin. This highly lethal tumor usually arises in skin nevi and has a strong predilection to metastasize to internal organs. Most of our patients had skin disease only, but 20 had metastases in lung, liver, bone and/or brain. We used BCG from two sources; the Glaxo strain supplied by Eli Lilly in the United States and the Chicago strain supplied by the Research Foundation of Chicago. In most of our patients, some lesions were left uninjected; many, however, had every visible lesion in the skin injected. As many as 55 lesions were injected in one patient in one day. Up to 150 million viable organisms were used at one sitting, but most patients received 20–30 million viable units (based on information of the suppliers).

Eighty percent of the patients were DNCB positive before and after therapy, confirming that melanoma patients maintain good DNCB reactivity, even when the disease is disseminated. The tests for preexisting immunity to unrelated antigens (candida, mumps, streptokinase/dornase) did not change. Sixteen of twenty-three previously negative patients developed a positive tuberculin skin test with a median time of about one month.

It is important to emphasize the side effects observed in these patients (Table 49). Many have suggested that immunopotentiators are less toxic than conventional cytotoxic agents used to treat patients with cancer. While the toxicity is different, it is probably not milder, and in some instances may be lethal.

Most patients developed fever within 2–3 days. Twenty-four had a syndrome of recurrent fever, malaise, nausea, vomiting and in some cases

TABLE 49
Side Effects of BCG Treatment

Manifestations of toxicity	Frequency in patients given BCG Number with symptoms/Total treated
Fever	42/55
Malaise, myalgia, etc.	24/53
Hepatic dysfunction	28/52
Hypersensitivity	3/55

myalgia and arthralgia. This appeared about two to three weeks after treatment and lasted, in some cases, up to 6 weeks, if not treated. In 2 patients, the influenza-like syndrome was so debilitating that isoniazid was given, with relief within one week.

At about the same time as the influenza-like syndrome appeared, 28 patients developed abnormalities of liver function. These also resolved spontaneously without treatment, unless there were progressive hepatic metastases. Six patients had liver biopsies and 5 revealed noncaseating granulomas. Of the 41 patients with serial liver scans, only 24 showed no change. The others had hepatomegaly, splenomegaly, or both.

The most serious toxic effect seen was severe hypersensitivity reactions occurring after either the second or third dose of BCG. Three patients developed severe chills, spiking fever, restlessness, bone pain, nausea, vomiting, and hypotension. Two became oliguric and azotemic, as well. All were treated with intravenous fluids, but two patients were treated with epinephrine as though they had anaphylaxis. One patient developed acrocyanosis at the tips of her fingers and toes which progressed to dry gangrene. In her case we added adrenocorticosteroids and isoniazid. All three patients recovered from the acute problems within two days. Gangrene, in the third patient, resolved within 6 months with no loss of bone or nail. Blood cultures in a few patients were positive for BCG up to 5 min after treatment, so it was no surprise that disseminated granulomata were found. Cultures obtained from the lesions some 2 months later still contained viable organisms.

Table 50 shows the antitumor effects. Forty-five of the 50 patients evaluated developed inflammation and, in most cases, ulceration of the injected lesions, but only 19 showed regression of every injected lesion. Only 4 of the 18 patients with internal metastases were in this group, and these regressions were all short lived, with no observed regressions lasting more than 6 months. Several patients are still free of disease, one over 3 years and one over 2 years.

TABLE 50
Antitumor Effects of BCG Treatment

Nature of tumor-modifying action of BCG	Frequency in patients given BCG number with tumor changes/ Total treated
Inflammation of injection nodules	45/50
Regression of:	
all injected nodules	19/50
internal metastases	4/18
skin metastases only	15/32
some injected nodules	16/50
noninjected nodules	2/29

These were the only 2 patients in the study in whom non-injected lesions regressed. These lesions were never more than 2–3 inches away from injected sites; we have no evidence of a distant effect. Sixteen patients had regression of some lesions, while others, that were also injected, progressed. This was not considered to be a clinically useful response. Finally, we attempted to correlate immune status and end result (Table 51). All patients with complete regression of tumor were reactive to DNCB, tuberculin or both.

CEPPELLINI: Is there any evidence that specific immunity is increased by this treatment? For instance, even if BCG gives equivocal effects against melanoma, is there any increase in immune reactions after the local treatment?

PINSKY: We have no information concerning specific reactivity against melanoma cell lines in these patients. Morton, who pioneered the intralesional injection of BCG in patients with melanoma, demonstrated increased antimelanoma antibodies in responders. Other workers have shown increasing cell-mediated antimelanoma reactivity in patients undergoing tumor regression.

CHAIRMAN GOOD: What do we know about the mechanism of action of BCG?

MACKANESS: Many of the side effects that BCG is said to have are not common features of clinical tuberculosis. One wonders, therefore, whether they are the result of properties peculiar to the BCG *vaccine* and not to the living organisms in it. Most BCG vaccines contain very few viable organisms relative to their content of dead organisms. What I suspect is even worse; most commercial vaccines also contain large quantities of soluble antigen. I wonder how many of the untoward effects of BCG are due to these extraneous constituents.*

TABLE 51

Correlation of Immune Status of Cancer Patients with End Result

Immune reactivity		Patients with complete regression
DNCB	Tuberculin	Total no. tested
+	+	8/19
+	−	9/21
--	+	2/7
−	−	0/3

Editors' comment: Questions have been raised regarding the efficacy of these and other sources of BCG used in immunotherapeutic protocols. Current data (as of July 1974) suggest that fresh frozen suspension-grown BCG is the preparation most likely to have an immunopotentiating effect on cancer growth in animal models.

Concerning the mechanism of BCG action, I recall data from the Zbar–Rapp model of a hepatocarcinoma in Strain 2 guinea pigs. Local infiltration of a line 10 tumor with viable BCG caused local regression, provided that the dose was large enough, that the organisms were alive, and that the host responded to it immunologically. Basically, local rejection of a tumor and its metastases in the regional lymph node appears to result from the cellular reaction against BCG itself.

Although the destruction of tumor cells is largely a fallout from the host's efforts to reject BCG, there is another, more enduring benefit. Following successful rejection of the tumor under the influence of BCG, a state of specific immunity remains. It is this aspect of BCG effect that we have studied: How does BCG enhance tumor-specific immune responses? We have approached the question in several ways, but I will start with a simple model involving the response to SRBC in lymph nodes responding to a primary dose of BCG.

Figure 49 shows that the lymph node draining the site of BCG inoculation responded by cell proliferation, measured as thymidine incorporation into DNA. The solid black columns represent the escalating cellular response to BCG alone. When the stimulus of SRBC was superimposed at different stages of this response to BCG, still using thymidine incorporation rates as an index of lymphoid cell proliferation, the combined response (black and white columns) became progressively augmented. The parameter that interested us most, however, in this modified immune response to SRBC, was the level of delayed-type hy-

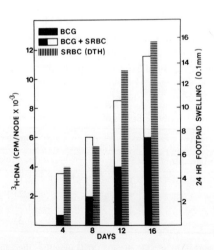

Fig. 49. Rate of DNA synthesis in lymph nodes at varying times after stimulation with BCG (black) or BCG plus SRBC (black and white). SRBC, given on the indicated day of the response to BCG, provoked an ever increasing T cell response as revealed by the resulting levels of DTH (hatched). (*J. Nat. Cancer Inst.*, **51**, 1669, 1973).

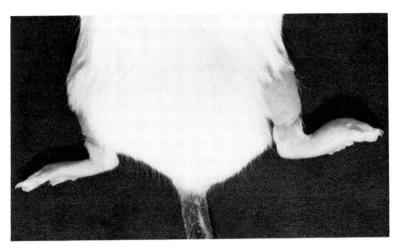

Fig. 50. DTH reaction in the footpad of a mouse sensitized to SRBC. The right test foot is only 1.5 mm thicker than normal. In this test for DTH, an increase of more than 0.1 mm is significant in groups of 5 mice (*J. Exp. Med.*, **139**, 1540, 1974).

persensitivity (DTH) developed against SRBC. This is represented by the hatched columns of Fig. 49. Early in the response to BCG, DTH was not augmented at all. But as the response to BCG mounted toward the end of the second week, the response to SRBC became greatly exaggerated, and the resulting state of DTH was increased out of proportion. The footpad reaction illustrated in Fig. 50 is comparable with reactions elicited in mice sensitized to SRBC on day 16 of the response to BCG (Fig. 51). The test foot appeared grossly swollen even though it was only 1.5 mm thicker than the opposite foot.

Using this information about the effect of BCG, it is possible to understand the observations of Hawrylko who studied the effect of BCG on the immune response to an experimental tumor—the mastocytoma P-815—which we know to be relatively nonimmunogenic in the conventional sense. When injected into the footpad in a dose of 10^6 cells, the tumor (MAs) grew as depicted by curve A in Fig. 52. It grew almost as fast in mice immunized 6 days previously with 10^7 irradiated tumor cells (curve B). However, when irradiated mastocytoma and BCG were mixed and introduced together into the footpad, a minor degree of tumor resistance developed (curve O).

When an interval was allowed for BCG to act on the regional lymph node before introducing the specific immunogen (irradiated tumor cells), tumor resistance became greater. The optimal interval in this experiment was about 10 days. In other words, it takes BCG about 10 days to modify the node to the point where irradiated mastocytoma cells become an effective stimulus for the production of antitumor immunity.

Figure 53(a) shows that these differences in the growth curves of the tumor

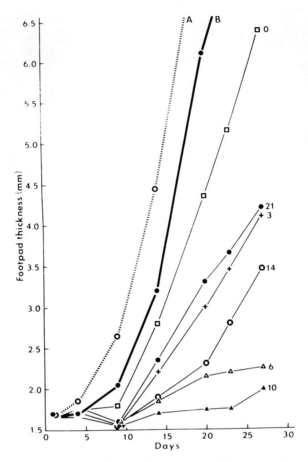

Fig. 51. Mean footpad thickness after challenge of 10^6 MAS in mice immunized with irradiated MAS, at varying intervals after BCG. Challenge was six days after the irradiated immunogen and is compared with the growth of MAS in control mice (A) and mice immunized with irradiated MAS alone (B). Time interval between the injection of BCG and irradiated MAS is indicated at the end of each curve. Each point represents the mean of six mice (*J. Nat. Cancer Inst.*, **51**, 1683, 1973).

were reflected in the ultimate survival rates. The observations imply that the adjuvant action of BCG takes time to develop, at least in this experimental system.

Figure 53(b) shows that the dose of BCG influences its modulating effect. Priming doses from 10^4 to 10^7 gave progressively more protection against local growth of the tumor and longer median survival times. The data also show that BCG alone gave no significant protection. Only the combination of BCG and specific immunogen gave an antitumor response.

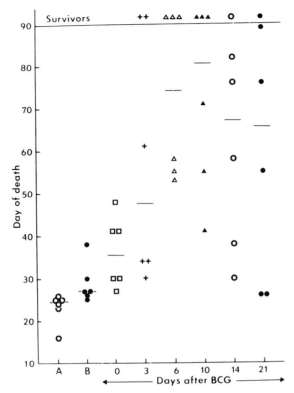

Fig. 52. Survival plot for mice given irradiated MAS at varying intervals after BCG (indicated on the abscissa) and challenged 6 days later with 10^8 MAS in the hind footpad. Group A shows the survival of the mice receiving the live MAS challenge only; Group B the survival of mice given only the irradiated MAS and then challenged six days later in the footpad. Horizontal bars indicate the median survival times (*J. Nat. Cancer Inst.*, **51**, 1683, 1973).

CHAIRMAN GOOD: So we have clear evidence, then, in animal tumor systems as well as in human tumor treatment, that BCG can have an influence on tumor growth. It has problems of side reactions, and we do not understand the mechanism very well.

STJERNSWÄRD: The situation in which Mackaness demonstrated no effect is closest to realistic clinical application, i.e., where we seek an anamnestic immunological response to a tumor *after* its removal.

MACKANESS: I agree. The situation that the clinician encounters is that of an established tumor which he hopes to destroy with BCG. While this may often be achieved by local infiltration, distant metastases cannot be so easily dispatched. Everything favors the effects of BCG in our experimental models, but,

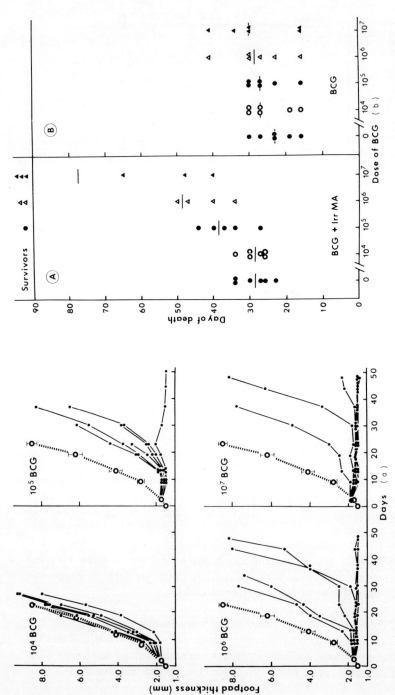

Fig. 53. Correlation between dose of BCG and specific protection immunization against MAS challenge. (a) Tumor growth in six individual mice immunized with 10[7] irradiated MAS at sites prepared 8 days previously with the indicated numbers of BCG. The challenge of 10[8] MAS was injected after another 6 days. Broken line indicates the mean growth curve ± SD for 6 controls immunized with irradiated immunogen only. (b) Survival plots of mice depicted in (A) and controls given only the priming dose of BCG (B). Horizontal bar indicates median survival time. Survivors at 90 days were tumor free. (*J. Nat. Cancer Inst.*, **51**, 1683, 1973).

326

unfortunately, in the clinical situations with which we must deal this is not the case.

WEISS: It is difficult to make the ultimate jump from any experimental animal system to man. One *can* learn a great deal, however, from systematic studies of animal models, defining the conditions and parameters which make for maximum immunotherapeutic efficiency and which avoid the dangers of enhancement and other risks. On the whole, these conditions have not been met for treatment of patients with living BCG. Most will recall the early and quite unfounded enthusiasm for living BCG as a vaccine against tuberculosis (Weiss, *Amer. Rev. Resp. Dis.* **80**, 340, 1959; **80**, 495, 1959; **80**, 676, 1959) which has now spilled over into enthusiasm for living BCG as a nonspecific agent. I suggest that it *is* possible to provide the basic laboratory and experimental animal information requisite to justifying clinical trials of nonspecific immunotherapeutic agents.

For some years now, we have studied the properties of a tubercle bacillus cell wall derivative of inactivated tubercle bacilli, the methanol extraction residue (MER). Some 30 publications have summarized the data obtained. Three basic points have arisen from our more recent studies with MER, and these paved the way for clinical investigation (Weiss and Yashphe, in Zuckerman and Weiss (Eds.), *Dynamic Aspects of Host-Parasite Relationships,* Vol. 1. New York: Academic Press, 1973, pp. 163–233; Weiss, *J. Nat. Cancer Inst. Monograph,* **35**, 157, 1972; Ben-Efraim, Constantini-Sourojon, and Weiss, *Cell Immunol.* **7**, 370, 1973; Haran-Ghera and Weiss, *J. Nat. Cancer Inst.,* **50**, 229, 1973; Yron *et al., J. Nat. Cancer Inst. Monograph,* in press; Kuperman *et al., Cell. Immunol.,* **3**, 277, 1972; Kuperman, Feigis, and Weiss, *Cell. Immunol.,* **8**, 484, 1973; Weiss, *Seventh Miles Inst. Symp. on Role of Immunological Factors in Viral and Oncogenic Processes,* in press).

The conclusions are as follows:

1. MER is a nonliving, wholly stable, and very much less toxic or allergenic agent than living BCG. It does not have to be given directly into the tumor focus in order to be effective. It is commonly more effective, both therapeutically and prophylactically, when given distal to the tumor site.

2. Under determined conditions of administration, this material favors cellular versus humoral immunological responsiveness. In recent studies in a guinea pig system, the animals are given different quantities of MER and sometime later immunized with protein–hapten conjugates in quantities, or of a kind, insufficient alone to lead to discernible responses. When, however, small amounts of MER were administered prior to this very weak antigenic stimulus, strong delayed hypersensitivity responses occurred in an appreciable proportion of animals. In contrast, larger amounts of MER and somewhat stronger antigenic stimulation led preferentially to the formation of circulating antibodies.

3. There is persuasive evidence from experiments with solid tumors in

inbred mice that the therapeutic effect of MER is consistently greater, additively or synergistically, when immunotherapy is accompanied by radiation and/or chemotherapy. It is erroneous, in the light of our experience, to consider immunotherapy and conventional therapy to be incompatible in cancer. Quite the opposite is true. MER in therapeutic doses prevents or reverses many states of immunosuppression, whether due to age, radiation, or treatment with different cancer chemotherapeutic agents (Kuperman *et al.*, *Proceedings of the Joint Meeting of European Soc. for Immunology*, 1973). Indeed, addition of MER to a treatment regimen permits more intensive standard therapy by affording protection against the immunosuppressive effects of irradiation and chemotherapeutic drugs.

An indication of the findings emerging from our current clinical trials is given in Table 52; the data show the present status of the first 15 patients with acute myelocytic leukemia. These patients were all given standard induction and

TABLE 52
Trial of MER in AML Patients also Receiving Standard Therapy[a]

Age	Patients Sex	Status	Survival (months) after Disease diagnosis	Survival (months) after Initial remission (complete or partial)	Time (months) treated with MER
			TREATED WITH MER[b]		
42	F	Alive, well	33	31	27
62	F	Deceased	17	15	8
28	M	Deceased	16	15	15
18	M	Deceased	15	14	8
26	F	Alive, well	11	10	5
44	F	Alive, well	9	7	4
16	M	Alive, well	8	5	4
34			15+	14+	
			CONTROLS		
22	M	Deceased	30	24	
38	M	Deceased	15	No remission	
63	M	Deceased	10	8	
38	F	Deceased	8	7	
62	M	Deceased	7	3	
66	M	Deceased	5	3	
36	F	Deceased	4	No remission	
33	M	Deceased	3	2	
44			10		

[a]Interim report Dec. 1973.
[b]1-2 mg, ID, in 5-10 distinct sites, every 4-8 weeks.

maintenance therapy; half are given MER once a month in addition. The data, although certainly still very modest, do indicate a therapeutic effect.

BALDWIN: Mackaness raised the point about the requirement for viable BCG in immunotherapy. Using transplanted rat sarcomas, we established that growth can be suppressed by BCG sterilized by γ-irradiation (1×10^6 R). Similarly, irradiated BCG will suppress pulmonary tumors produced by intravenous injection of tumor cells.

TERRY: Can Weiss tell us which animal model gives the best results with MER?

WEISS: Striking results are obtained with certain leukemias. A radiation-induced leukemia in C57BL/6 mice gives a background of 95–100% deaths in controls. Life-long prevention of any evidence of leukemia occurred in up to 60% of MER-treated animals (Haran-Ghera and Weiss, *J. Nat. Cancer Inst.*, **50**, 229, 1973).

CHAIRMAN GOOD: Did you ever cure leukemia after establishment of the disease?

WEISS: We could effect a cure after some leukemic cells have already appeared in the circulation. Spontaneous mammary tumors were never cured, but in combination treatment with irradiation or chemotherapy, significant retardation of tumor growth did occur. Other solid tumors give results which fall in between.

CHAIRMAN GOOD: It seems to me that the only controlled study of BCG in man which shows real value is when BCG and leukemia cells are used together in an effort to decrease the frequency of recurrences of acute myeloid leukemia in man. Powles and Crowther show that BCG can have value in this form of human cancer. The initially impressive data have continued to hold up and show promise.

WEISS: When BCG trials were started in man, there was, as far as I know, hardly a shred of information suggesting under what kind of circumstances the likelihood of enhanced tumor growth could be avoided or reduced. Animal models had shown clearly that both enhancement and heightened resistance are a possibility. The rationale seemed to be that it was permissible to attempt to benefit some patients and to ignore the likelihood that others would be harmed. I disagree with this approach because it is possible by animal models to define basic parameters under which enhancement is least likely to occur. With regard to MER, one finds that combined treatment with the agent plus radiation or chemotherapy largely avoids enhancement. The potential danger inherent in using a living, still partially pathogenic preparation was similarly ignored. The necessary background information should have been a precondition for the initiation of the trials with living BCG in man.

CHAIRMAN GOOD: I would press onto laboratory scientists the fact that when human disease is bad, as in acute myeloid leukemia and melanoma, the clinician and the clinical investigator feels the pressure of the bad prognosis. He is not willing to stand around and wait for the animal models to be perfected before beginning carefully conceived efforts to use the current best ideas in therapeutic trials. Indeed, to begin as has been indicated here with toddling steps, even though many falls are certain, is a better and a more certain way toward ideal treatment and prevention than waiting until the ideal approach has been thrashed out in the laboratory. The real issue is that without new approaches, the great majority of patients being treated only by conventional modalities of therapy will die.

COHN: Does Good have a general conceptual formulation which would permit him to propose rational ways of analyzing the relationship between delayed hypersensitivity to BCG and DNCB and to tumor rejection? At the moment I discern no general concept, and one is needed.

CHAIRMAN GOOD: There are numerous theoretical explanations of the effect. Mackaness thinks that to get a vigorous rejection reaction one must help the host to look upon weak antigens in the same way as he otherwise looks upon strong antigens. To do this effectively, one must facilitate removal of antigen–antibody complexes that seem to interfere with effective antitumor immunity. This is the kind of theoretical model one can strive to achieve in the clinic to improve one form of immunoprophylaxis or immunotherapy.*

CEPPELLINI: I would like to clarify the real issue. When one is using BCG or MER, are we potentiating the immune response in a general sense, or the phagocytic cells? Are we merely giving an adjuvant which increases the antigenicity of some antigens that may be present in normal tissues?

*Editors' note: Possible theoretical explanations for the DNCB and the BCG effects were discussed around a list (Table 22) formulated by Mitchison at the 1970 Brook Lodge Conference on Immune Surveillance (in Smith and Landy [Eds.], *Immune Surveillance*, New York: Academic Press, 1970). Data accumulating since that time have not substantially reduced or more sharply defined that array of seven possibilities.

SMITH: I would like to describe, especially for Ceppellini and Cohn, *in vitro* correlate of what Mackaness has shown us so clearly. In multiple strains of congenic and syngeneic mice, Forbes, Nakao, Konda, and I (in Lindahl-Kiessling and Osoba [Eds.], *Proceedings of the Eighth Leucocyte Culture Conference,* New York: Academic Press, 1974 p. 673) have examined the effects of BCG, both locally and systemically, on the total lymphon, if I may use that term.

A single injection of living BCG causes a great increase in the numbers of cells in the regional lymph node mass (Table 53). The number of Θ-bearing cells and the number of Ig-bearing cells increases likewise, together with responses to PHA, alloantigens, and to LPS. This increase in response to LPS is far out of proportion to the increase in the numbers of cells expressing Ig on their surface.

PHA stimulation, on the other hand, is increased in approximate proportion to the number of theta-bearing cells. The alloantigen-responsive subsets are augmented out of any proportion to the number of theta-bearing cells. Figure 54 shows data obtained by inoculating congenic lines with BCG. The response of treated animals' lymphyocytes in MLC to both the K- and D-end antigenic differences is greatly augmented over that of controls. These findings suggest that either the numbers in each responsive subset are selectively increased through proliferation induced by BCG, or that some kind of heightened reactivity of each individual subset has been induced by BCG. The former seems more plausible and may ultimately have an explanation in terms of amplification of self-responsive subsets through the local inflammation and necrosis established by BCG.

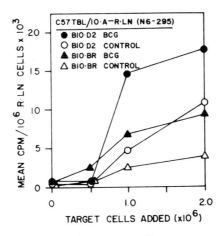

Fig. 54. Augmentation by BCG of T cell responses to alloantigens.

TABLE 53
Effect of Single BCG Inoculation Upon
Lymph Node Cell Function in C57BL/6

Organ and attribute assayed	Control (no. =10)	BCG-19 days (no.=20)	BCG/control
LNC			
Cell mass – no. ($\times 10^6$)[a]	6.0	49.7	8.34
Cell mass killed by Anti-θ + C' ($\times 10^6$)	2.6	15.9	6.12
^{3}H-thymidine incorporation (CPM/cell mass $\times 10^3$)			
unstimulated	1.3	76.1	58.54
PHA	514.2	2,885.1	5.61
CBA M	225.0	3,549.5	15.78
LPS	2.8	196.0	70.00
PPD	2.0	948.9	474.45

[a]Brachial and axillary nodes 19 days after single injection (F174-2).

As expected, the PPD response in an immunized animal is larger than that given by the known mitogenic effect of PPD. The effects observed are always greatest in the regional lymph node but are detected in spleen and nonregional node masses. This feature distinguishes the impressive stimulatory effects observed in the tumor-bearing animals from those in BCG-inoculated ones. In the latter, the effect in the regional node is sustained, whereas in the tumor-bearing animal the regional node effect wanes as spleen and nonregional nodes become involved.

The effect, in summary, is that of an adjuvant and not unlike that of tumor-bearing, with the exception that BCG sustains the local response which tumor bearing soon overcomes. Perhaps one of the mechanisms by which BCG might operate in controlling tumors is to sustain or concentrate T and B cell subpopulations in the draining regional lymph node.

CHAIRMAN GOOD: Another mechanism associated with BCG experimentally is augmented lymphoreticular activity. Mackaness also has some data on this point.

MACKANESS: SRBC given intravenously in sufficient dosage will prevent the induction of DTH, as measured by a footpad reaction. If one begins with the optimum dose of 10^5 and progresses to the fully blocking dose of 10^9, one finds that the responses of normal and BCG-infected mice are quite different (Fig. 55). Even the highest dose of SRBC produces DTH in BCG-infected mice. It seems that this effect lies in the ability of BCG-infected mice to clear the circulation of whatever it is that blocks T cell activity in normal mice. As we saw in an earlier session, absorbed immune serum contains factors which blocked both the induction and expression of DTH to SRBC. But the same blocking serum failed to interfere with either function in BCG-infected mice (Fig. 56). This suggests that an activated lymphoreticular system, which is characteristic of BCG-infected animals, is able to remove immune complexes from circulation. If these are indeed the blocking factors that interfere with T cell induction, their accelerated removal from circulation would free the T cell response from feedback inhibition and allow cell-mediated immunity to reach normal levels.

CHAIRMAN GOOD: Can you manipulate that by splenectomy; and what is the time course of the BCG effect?

MACKANESS: Splenectomy produces a similar effect by minimizing antibody production, thereby reducing complex formation. Modified response to immunization with SRBC appears within a week of injecting an adequate dose of BCG; the effect is at a maximum in about 21 days and then diminishes gradually. The changed responsiveness runs parallel with the growth and subsequent death of BCG in liver and spleen.

CHAIRMAN GOOD: With respect to BCG or similar agents such as MER, the real hope lies in creating new approaches. We must look in the clinic for

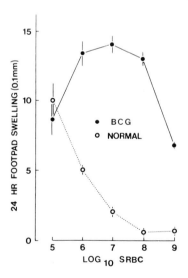

Fig. 55. Levels of DTH present in normal (O----O) and BCG-infected mice (O—O) 4 days after i.v. immunization with varying amounts of SRBC. Sensitization was initiated 20 days after i.v. inoculation of 9×10^7 BCG Montreal. Means of 5 ± SEM (*J. Exp. Med.*, **139**, 1540, 1974).

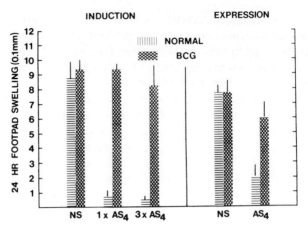

Fig. 56. Reversal of immune serum blocking of DTH in BCG-infected mice. Left: Effect of absorbed 4-day immune serum (AS4) on the induction of DTH to SRBC in normal or BCG-infected mice. DTH was measured 5 days after a footpad sensitizing dose of 10^8 SRBC, in animals (NS) given 0.2 ml of normal mouse serum absorbed with an equal volume of SRBC and in similar animals which had received one ($1 \times$ AS4) or 3 ($3 \times$ AS4) doses (0.2 ml) of AS4. The latter were given intravenously 12 hours before, together with, and 12 hr after the sensitizing dose of SRBC. Right: Effect of AS4 (0.2 ml) on established DTH in normal or BCG-infected mice. BCG was given intravenously 12 days before a sensitizing footpad injection of SRBC (10^8). Footpad tests for DTH were performed 5 days after sensitization. Controls received 0.2 ml of normal serum (NS) which was also absorbed with SRBC. Means of $5 \pm$ SEM (*J. Exp. Med.*, **139**, 1540, 1974).

applicability first in hopeless situations, while we develop appropriate animal models, perfect animal models, then take the fruit of the perfections back to the clinic. The product of this interaction will be improved prophylaxis and improved treatment. Other immunopotentiators have worked well in certain experimental systems and already have a clinical beginning. Corynebacteria were shown to have immunopotentiating effects by Halpern in France. From the point of view of immunotherapy, the definitive experiments have been performed by Currie and Bagshaw. These investigators showed that when one gave *C. parvum,* following treatment of a transplanted tumor with cytoxan, the tumor regressed—an effect exceeding that of *C. parvum* or cytoxan alone. The time administration of *C. parvum* seemed crucial, for prior to the cytoxan treatment, or at other intervals after treatment, the material had little or no influence on the course of the tumor. These data have been largely confirmed. Old, Stock, Oettgen, and others have used Meth A and Sarcoma 180 as screening systems in search of agents that have similar immunopotentiating influences on cancer. Israels and his coworkers in France have shown, in randomized controlled studies of a variety of human sarcomas and carcinomas, that survival was longer and regression of disseminated human cancers occurred more frequently when *C. parvum* was combined with chemotherapy, as compared with chemotherapy alone.

Some of Coley's early dramatic responses in human tumors are more well known. When mixed bacterial vaccines were studied in experimental animal systems, they were shown to have a capacity to eliminate very extensive malignancies. Shear kept this field alive by his studies focusing on endotoxin from *Serratia marcescens*. Endotoxin and mixed bacterial vaccines have now been investigated in many experimental systems, using both transplantable and spontaneous tumors in animals. In one spontaneous tumor in dogs, a disease very reminiscent of human eosinophilic granuloma, mixed bacterial vaccines sometimes cure the disease without other therapy. In some instances, mixed bacterial vaccines produced regression of transplantable chemical carcinogen-induced lesions. Plasma taken during such a period of regression also caused dramatic tumor regression. Perhaps Pinsky will summarize the experience with mixed bacterial vaccines in human tumors.

PINSKY: By now there is enough anecdotal information about mixed bacterial vaccines in the treatment of human cancer. We are now attempting to define, in controlled studies, the optimum dose, route, and schedule for both immunopotentiating and antitumor effects. Immunologic reactions are assessed *in vitro* and *in vivo*. Where available, assays for specific antitumor immunity are performed. In 22 patients studied to date, convincing antitumor effects have been seen only after repeated intralesional injections of a mixture of heat-killed streptococcus pyogenes and *Serratia marcescens*. This vaccine corresponds to the Tracey XI formula of Coley's Toxins, previously described by Nauts (*Acta Med. Scand.*, Suppl., 256, 1953) to be clinically effective with minimal toxicity. One large batch was prepared, obviating previously encountered difficulties in interpreting results when patients received different lots with varying potency.

The only *in vitro* parameter affected, related to immunologic function in these patients, is an increase in nitroblue tetrazolium reduction in granulocytes. Most of the patients were terminal at the time of treatment. As we gain more experience, we hope to study patients who are not so desperately sick.

WEISS: Is there anything that mixed bacterial vaccine will do that endotoxin preparations, such as the detoxified lipid A component especially, will not do?

CHAIRMAN GOOD: This is in the process of being investigated, but I have the impression that the mixed bacterial vaccine has effects that cannot be reproduced with a purified endotoxin.

SMITH: That was not Shear's finding some years ago.

CHAIRMAN GOOD: Shear thought he could reproduce all of the effects of mixed bacterial vaccine with a product from *Serratia marcescens*. As I understand the studies by Old and Hardy, they are not confident that all the effects of mixed bacterial vaccine can be attributed to conventional influences of bacterial endotoxin. Recently Kim, working with Watson at Minnesota, found that combinations of streptococcal toxin and endotoxin enhance each other's effect many fold. In some experiments, enhancement of endotoxin influence by streptococcal exotoxin was as much as a millionfold.

Hyperimmune sera also appears to affect favorably the course of experimental tumors in certain situations, as Sjögren will relate.

SJÖGREN: Treatment with hyperimmune sera has not given very positive results, especially not with solid tumors. When the unblocking phenomenon was discovered, it was natural to ask first whether we could counteract blocking *in vivo*. What was the effect on tumor growth by treatment that really abolished blocking in the tumor-bearing animal? Bansal and I studied this in different situations, including the primary tumor-bearing animal. We infected newborn rats with polyoma virus; five weeks later these animals all developed kidney tumors. At that time, we made laparotomies and checked the animals for macroscopically visible tumors. The animals at laparatomy were divided into two groups. One got control serum treatment; the other got "unblocking" serum in large quantities over a fairly long period of time after splenectomy. The tumors of the control animals grew rapidly. Fifty percent were dead within 5 weeks, and all were dead within 8 weeks. Tumors in 3 of 11 treated animals grew at about the same rate as the controls, but 6 had delayed growth. In 2 animals, tumors actually disappeared macroscopically, although by histology the kidneys were found to contain some tumor cells. The inhibitory effects on tumor growth were thus clear-cut. Lymphocytotoxicity, serum blocking activity, and complement-dependent cytotoxicity were assayed in all the treated rats. Decreased blocking activity was demonstrated in all the treated rats, even in ones without tumor growth inhibition. However, the decrease was most definite in the 2 rats that showed greatest tumor inhibition. It was soon increased in those 3 that showed no significant growth inhibition. Passive transfer of antitumor serum with unblocking activity has also been tried in metastatic models, with similar partial effects. We did not get a complete 100% effect; about 50% of the animals showed growth inhibition.

CHAIRMAN GOOD: Has anyone used unblocking sera, as you defined it, in a clinical situation?

SJÖGREN: The Hellströms have studies going on in melanoma patients right now, but it is too early to say anything about the results. It is possible, in human patients, to counteract blocking activity, as assayed *in vitro*. Although they still have the tumor, their serum blocking activity disappears.

CHAIRMAN GOOD: Another new way to achieve regression of tumors was recently discovered by Old, Kessels, Hardy, and others. This phenomenon could have been anticipated by clinical observations made in the late 1940s and early 1950s. Moore was trying to treat leukemia by giving exchange transfusions. The basis of this endeavor was that after blood transfusions, leukemia patients occasionally experienced a remarkable regression of their disease. Moore extrapolated this anecdotal experience by exchange transfusions of leukemics with fresh blood from volunteers. Without question, short-lived remissions were obtained. This approach would certainly have developed further had not Farber discovered the remarkable capacity of amethopterin to induce remissions in leukemia patients. Bessis and Dausset subsequently published several extensive papers describing inconsistent but occasionally dramatic consequences of exchange-transfusion therapy of human leukemia.

More recent studies began as an effort to use interferon to treat mouse and cat leukemia. Old and his coworkers discovered that administration of fresh normal serum or plasma to AKR mice bearing their spontaneous leukemias regularly induces destruction of leukemia cells. The responses are short lived but substantial. An explanation of the phenomenon may be that AKR mice are deficient in the fifth component of complement. Highly purified preparations of this complement component will produce similar remissions of leukemia in AKR mice. Hardy and Old have extended these findings to cats in which lymphoma and leukemia may also regress after administration of normal cat serum. Normal cat serum but not leukemic cat serum produces the effect.

Another recent approach to immunostimulation which merits discussion is related to the use of the antihelminthic agent levamisole, which Renoux and Renoux found to have both antitumor and immunostimulating effects. Antitumor activity has been described in the Lewis transplantable lung carcinoma system, and distinctive effects upon immunological functions have been produced with this relatively simple chemical compound.

PINSKY: Levamisole is an agent used for some time in Europe as an antihelminthic. It has not been on the market in the United States. A single oral dose of 150 mg has rather remarkable effects. Quite by accident, it was found to be an immunopotentiator, first in an antibody producing system, but later work has suggested that it may have activity in cell-mediated systems, perhaps in T and B cell interaction. Other investigators have used it clinically to reverse negative DNCB skin reactivity in patients with cancer. The dose was 150 mg per day for 3 days, with application of the skin tests on the first day and reading on the last day.

We have performed a similar study in 100 DNCB-negative patients. All patients received conventional antitumor therapy. The patients were randomized, 50 to receive levamisole and 50 were controls. One week after anergy to

DNCB had been demonstrated, the treated group received levamisole and both groups had DNCB rechallenge. Ten patients treated with levamisole and 7 control patients had conversions to DNCB positivity.

At this dose, there is no significant difference between the treated and the control patients. Because there are potent effects in animal systems, both T and B cell effects, further investigation with this agent is necessary in order to determine an effective schedule of administration. Indeed, some preliminary data have come to us from the manufacturer, suggesting that the schedule we used is not optimal, and further studies are under way.

BALDWIN: We have recently been screening levamisole against a number of transplanted rat tumors. At 5 mg/kg, either as a single or repeated treatment, this drug has not influenced the growth of local tumors. It has also failed to modify the growth of pulmonary metastases either arising by spontaneous shedding from one tumor (epithelioma Spl) or from intravenous injection of tumor cells (MCA sarcomas).

MARTIN: I wish to add one other immunotherapeutic possibility to this long and growing list. The possibility that spontaneous tumors need not necessarily express tumor-specific antigens has been discussed in detail earlier in this conference. These tumors may, however, continue to express differentiation antigens characteristic of the organ origin of the tumor. For tumors of nonvital organs (e.g., breast, prostate, uterus, thyroid), an organ-specific antigen may be an acceptable target against which one could attempt to generate effective immunity.

The problem is, then, how to generate cellular immunity against a tumor or organ-specific antigen in a tumor-bearing host. Wunderlich and I initiated studies on this issue to ascertain the way in which we can generate cytotoxic lymphocytes in C57BL mice against EL-4 leukemia cells. The spleens of tumor-inoculated mice were tested *in vitro* against ^{51}Cr-labeled EL-4 cells in a 4 hr assay for cytotoxic lymphoid cells. No response was detected in mice given untreated EL-4. A small anti-EL-4 response was detected in spleens of mice given Con A-coated EL-4 (0–5% specific lysis). Relatively high levels of activity were present against Con A-coated EL-4 or Con A-coated LSTRA control target cells, suggesting that the mice were, in fact, immunized but that the main response was not directed against the tumor-specific antigen. If mice were simply primed with a single injection of Con A-coated EL-4 and boosted with uncoated cells, a consistently good anti-EL-4 response was generated (20–80% specific lysis at a 100:1 ratio of lymphocytes to target cells). This response was associated with discernible resistance to *in vivo* challenge with live tumor cells.

Various cell lines of EL-4 express somewhat different tumor antigens, either as the result of the loss of antigen or the contamination of the tumor cells by laboratory viruses. Treatment with Con A did not render one EL-4 cell line, obtained from Boyse, capable of evoking cytotoxic cells in syngeneic mice. This cell line did not express the tumor antigen against which mice successfully immunized with the NIH EL-4 cell line responded. Mice immunized with irradiated untreated EL-4 of the NIH cell line have lymphoid cells active in the colony-inhibition assay against EL-4. Further, when spleen cells of these mice are cultured *in vitro,* anti-EL-4 specific CLC develop. Thus, the tumor antigen on this EL-4 is immunogenic but appears to evoke an ineffective immune response in the sense that no cytotoxic cells nor discernible *in vivo* resistance develops. Treatment with Con A renders the immunization more efficient as regards the generation of cytotoxic cells. We have no evidence that Con A can render a nonimmunogenic tumor antigen immunogenic.

NOTKINS: There is some evidence, primarily from the experiments of Lindenmann and P.A. Klein (recent results in *Cancer Research,* vol. 9, Springer Verlag, Berlin, 1967) that viruses can also increase the immune response to certain tumors. The idea is that when a virus (e.g., influenza) infects a tumor cell, viral antigens become associated with the weaker tumor antigens. The viral antigens then act as a "helper" determinant resulting in a more effective immune response to the tumor antigens.

CHAIRMAN GOOD: Two additional forms of immunotherapy have been used in treatment of cancer in man and experimental animals. Voss and his co-workers some time ago cured leukemia in mice by fatally irradiating them and restoring with transplantation of bone marrow from an allogeneic donor, but one matched to the recipient in terms of major H-2 determinants. Some bone marrow, used for "rescue" of the hematopoietic system from irradiation damage, did not cure the leukemia. Similar cellular engineering has been used more recently to treat aplastic anemias in man and to produce prolonged remissions in human leukemias. Oettgen and others have, from time to time, observed regressions in human tumors after Lawrence's transfer factor was given.

In our laboratories, and in the laboratories of Yunis, Dupont, Jersild, and Svegaard, there is evidence which permits us to consider the possibility that these lines of evidence are related. If so, a powerful approach to manipulating human disease may be available. Briefly, the development of this approach began five and one-half years ago when we did the first successful marrow transplant to correct severe combined immunodeficiency disease. We encountered a peculiar immunogenetic situation. The marrow donor was female and the recipient was male, and they matched at the Four locus and by MLC but were mismatched at the LA locus. Because the donor was of blood group O and the recipient of blood group A, and the donor lacked an LA determinant possessed by the recipient, we used two bone marrow transplants to completely correct the primary, severe combined immunodeficiency. Neither marrow transplant produced serious GVH reaction. It was thus possible to separate capacity to produce severe GVH reactions from an influence of the ABO system and from the LA locus.

With Meuwissen, Yunis, and Terasaki, it was possible to show that "full house" HL-A matching in the general population was only rarely associated with a match in the MLC reaction. By contrast, HL-A matching in siblings regularly yielded unresponsive or minimally responsive MLC. This suggested dissociation of MLC and serologic typing data.

Studies with several large Minnesota families and one crucial North Carolina family led Yunis and Amos to conclude that the MLC reaction was under separate genetic control from the HL-A system. Of course, this fit the observation that HL-A typing was of little value for improving organ transplant survival when a donor from the general population matched the recipient, in contrast to HL-A matched siblings.

The next step involved a Danish child who had severe combined immunodeficiency but no siblings. The child's leukocytes did not stimulate either of two uncles in MLC, even though they were a double HL-A haplotype mismatch. The mother was a single haplotype mismatch and did not stimulate. We reasoned from our prior experience to the effect that if the Four locus did not determine GVH anymore than the LA locus, the correction should be successful and GVH should not be a serious problem. The uncle's marrow produced minimal not fatal GVH and the child was cured. Moreover, it was possible to dissociate GVH and MLC reactions from both the Four and the LA locus of the HL-A system.

In Minnesota, Dupont, Yunis, and I studied a series of families that established the dissociation of HL-A from strong MLC reactions and located the MLR-S locus outside of and probably to the right of the Four locus on the HL-A system. Already Dupont, Jersild, Svegaard, Southwick, O'Reilly, and I have transplanted marrow from a healthy unrelated donor in Copenhagen to a child with severe combined immunodeficiency. These data extend the possibilities of cellular engineering from matched sibling donors to suitably matched donors from the general population, and thus enhance the possibilities for treatment of leukemia with replacement marrow.*

*Editors' comment: Immunologic reconstitution through bone marrow transplantation after lethal X-irradiation is theoretically an attractive therapeutic goal in certain forms of radiation sensitive malignancies. It has rarely succeeded in curing the patient when actually attempted, however. The guiding principle in this approach has been to select as marrow donor an individual whose HL-A type and MLC reactivity are as nearly identical to the recipient as possible, in order to avoid fatal GVH reactions. While the principle is correct when the goal is to replace an acquired or genetic defect in marrow function, the goal in the case of destroying malignant growths may be quite different.

Additional possibilities of this approach come from recent work of Dupont, Ballow, and Biggar in our laboratory. Transfer factor was given to an immunologically normal child matched with his mother at HL-A and MLR-S. After treatment with transfer factor (third party), his lymphocytes responded to the mother's in a one-way MLC and stimulated her cells when blocked. Transfer factor apparently activated the response of the recipient cells nonspecifically and induced a stimulatory effect as well. Ballow, Dupont, Biggar, and I, and Griscelli and Seligmann have also found that transfer factor exerts a nonspecific influence. It renders recipients capable of expressing preexisting sensitivity to DNCB, even if the donor was not sensitive to this compound.*

Dupont, Jersild, and others established that ankylosing spondylitis and Reiter's syndrome are closely linked to the W27 allele of the Four locus. Multiple sclerosis (MS), coeliac disease, and lupus erythematosus seem to be more loosely linked to the same locus. Four-locus alleles are associated with MS, for example, about twice as frequently as in the general population. Dupont and associates have developed a set of reagent lymphocytes (cousin marriages backtested to parent) which detect some alleles in the MLR-S locus. One hundred percent of patients with rapidly progressive multiple sclerosis had the 7A allele. Furthermore, MS has long been linked with measles and distemper virus infection (Adams and Imagawa). These two viruses produced identical intranuclear and intracytoplasmic inclusions and cross react immunologically. Antibody titers to measles virus were high in MS spinal fluid. Circulating antibodies to measles virus were very high. Measles virus, therefore, seemed associated in some way with MS. Jersild, Dupont, and their coworkers have now tested re-

---

As Klein emphasized, an important factor in tumor cell selection may be nonrecognition of critical tumor antigens by specific Ir gene products. The practice of matching carries with it the probability of reconstituting the host with Ir-gene-carrying stem cells identical with those already manifestly unable to cope with such antigens—that is, they constitute an I region match. In view of the success with which even weakly allogeneic tumors are brought under control through immune attack, both experimentally and in man, a case can be made to the effect that the guiding principle in tumor therapy involving reconstitution should be to provide Ir gene products *not* naturally possessed by the tumor host. Such an approach comes headlong against the almost impenetrable barrier of GVH induction, at least on the basis of current information. Unfortunately, mismatching in order to provide appropriate Ir gene products will very likely carry with it the necessary MLC or LD nonidentity for GVH to occur. Methods of immune intervention are needed which will permit concomitant tolerance of nontumor structures or perhaps selective blocking of GVH potentiality. This seems at least as likely to become a reality as current efforts to convert syngeneic tumors into allogeneic ones.

Editors' comment: This apparent demonstration of conversion of an MLC-negative individual (presumably immunodeficient) to positive reactivity after transfer factor administration, if confirmed, is of great potential importance, regardless of the mechanism shown ultimately to be involved. As Good points out, it appears to convert a nonresponder to responder status. Because of time constraints the issue received no formal discussion, but many questions are raised. Does it work by conveyance of Ir gene products? By enhancing effector function? In either context, is the effect specific or general? Would the recipient then reject allografts?

sponses of lymphocytes of MS patients to antigens of measles, mumps, and paramyxo 3 viruses. MS patients showed no evidence of cell-mediated immunity to these paramyxo viruses. They then gave MS patients transfer factor from indifferent donors. The responses to irradiated measles and mumps virus in the Bendixen assay of cell-mediated immunity were restored. Clinical extension of these findings suggests using transfer factor as a possible modality for treatment of MS.

In summary, this long train of studies has led to analysis of the major histocompatibility matching for transplantation with respect to MLR-S, a relationship between alleles of the MLR-S region and susceptibility to specific disease, and the wherewithal to manipulate susceptibility through transfer factor. Lepromatous leprosy, cutaneous Leishmaniasis, chronic active hepatitis, subacute sclerosing panencephalitis, and cancer, all related to unusual susceptibility to viruses and other microorganisms, ought to be approachable with these new instruments. Possibly, a modality exists now for correcting lacunar immunodeficiencies. This powerful immunologic approach to human disease may also be applicable to cancer immunotherapy and immunoprophylaxis.

Translating into specific experiments that involve immunotherapy, I propose that transfer factor type preparations be used to abrogate susceptibility of mouse strains that show unusual susceptibility to a particular oncogenic virus.

BACH: The real question with the transfer factor experiments Good describes is: Is he giving the LS stimulant with transfer factor? Is this another nonspecific way to boost immunity? The reaction observed may be to the SD region. We can induce a cellular reaction to SD antigens if we have the LD stimulus factor there. You may be bypassing that.

CHAIRMAN GOOD: Bach is focused unduly on technical issues and terminology which are certainly important but rather aside from the larger issues I sought to emphasize.

BACH: Our Chairman is using the terminology MLR-S to stand for what I have been calling LD; I hope everybody will be clear about that. In mice, we can analyze in congenic strains, strains that differ presumably only within the H-2 locus, what the effect of LD is and what the effect of SD is. In the mouse, I remind you, we know that there must be a minimum of two LD loci. In fact, the work of Meo, Shreffler, and their group has suggested that it is a bipartite distribution; we know now that there are three SD loci.

In the mouse, LD disparity is overriding if you test LD or SD alone. SD is difficult to evaluate, but it is clearly much weaker than LD in determining MLC responses. It may be that the SD antigens are not at all stimulatory in the absence of an LD difference. In GVH assays, our two studies presented here, one with Jan Klein and the other by Elkins, give the same results. The LD differences are of great importance; the SD differences, just as in MLC, are relatively unimportant.

The possibility of adoptive cellular immunotherapy, where one is worried about fatal GVH response, has been examined by Rodey, Bortin, Rimm, and myself, looking at mouse strains which are not congenic. These strains differed in many loci but all were SD identical in the H-2 regions, i.e., they all had the same H-2K and H-2D antigens. We obtained significant correlation between MLC activation and percent mortality as done in two different laboratories, double blind. The greater the MLC activation observed, the higher the mortality measured at 100 days. It is also clear that one can obtain moderately rapid skin graft rejection associated with LD differences in the I region. These differences will lead to skin graft rejection in the range of 14–19 days. Skin grafts are also rejected in similar lengths of time with K region difference. In this case, we are not clear whether this is due to LD components in the SD region, the SD antigens, or the combination of LD and SD.

NOTKINS: The linkage Good attempts to make may not be related at all to an immune deficiency.

CHAIRMAN GOOD: Data are not yet sufficient to choose; however, it seems irrelevant whether the susceptibility to a virus is the consequence of a receptor being there, so the virus can produce a lacunar immunodeficiency, or whether the genetic characteristic leads to a specific lacunar deficit. This analysis may become the cornerstone of really rational immunotherapy of malignancy, where immune responses to the oncogenic agent or oncogenic cells can be controlled.

NOTKINS: Are you saying that MS could be due to mumps, measles, or para influenza? Does that follow?

CHAIRMAN GOOD: Because of the antibody data, I would conclude that is consistent.

We have now had much analysis of the tumor–host relationship as a basis for immunotherapy. A series of questions are raised in my mind from these discussions. Are we satisfied with the general hypothesis that a major approach to cancer can involve immunological analysis and efforts at immunomanipulation? Are we satisfied that this direction can improve our diagnosis, analysis, and treatment of cancer? I sense that our answer is affirmative. Nonetheless, we have heard over and over again outcries against the original immunosurveillance concept. It is my interpretation that the immunosurveillance concept still has viability. My confidence in its usefulness as a hypothesis is not at an end. Already the concept has shown its value for generating new data and new approaches, and strengthening of older approaches can derive from continued investigation in light of this postulate. However, I doubt very much if any of us would now restate the case for surveillance as Lewis Thomas did in 1958. We need to modify our hypotheses to make them more useful. Hypotheses are neither right nor wrong. For this to be a useful hypothesis, it needs some retooling.

PREHN: I think we should make it clear that even if immunosurveillance were not to turn out to be all that it was originally cracked up to be, that there is no question in anybody's mind that immune mechanisms impinge on cancer. Then too, the very fact that immunosurveillance may not be as good as we thought it was provides us with a tremendous therapeutic challenge.

CHAIRMAN GOOD: I believe Prehn is stating, in perhaps another way, that the hypothesis has generated much useful information.

What particular experiment would Smith propose as likely to eliminate virus infection that some here have used to explain his findings of cross-reacting specificities or the allogeneic influence of Lafferty? How then does he visualize the tolerant state? If there are subsets of lymphoid cells capable of reacting to the components of the histocompatibility complex inherited from each parent, is there then no such thing as true tolerance viewed in the old Billingham, Brent, and Medawar perspective?

SMITH: I believe that the virus and allogeneic questions must remain open ones, subject to experimental approach. The tolerance question is one I pondered, not only in terms of the design of further experiments, but also in terms of the biology of cancer. In this disease, the lymphoid system must deal with multiple antigenic ligands on the tumor cell which are not necessarily associated with the transformed state. This involvement must have an effect on concomitant responses to "non-self" tumor-borne antigens, when they exist. The immunotherapeutic implication is that the host might require conversion, essentially toward a type of controlled self-destruction in order to deal with tumors most effectively if they are largely "self," in the original sense.

HOWARD: One is always told that we are going to *immunize* against tumors by using virus vaccines. This has never come up during this conference. I wonder why.

CHAIRMAN GOOD: This is a fair question. Current thought concerning cancer vaccines is no longer limited by the biologic impossibility derivative of a central mechanism involving vertical transmission and the oncogene theory of

Huebner, Todaro, and Temin. From a famous cat house of New York, clear evidence has now come through Hardy and Old that horizontal transmission occurs in the case of an RNA tumor virus causing leukemia in cats. The many skips of leukemia through infected but not leukemic cats confounded the epidemiologist and supported the contention that horizontal transmission could not be implicated. Yet, when the serological tools were perfected to permit tracing the virus and recognizing the immunologic footprints of its horizontal spread, it became clear that a major mechanism for development of leukemia, with this oncorna virus, was horizontal spread from cat to cat through close contact. Accordingly, Hardy and Jarrett are absolutely convinced a vaccine to prevent cat leukemia can be developed. I do not believe that cats and chickens are biologically unique. I take seriously the imperfect epidemiological evidence that certain human lymphomas may be horizontally transmitted to few among many contacts.

KLEIN: One situation where vaccination has been carried out successfully is Marek's disease. This was the largest economic problem for the poultry industry. A closely related, apathogenic turkey virus protects susceptible birds quite efficiently from Marek's disease. Another case where vaccination might be feasible is cat leukemia, since it becomes more and more clear that this is due to a horizontally spread C-type virus.

As far as man is concerned, EBV is the only human tumor-associated virus that can be identified so far. Here, I think, vaccination would neither be necessary nor feasible. Eighty-five percent of us have the virus already, and we are thereby efficiently protected from infectious mononucleosis. What makes the occasional clone slip through and grow into a tumor, an event that we know happens in African Burkitt's lymphoma, is not clear. It could well be due to cofactors, including immunosuppression, for example, associated with chronic holoendemic malaria. If that were the case, it might be much simpler to get rid of malaria than to vaccinate against EBV. Another difficulty in vaccination is inherent in the very unusual properties of this virus, and it would not be feasible to develop an adequate safety test for vaccine virus inactivation. In other words, in spite of the impression one gains from discussions in the mass media, vaccination against tumor viruses is neither simple nor feasible right now. Nor is it necessarily true that vaccination will be the right approach after more viruses have been defined. This depends entirely on the details of the virus–cell–host interaction in a given system.

CHAIRMAN GOOD: Does Klein think it impossible, in light of our information on the Ir genes and the histocompatibility region, that those few among many children who are destined to develop cancer from the EBV infection can be identified? Might their susceptibility be defined, and then manipulations be initiated to alter their susceptibility with either killed vaccine, administration of macromolecules such as transfer factor, or some day, perhaps, small molecule pharmacology?

KLEIN: If Ir genes are responsible for susceptibility variations to the oncogenic effect of the virus, and if this susceptibility could be identified, these would be very interesting approaches.

CHAIRMAN GOOD: And now a few final impressions of our full and active week. After much discussion seeking more precise definition of *in vitro* models, we understand better the relationship of the different kinds of killer cells and the different models in which they are studied. What we need desperately, however, is to define in molecular terms the basis for T cell and for B cell killing. How does the T lymphocyte kill a tumor cell? Are several killer T cells required to make the hit? More specifically, how does the T lymphocyte in the Brunner–Cerottini assay actually kill the target cell? How does the B lymphocyte do its work in the Klein model? Does it act entirely by classical antibody activation of complement, or are there other components to these killer actions?

How important is the role of the so-called nonspecific cells in tumor destruction? These cells need not act nonspecifically, but can probably be armed by antibody of a special kind and presented in a special way. We need a better definition of the molecular basis of this communication.

How is the "activated" or angry macrophage differently armed to kill other cells? It becomes capable of doing in any tumor cell, but is apparently also capable of distinguishing tumor cells from normal cells. We must seek to analyze this model in molecular terms. Is Djerassi correct when he designs an instrument to obtain macrophages in large amounts and treats tumors with monocytes or macrophages in enormous increments? Does he not need first to "activate" these monocytes before expecting them to do much of a job on tumor cells? Uhr said that it was clear to him that antibody-like macromolecules were *not* involved in this recognition process. Perhaps a different class of macromolecules *is* involved and is of every bit as great an interest. We need to begin to be able to decipher and then read the biologic language of the cell surface and learn the surface to nuclear signals much better than we know them right now.

The knowledge we seek must be a succession of questions, intelligent answerable questions that bisect the remaining field, or we flounder in description and detail. I look at each presentation of our conference in this way. Hopefully, that is the business of a nonstructured conference such as this one has been. I would urge that all of us accept this exercise as the *real* work of the conference and not be satisfied with the way things are going. We are making real progress, but to those facing cancer at the bedside, the pace is too slow. We need better questions, not just more research. Howard urged us to dissect cancer immunity with *in vitro* models. We should be highly critical of each one, and be certain that in exploring it, we are seeking fundamental information, that we are satisfied with only incisive molecular definitions, that we are constantly inquiring as to whether the *in vitro* assay will help us bring more quickly an effective immunobiologic approach to treatment or prevention of cancer.

The turtle has taught us that we cannot make progress without sticking the neck out. Perhaps, to the extent to which many here have done just that, the next such conference will unveil much greater progress towards acquiring the basic knowledge for meaningful immunotherapy and immunoprophylaxis.

ABBREVIATIONS

AAF	2-acetylaminofluorene
ALL	acute lymphatic leukemia
AM	activated macrophage
BCG	Bacille Calmette-Guerin
BL	Burkitt's lymphoma
BSA	bovine serum albumin
BUdR	5-bromodeoxyuridine
CMI	cell-mediated immunity
CML	cell mediated lympholysis
CTL	cytotoxic thymus-derived lymphocyte
Con A	concanavalin A
CRBC	chicken red blood cells
DMBA	dimethylbenzanthracene
DNCB	dinitrochlorobenzine
DNP	dinitrophenyl
DTH	delayed type hypersensitivity
EA	EBV early antigen
EBNA	EBV-determined nuclear antigen
EBV	Epstein-Barr virus
ENU	1-ethyl-1-nitrosourea
Fab	Ig fragment with one antigen binding site; one L chain and amino-terminal half of H chain
F(ab')$_2$	two Fab fragments attached to each other

Fc	carboxy-terminal halves of two H chains from same Ig molecule
GVH	graft-versus-host
H-2	the major system of mouse histocompatibility antigens
HD	Hodgkin's disease
HL-A	the major system of human leucocyte antigens
HLV	helper leukemia virus
HSV	herpes simplex virus
HVS	herpes virus saimiri
^{3}HTdR	tritiated thymidine
HuLCL	human lymphocytic cell lines
Ig	immunoglobulin
IgA IgG IgM	standard nomenclature for human-globulin classes; also used here to name analogous proteins in other species
IM	infectious mononucleosis
IUdR	5'-iododeoxyuridine
LALI	lymphocyte antibody lytic interaction
LD	lymphocyte defined antigen (allogeneic difference in lymphocytes)
LDA	lymphocyte-dependent antibody
LPS	lipopolysaccharide
MA	EBV membrane antigen
MAS	mastocytoma
MCA	methylcholanthrene
MER	methanol extract residue (of M. $tuberculosis$)
MHC	major histocompatibility complex
MIF	macrophage inhibitory factor
ML	mammary leukemia (antigen)
MLC	mixed lymphocyte culture

MLV	Moloney leukemia virus
MS	multiple sclerosis
MSV	Moloney sarcoma virus
MTV	mammary tumor virus (Bittner agent)
MuLV	murine leukemia virus
MuSV	murine sarcoma virus
NM	normal (resting) macrophage
NPC	nasopharyngeal carcinoma
PBL	peripheral blood lymphocyte
PEC	peritoneal exudate cell
PHA	phytohemagglutinin
PPD	purified protein derivative, an extract of *M. tuberculosis*
PWM	pokeweed mitogen
Rgv-1	locus for *R*esistance to *G*ross *V*irus
RSV	Rous sarcoma virus
SD	serologically defined antigen (allogeneic differences in lymphocytes)
SRBC	sheep red blood cells
Suc Con A	concanavalin A modified by succinylation
TATA	tumor-associated transplantation antigen
Thy-1	thymus isoantigen expressed on murine thymus-derived lymphocytes
TL	thymus leukemia (antigen)
TSAA	tumor susceptibility alloantigen
TSTA	tumor-specific transplantation antigen
VCA	EBV late capsid antigen

AUTHOR INDEX

SUBJECT INDEX

A 5
B 6
C 7
D 8
E 9
F 0
G 1
H 2
I 3
J 4